The Cure And Prevention Of All Cancers

ISBN 978-1-890035-58-7

Re-Printed 2010

Published in the United States by:
New Century Press
1055 Bay Blvd., Suite C
Chula Vista, CA 91911
1 800 519-2465
www.newcenturypress.com

Other books by Dr. Clark available from New Century Press:

The Cure For All Cancers
(English, Bulgrian, German, Italian, Mongolian, Russian)

The Cure For All Diseases
(English, Bulgarian, Dutch, Finnish, French, German, Hungarian, Italian, Lithuanian, Polish, Portuguese/Brazilian, Russian, Serbian, Slovenian, Spanish)

The Cure For All Advanced Cancers
(English, French, German, Italian, Russian)

The Cure For HIV And AIDS
(English)

The Prevention Of All Cancers
(English, Italian)

Syncrometer® Science Laboratory Manual
(English, French, Spanish)

Syncrometer® Science Laboratory Manual 2
(English)

Dr. Clark's Healthy Recipes
(English)

What Is A Cure?

The word "cure" in the title was chosen, rather than "treatment," because it is scientifically accurate.

When the true cause of an illness has been found and, by removing it, the illness can be stopped or prevented, a true cure has also been found. When the cause is not found but the symptoms can be removed, helpful as this is, you have only found a treatment.

New and more effective ways to kill cancer cells, however important, are merely treatments. My research was a search for the causes of cancer. I searched for ways to remove these causes. Then I observed whether this would actually lead to relief from these diseases. I did not search merely for relief from the diseases as regular clinical research does.

Syncrometer® technology makes such searches for causes and cures possible. Hopefully, others will repeat my investigations and extend my findings. The new technology is described in the *Syncrometer® Science Laboratory Manual*, available from the same publisher.

Is This Really A Cure?

Cancer can now be cured, not just treated. The finding that cancer is caused by a cluster, not a single item like a carcinogen, is what shortened the *Curing Program* to two weeks instead of three. In this book you will see how you can break up this cluster so it can never be formed again. The components of this cluster get trapped in your tooth fillings as they harden and establish the main source of metastases. But these can be replaced. For the first time in history you can walk away from a dental office with complete certainty of a cure.

You may not have time…

…to read this entire book first if you have cancer and are scheduled for surgery, chemotherapy or radiation treatment. You may wish to skip the first pages, which describe how a parasite and a cancer-complex in your drinking water cause cancer to develop. Go directly to the instructions on eliminating the parasite with herbs and with electricity. Using the herbal recipe along with the zapper is best. It only takes days to clear your teeth and gums of the radioactivity that supplies the cancer-complex with polonium. It does not matter what kind of cancer you have or how far progressed the cancer is—you can still stop it immediately.

After you have stopped the cancer, you can turn your attention to getting well.

Does this mean you can cancel your date for surgery, radiation, or chemotherapy? Yes, but only <u>after</u> curing your cancer. Your doctor would be the first to agree. But he or she should have proof. You could provide this. Set yourself a goal of providing proof to your doctor before your admission date to the hospital. This is not a treatment for cancer: It is a cure! The cure does not interfere with the treatment because it is mainly <u>removing</u> things, not <u>giving</u> things. Removing causes with noninvasive methods cannot interfere. Feel free to discuss this concept with your doctor.

Remember that oncologists are kind, sensitive, compassionate people. They want the best for you. They have no way of knowing about the true cause and cure of cancer since it has not been published for them. I chose to publish it for you first so that it would come to your attention faster. The program starts on page 355.

Acknowledgements

It was the microscope slide of Fasciolopsis buski, made by Frank Jerome, D.D.S that turned out to have the parasite responsible for causing malignancy in cancer. The generous loan of his parasite slide collection, around 1990, made this discovery possible. Now four more slides that were in his collection will take part in finding the true beginning of all tumors. Thank you, again, Dr. Jerome!

As a student he had mounted and stained the entire adult Fasciolopsis buski fluke. It was not shipped in from China or India. It was obtained from the local abattoir on a day when hog slaughtering was done and the same day as his parasitology class. All flukes needed to be very fresh and alive in order to be mountable on a glass slide. It would need to be pressed flat while alive; otherwise it would be too hard to make into a thin specimen. Only a very thin specimen, perfectly expanded to show all details and beautifully stained would garner an "A" grade in this class. Pigs yielded handfuls of these slithery parasites, besides Ascaris worms, which filled buckets. Other animals could yield a few flukes, but not as many as pigs or a wild deer or moose that was accidentally killed on a highway.

Other flukes, especially lung flukes (Paragonimus) were plentiful, too. Pancreatic flukes (Eurytrema) were easy to pick out, as, of course the ever present Fasciola hepatica.

Later, when dissecting the frog, some of these same parasites were encountered again in smaller versions. They were not too strict about their host.

In 1999, the collaboration with Erika Hüther, M.D. made possible our discovery of mercury, thallium and phenylalanine in every malignant melanoma and the **tumor nucleus**.

Thanks are due the entire staff of Century Nutrition of Mexico, whose personal dedication to the salvage of advanced cancer patients was inspirational.

I gratefully acknowledge the help of my son, Geoffrey A. Clark, as provider of toxin-free food, environmentally safe lodging, and as computer editor of this book. This project could not have been done without him.

I am deeply grateful to Barbara and John Crook for procuring rare products for Syncrometer® analysis.

Thanks are due Kirk White who helped develop our automatic hot-backwash filter that removes the cancer-causing complex from water.

I am grateful to our oral surgeon, C.D. Benjamin Arechiga, C.M.F. Without his expertise our terminally ill cancer patients could not have recovered.

I also thank our innovative dentist, Dr. Virgilio Oscar Solorio U.A.G., who has stepped up to the challenge of removing past radioactive dental work from patients' mouths. It takes priority over earlier dental goals. His replacements are non-radioactive and bring the success rate to 100%.

Thanks are due my financial supporters, as well as Tim Bolen and those attorneys who protected me from the legal onslaughts of vested interests who would incarcerate me for publishing these findings. The individuals involved are in the public record and can be freely studied as judges, attorneys, expert witnesses and the corporations that sued me. It is an important social phenomenon and should be studied.

And finally, Mexico itself is to be commended on its research-friendly climate. I am truly grateful to this forward-looking country that made this venture possible.

Notice to the Reader

The opinions and conclusions expressed in this book are mine, and unless indicated otherwise, mine alone. They are based on my scientific research and on specific case studies involving patients. Be advised that every person is unique and may respond differently to the treatments described in this book. On occasion I have provided dosage recommendations. Again, remember that we are all different and any new treatment should be applied in a cautious, common sense way.

The treatments outlined herein are not intended to be a substitute for other forms of conventional medical treatment. In fact, they are completely compatible. Please feel free to consult with your physician or other health care provider.

I have indicated throughout this book the existence of pollutants in food and other products. These pollutants were identified using a testing device of my invention known as the Syncrometer®. It uses an oscillator circuit in conjunction with open capacitor plates. Complete instructions for building and using this device are contained in the *Syncrometer® Science Laboratory Manual*. Therefore anyone can repeat the tests described and verify the data.

The Syncrometer® is more accurate and versatile than the best existing testing methods. A way to determine the degree of precision is also presented in the laboratory manual. However, at this point it only yields ***Positive*** or ***Negative*** results, it does not quantify. The chance of a false ***Positive*** or false ***Negative*** is about 5%, which can be lessened by test repetition.

It is in the public interest to know when a single bottle of a commercial product tests ***Positive*** to a serious pollutant, such as benzene or asbestos or polonium. If one does, the safest course is to avoid all bottles of that product entirely, which is what I repeatedly advise. These recommendations should be interpreted as intent to warn and protect the public, not to provide a statistically significant analysis. It is my fervent hope that manufacturers use the new electronic techniques in this book to make purer products than they ever have before.

And it is my hope that researchers, including the layperson will advance toward use of the oscillator technology described here to study high frequency-related phenomena in living animals and plants.

Today, in 2007, the Syncrometer® is still operated manually 15 years after my invention. Hopefully a research budget will soon become available to find a way to automate it.

Contents

Figures

Your Invitation

This book is about a completely self-sufficient cancer-curing therapy. It can be carried out by the patient at home at fairly low cost if it is not too advanced. It seldom requires medical care before it is diagnosed. Don't hide from it nor take a casual attitude. It can be detected before it is diagnosed and therefore is the first true preventive cancer therapy.

Scurvy was once a dreaded disease, as much as cancer is today. Even the CA-word strikes terror in many of us. Now we know that scurvy is a simple vitamin C deficiency disease. It doesn't even require medical care as it always did in the past. It is noteworthy that all the medical care given at that time did not save the scurvy patient. It was terminal. But the women of a Native American Indian tribe, the Iroquois, knew how to prevent and **cure**, not just treat this disease, and to do it quickly, in days. This is an excerpt from the personal journal of Jacques Cartier, the early French explorer.

> *Thus it was that we lost 25 of our best men to the dreaded sickness. There were another forty who were at the point of death and the remainder, except two or three, were all gravely ill... People from Stadacone... among whom was Agaya... responded that... the liquid and residue from the leaves of a tree... was the sole cure for the illness... Two women... gathered nine or ten branches... to boil them in water... Drink the water every other day... It... turned out to be a miracle... they were cured and restored to health after having drunk the brew only two or three times... After all that, the crew was ready to kill to get to the medicine. This wonderful tree has done in less than a week what all the physicians of Louvain and Montpellier, using all the drugs of Alexandria, would not be able to accomplish in a year...*
>
> *Cartier, Jacques. Winter–1535.*[1]

---

[1] Cartier, Jacques, 1491-1557 *Voyage de J. Cartier au Canada Relation originale de Jacques Cartier,* (French) not copyrighted in the U.S. www.gutenberg.org/etext/12356

It took 400 years from the discovery of its cure (1535) to the use of the cure by the public in the early 1900's. Yet it had even been published in medical journals many times.[2] Today, we all know how to prevent, not just cure this dreadful disease: eat fresh fruit and vegetables. It is not medical advice. It is nutritional. It took the unrelated orange juice industry to bring it to the public's attention in the early 1900's. It was not the medical profession! That should be a lesson to us to be wary of professionals.

Why did it take so long to put into practice a simple cure, the eating of fresh fruit and vegetables? The medical profession was waiting for absolute "proof" on its own "scientific" terms. The cure was called "controversial" by medical professionals, giving it a bad reputation. Sick persons and their families would not have waited to resolve professional or commercial conflicts. Their priorities hold life dearer than financial interests, or analytical reasoning. And ordinary people, not able to read the medical journals, had no way to even learn about the controversy.

If they had, they would have tried the controversial cure, as any intelligent being would, since that could do no harm and in a few months would have resolved the controversy. Why didn't the doctors do this, just try it? Success would have meant an instant reduction in the number of doctors per ship, from a minimum of two, to one.

It was in the professionals' interest to keep the cure and even the controversy over it out of the hands of the public, "lest they injure themselves with an unproven treatment". The public was held hostage by its medical professionals.

Unless the public has access to the great truths uncovered by scientists, they cannot learn them even now. Computers are making it possible for the first time in history.

In this book the true beginning of cancer will be described. From this the first true prevention program can arise.

---

[2] Davies, M.B., Austin, J., Partridge, D.A., *Vitamin C, Its Chemistry and Biochemistry,* Royal Society of Chemistry, 1991, chapter 2 www.rsc.org

Cancer as an epidemic is now 100 years old. Some of its true causes were already known 100 years ago, like parasites (in several animals),[3] coal tar,[4] synthetic dyes,[5] and improperly prepared foods.[6] But these discoveries have been ignored rather than treasured, as befell the scurvy cure. Every spontaneous remission should have been carefully studied instead of discarded.

Scientific research pursued a course of finding carcinogens for animal and bacterial models instead of in its real victims, the human race. This was in spite of a warning by Jesse Greenstein, a widely respected cancer researcher, and others in the 1940s not to pursue carcinogens because it would be endless and useless. It certainly did lead to an explosion of research data, altogether overwhelming with promise, but none of it really relevant. By implanting or injecting tumor cells or by working with special transformed culture lines, the beginnings of cancer were already lost. This is not how we get our cancers. Hopelessness then gave birth to the current new direction in research, supplying corrective genes. This in itself is a huge, population-wide human experiment. This time it misses not only the true cause of cancer, but also the mutagens that damage the genes. It seems unwise as an overall strategy.

Hopefully the age of computers will now set free the bird of truth as was never before possible. Patients and their families have easy access to information just like doctors and researchers do.

Only when each layperson and common laborer possess the knowledge about cancer prevention, as they already do for scurvy prevention, will the medical profession stop claiming an exclusive right to cancer treatment. It will no longer be

---

[3] A good discussion of this topic (more than just dogs) is by Bailey, W.S., *Parasites and Cancer: Sarcoma in Dogs Associated with Spirocerca lupi,* Annals of the New York Academy of Sciences, v. 108, 1963, pp. 890-923

[4] Greenstein, Jesse P., *Biochemistry of Cancer,* 2nd ed., Academic Press Inc., 1954, pp. 44-56

[5] Ibid., pp. 88-96

[6] Lane, A., Blickenstaff, D., and A.C. Ivy, *The Carcinogenicity of Fat "Browned" by Heating*, Cancer, v. 3, 1950, pp. 1044-51

lucrative. Till then its power to restrict and hold hostage the patient will continue. At present this power seems quite misplaced, since medical professionals know neither how cancer begins nor how it progresses. In the future, preventing cancer, like preventing scurvy will not generate high incomes for anybody. Nor will herbal and natural treatments. These therapies will fall to lay health advisers and lay nutritionists. It will be a huge step of progress for humanity.

But making practical use of this new knowledge still depends on wisdom, something that we all have and all lack to some degree.

An example of wisdom for an individual might be moving the home to a safer location, improving diet, and stopping addictions.

An example of wisdom for the medical profession would be analyzing tumors for the radioactivity and immunity destroyers they contain. Then searching for the same items in the patient's environment, the water, food, cookware and dentalware. Such tests were prohibitively expensive even 10 years ago. Now they are not. A test for radioactivity in the drinking water can cost less than $100.00.

The dye, DAB (butter yellow), is known to cause much too high alkaline phosphatase levels in animals. Many cancer patients show high alkaline phosphatase levels. The dye has accumulated in the white blood cells. An example of wisdom would be to search for this dye in the food, water and dentalware of these cancer patients. The LDH enzyme can reach sky-high levels in cancer patients, too. This is due to Sudan Black B dye accumulated in the red blood cells. When cobalt has accumulated in any organ, these enzyme levels are too low instead of too high. With so many dyed foods in the market place and so many heavy metals in our drinking water, cancer patients should be studied for their dye and metal exposure.

To my knowledge such studies have not been done, nor do I see evidence of these rational approaches. Here is another example. Scientists know that mutations and broken chromosomes are characteristic of nearly every cancer.[7,8] This means there is severe genetic damage. They also know that heavy metals, like copper, cadmium, the lanthanides ("rare earths") and alpha radiation from polonium could cause chromosomes to break.[9] Yet doctors do not send biopsy specimens to a lab for radioactivity or heavy metal analysis! If they did, they would be in a position to search for the patient's source of these mutagenic metals and to advise chelation therapy or at least avoidance. EDTA (ethylenediamine-tetraacetate) chelation removes heavy metals from the body. Patients should remove heavy metals from dentalware, cookware, plastic ware used for food, eyeglass frames, wristwatches and jewelry, water pipes, and the water itself. The cost of metal analysis is now so low and the test itself so sensitive, no biopsy specimen or drinking water sample should be untested.

Ordinary laypersons have a great deal of wisdom. This book will help you to practice and express your own wisdom. Your instincts and questions are well worth pursuing. You can build the same investigative tool that I have used: instructions are in *The Cure for all Cancers* and the *Syncrometer® Science Laboratory Manual*. Your discoveries and experience, together with others', are valuable and very much needed. When wisdom is accumulated, it can contribute to a new bank of information for persons in the future that face the same dilemma that you may have faced. Solutions can be found by communicating and listening to others in similar predicaments. It is my cherished belief that in this way you and others can

---

[7] Weiss, L.M., Warnke, R.A., Sklar, J., Cleary, M.L., *Molecular Analysis of the Chromosomal Translocation in Malignant Lymphomas, (14;18)* N. Eng. Jour. Med., v. 317, no. 19, 1987, pp. 1185-89

[8] Warrell, R.P., et al., *Differentiation Therapy of Acute Promyelocytic Leukemia with Tretinoin (All-Trans-Retinoic Acid),* N. Eng. Jour. Med., v. 324, no. 20, 1991, pp. 1385-93

[9] Komiyama, Makoto, *Sequence-Specific and Hydrolytic Scission of DNA and RNA by Lanthanide Complex-Oligo DNA Hybrids,* J. Biochem, v. 118, no. 4, 1995, pp. 665-670

solve human health problems that lie languishing as orphans as well as our most common ones.

I invite you to do so.

And a special invitation goes out to younger readers. Building the electronic device and searching for cause and effect in all the health problems your family suffers from could stir the heart of any of us who are detectives in spirit. It is much more important than finding a name for an illness. Finding a name is diagnosis. That can be left to doctors. It does not contribute to the study of health. We will be analysts: nutritionists, chiropractors, homeopaths, massage therapists, engineers, biologists, naturopaths, cell physiologists, veterinarians, medical doctors, physicists, dentists, and plain hobbyists, all with a common goal: to analyze our problems, find causes that can be removed, and improve the health of others and ourselves. That is the essence of curing.

Challenge to Students

This whole book is just one chapter of a very long detective story that began over 100 years ago. Nobody knows why we suddenly develop a lump, then more lumps, all of them growing and spreading like mold in a loaf of bread. This book is about detecting parasite eggs and stages in these lumps, of the most unexpected varieties. Imagine finding a coiled up filaria, such as dog heartworm in every chest mass and Hodgkin's lymphoma! Imagine finding aluminum holding it all together…and another filaria, Onchocerca, in similar abdominal masses, called non-Hodgkin's lymphoma.

We can detect parasites, bacteria and viruses in many places inside our own bodies, which we always thought was nearly sterile! Some of these cause cancers. Some cause other health problems, commonly called diseases.

But can't this be done everyday by any doctor or scientist in a laboratory? Yes! But for them it is laborious, costly, and takes years. Their results are unreliable and must wait to be repeated for about another 10 years! They are based on chemistry, immunology, and microbiology, all very difficult and expensive techniques. The electronic method we will use in this book takes minutes and is highly reliable. But you must train yourself, just as you once did to use a computer or to ride a bicycle.

Present day medical science does not approach cancer or other disease in the rational way described here, partly because it involves study of a new technology and the cost with the old technologies.

So, instead, chemicals are snatched off the shelves, and tried one after another, to see "what they can do" for some disease! This is inefficient to the extreme and ultimately much more costly. There is almost nothing to show for 100 years of such random research when true detective work could have yielded much more.

My detective device is a new invention. It is an electronic circuit that detects resonance in much the same way a radio does. In your radio a distant frequency produced in a studio is matched to a frequency you produce with an oscillator circuit in your radio at home. The new device used for these experiments matches a frequency produced in your body with one after you place an object on a capacitor plate. Although the new device is simple to build it is much more advanced in principle than other devices. A voltmeter is almost the only device that has ever been used to make electrical measurements in the body. Electrical studies of the human body have lagged far behind other fields. Measuring the voltages of the heart gives us the EKG. Voltages of the brain give us the EEG. There is also a magnetometer that can make magnetic measurements of the body. The newly invented device described here scans for anything—be it an object, an organ, a chemical, or virus, even a gene, because everything has a characteristic frequency or set of frequencies. And the capacitance and inductance of any body part is easily influenced. The device is so simple to build that even girls and boys can build it. And I hope you do.

Girls and boys have often become radio amateur operators in their teen years. It is not beyond your skill level. Nor beyond your level to learn its uses. With this new technology you will be led into the secret world of the inner body. Not it's outside appearances but the strange inner workings. These have never been seen, heard or measured before. A whole inner world is waiting to be explored. Whether it's the brain or heart or skin, you can go on a detective hunt for what is really going on there. You can search for answers to profound questions. Why did your brother or sister develop a "bad gene"? Why did you develop a little brown spot on your face—or a little red blister on your leg? What is a freckle? Why is your dad beginning to go bald? Why is your grandmother getting pain in her fingers? These are all detective stories waiting to be told, waiting for the detective in you to feel the urge to find the villains.

I call my new device a Syncrometer®. You can build it or buy it. Building it is by far the best. Then you know how it works and can troubleshoot it in minutes at no cost.

You put yourself into the circuit and hear your resistance change as you tune the circuit to different frequency patterns. When you find a pattern that matches yours, your resistance drops and a huge current will flow. A resistance change can be heard. Any place you touch on the body can be eavesdropped. It does this by amplifying a signal through an ordinary, inexpensive PNP transistor.

You can tune your Syncrometer® to any organ by placing it (the organ) on the open capacitor plate, even the genes themselves. You can hear a Herpes virus coming out of a chromosome. You can hear an enzyme coming out of a gene. You can hear DNA going about its business of transcription. You can hear a CD4 type of white blood cell capture an HIV virus. Will the virus get killed or the cell? Or will it be a standoff? There are telltale signs you can use to eavesdrop on this battle. Simply listening gives data beyond anyone's imagination.

You can learn the new Syncrometer® mathematics and find that frequencies rule your body in some yet mysterious way. Maybe you will find the energy sources of these frequencies. Maybe you will find the perfect antidote against any intruder in your body by using this arithmetic. Why does your body add, subtract, multiply and divide these frequencies like regular radio signals? Why does all life come from life? Is the secret in these frequencies? Can they only be handed on (transmitted), not created? Or are they created in the recesses of our mitochondria? Could they have come from outer space? Could they be replaced or duplicated, or at least patched up when the body is sick? Could you find the antidotes to new diseases appearing in our population by searching for missing frequencies?

The world of life is full of too many mysteries to even ask the right questions. But those who think and explore will be rewarded. Applying chemistry was once very rewarding to biologists when it first began. But now it is a slow and costly pathway to find truths. The electronic method gets a whole host of research results in an afternoon. Best of all, you can make all the research plans yourself.

You are invited to become a Syncrometer® detective. Learn basic electronics from a beginner's amateur radio manual. Scout out this hobby at a Radio Shack store. See how easy it is. Get an amateur radio license while you're at it, though it is not essential. Start building electronic kits, and build from scratch. This is a hobby that reaches ages 18 to 80. Use the *Syncrometer® Science Laboratory Manual* to launch your new detective profession. Maybe you can move this beginning science forward to automation or to a whole new application.

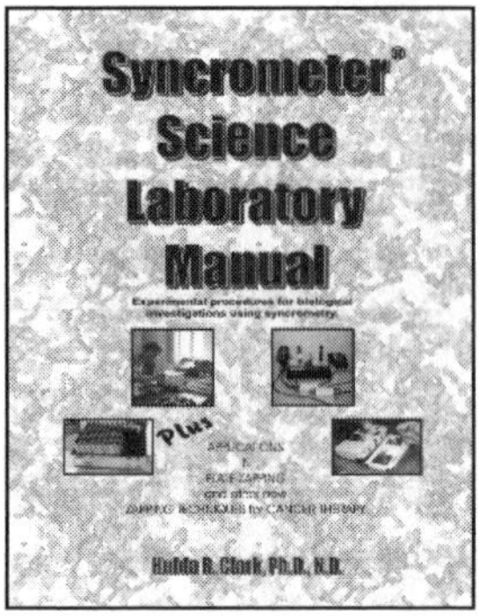

ISBN 1-890035-17-3

*Fig. 1 The underlying science for my **"curing"** books*

Just be sure to write your detective story in a notebook as you unravel mysteries, the way I have done. If 10 students with 10 home-built Syncrometers® wrote 10 such detective stories, and one of them contacted the other nine to form a special Syncrometer® club for students, you could REALLY begin to rescue this planet!

Keep in mind a quote from the discoverer of vitamin C:

"Research means going out into the unknown with the hope of finding something new to bring home. If you know in advance what you are going to do, or even to find there, then it is not research at all: then it is only a kind of honorable occupation."

—Albert Szent-Györgyi (1893-1986)

RSVP - *The author*

To the Cancer Patient

This book is meant for the complete novice.

Even though you have never taken an herb, never used a "bioelectrical" device, never taken supplements, and know nothing about homeography, you can protect yourself and even get yourself well from this dreadful disease.

All you need is a determination to get well and keep well. You need the intelligence to follow instructions carefully, and the good fortune to have a friend or family who loves you and will help.

It is not incompatible with any other method, clinical or non-clinical. In fact, it would be profoundly helpful.

This book does not have detailed explanations for the advice given, only general explanations. For the details go to *The Cure For All Cancers* book and *The Cure For All Advanced Cancers* book, as well as *The Prevention Of All* Cancers and the *Syncrometer® Science Laboratory Manual*[10], all by this author.

Although this book is non-technical, details can be important, especially if you have scientific-minded friends and doctors, who would like to understand why you are advised to make certain changes or take certain things. The underlying science has been recorded in the *Syncrometer® Science Laboratory Manual* so others can repeat it. The essence of

[10] New Century Press, 800 519-2465, www.newcenturypress.com

science is repeatability. They, as well as you, may wish to analyze and compare my interpretations with others'.

It is important, too, to have some perspective on the last 100 years of cancer treatment. Reading books like *The Cancer Cure That Worked* and others[11] will give you this perspective.

In reading these books you might feel frustration, and wonder how so many alternative therapies could exist, with such widely different approaches, and yet each one seeming to claim they had found the one cause and solution for cancer. They saw their patients recover by removing this one cause. And when a **chain** of causes is responsible for a disease, removing a single one can be so helpful it seems to be the only one. Of course they had also changed the diet, water, and residence of their patients. Today, we can fit their findings into this chain because they are science and experience based. The concept was certainly flawed, that for every single disease there is a single cause, but it seemed so to them, because it worked! Many of us still suffer from the same wrong concepts today. When you read this cancer book you will be in awe of cancer's great complexity. I could easily see how very important each early therapist's contribution was. Each helped to shape my ideas as well as others'. They gave a lifetime of dedication and service to American society and science. They did it without a research budget, without a Syncrometer®, and often harassed and scorned. Their writings should be gathered

---

[11] Lynes, Barry and Crane, John, *The Cancer Cure That Worked!* Marcus Books, 1987; Livingston-Wheeler, MD, Virginia and Addeo, Edmond G., *The Conquest of Cancer, Vaccines and Diet,* New York, F. Watts, 1984, Chicago, Advanced Century Pub. Co. 1978; Manner, Harold W., DiSanti, Steven and Michalsen, Thomas, *The Death of Cancer*, Cancer Book House, June 1979; Koch, William F., *Natural Immunity, www.williamfkoch.com;* Gerson, MD, Max, *A Cancer Therapy, Results of Fifty Cases,* New York, Whittier Books 1958; Bradford, R., Culbert, M.L., Allen, H.W., *International Protocols For Individualized, Integrated Metabolic Programs In Cancer Management,* 2nd ed., The Robert W. Bradford Foundation, 1983; Krebs Jr, Ernst T. *A collection of papers bearing on the Unitarian or Trophoblastic Fact of Cancer and related works on Metabolic Therapy*, http://www.navi.net/~rsc/krebsall.htm

up to be commemorated for their true worth. Their contributions are priceless.

Succeeding with a natural method like mine, and those of earlier therapists, is vastly more important than simply using a clinical method, even though the clinical method is quicker and does not interfere with your lifestyle. A natural method puts you in control of your own health. It reaches into your lifestyle to show you causes of your diseases, causes that you could abolish. It reaches into the environmental causes that need change. It gives you the confidence that you are not just relying on a doctor's promise that "he got it all" in surgery, and his or her implication that you could not be struck again.

You may wish to combine this natural method with other natural methods or with a clinical method. There is no conflict between natural and clinical methods. In fact, a natural method added to a standard clinical method should raise the success percentages of clinical treatments astronomically. But your clinician may prefer that you do not take vitamins or herbs or other alternative treatments. This is usually advised from a position of ignorance. We must never lump "vitamins" or "alternative treatments" together as if they did the same thing. Each has individual action and should be individually evaluated for your situation. You could copy the page from the earlier book, *The Cure For All Advanced Cancers,* with the reference cited that discusses the issue of vitamin taking, and even provide a copy of the research article.[12] Your oncologist may appreciate this gesture. He or she will have a better standing with their peers with this new knowledge, especially after you recover.

One of the main objectives in this book is to reach as many persons as possible with the new knowledge about preventing cancer, and reaching those without access to natural health care, without access to the accumulation of health-related knowledge that already exists. It stretches back over thousands

---

[12] Jaakkola, K., et al., *Treatment with Antioxidant and other Nutrients in Combination with Chemotherapy and Irradiation in Patients with Small-Cell Lung Cancer,* Anticancer Research, v. 12, 1992, pp. 599-606

of years! They need to hear the good news that the true causes of cancer have been found, although not published in the standard scientific journals. Publishing here must wait till the subject is returned to the realm of science, rather than emotion and economics. People need to hear that a recipe for prevention as well as cure has been developed that is within their reach, their capability and their finances. These recipes invite innovation; they are open to change as experience is gathered.

The discoveries described in this book create a scientific basis for a cure, in fact, more than one cure. There are always more ways than one to accomplish a task.

Now that health has a scientific path to follow and a device to monitor it, health could become a reality for all of society. We could put cancer "to rest", beside scurvy. Only reaching the afflicted, far and wide, will accomplish this.

CHOOSING YOUR PROGRAM

For Beginning Cancers

If you now have a beginning cancer, with just a small tumor, less than the size of a marble, you may be able to clear it up with the simple program given in the first book, *The Cure For All Cancers*. Many patients reported that they did. But in that program we stopped only the malignancy part of the tumor. Then we went on a major clean up program for your lifestyle. Your teeth, your diet, your home and your body products were all cleared thoroughly from those things that burden your immune system. After this your own immune power returned to remove the tumor without clinical help. You were advised to stay on a *Maintenance Program* of killing parasites regularly and keeping a clean environment. That was in 1993.

If you once had a beginning cancer and tumors went away without help from a more drastic, clinical method, you know you did the right things then. Nevertheless, you should remember that you WERE TARGETED. You were targeted by a specific parasite, specific bacteria and a specific virus, as you will see. None of us knew the specific radioactive element, **polonium**, or its partners that make up the **cancer-complex** or cluster that starts your cancer. Your immune system rescued you even while you neglected many important things. That is the magic (not yet understood) power of the immune system. But once targeted, you can never be "untargeted". To live safely past the five-year mark and have a NORMAL lifespan you will always need to kill these former invaders regularly and protect your immune system. You may have done nothing about your dentalware or water supply or house-radioactivity. But luck is not dependable. It is an insecure way to live. You should add the new prevention path described in this book.

If you did require the help of clinical doctors at one time, you are even less secure. As you continue to drink polonium-contaminated water cancer is bound to find a new organ to grow in. Use all the advice in this book to prevent a recurrence.

Cancer recurs because it is a systemic disease caused by a chain of events that has eluded us till now. It can be compared to mold developing in a loaf of bread or termites entering a house. They will never leave on their own. Once you see these, it is already far past the beginning and almost too late. The whole loaf and the whole house are at risk, not just where the trouble is spotted. Organ and body destruction, which happen in cancer, may appear to be stopped. But they may have merely moved to another location or be having their ups and downs. The disease can never be trusted even if you were told by the surgeon "they got it all". The recurrence will not be noticed until it has become advanced. Hurry, to put your prevention program in place before cancer surfaces again.

If you choose the beginners' program from *The Cure For All Cancers*, be sure to add the prevention program described in this book. It is newly discovered. Never before has there been a way to prevent cancer with certainty.

Also be sure to give yourself time limits and objective tests, such as cancer markers and scans, so you know with certainty how effective your chosen program is for you. Avoid x-rays if possible, they are too damaging. Substitute ultrasounds where possible. If x-rays are necessary, use as few exposures as possible, not dozens. If scans are used avoid being injected with dyes, lanthanides (like gadolinium), or radioactivity (like technetium) to make you "glow" on the *Negative*. It makes no sense to apply more radiation, even though it is not the alpha type (most harmful), when radiation is at the root of the whole disease! The scanning industry has taken on a life of its own, with less regard for yours. Certainly, it is easier to see a detail, but minute details seldom count. Find a cooperative doctor with conservative, least invasive methods, but with realism. In other countries (Europe) you can request these tests yourself. Society's health is better served with such freedoms, without paying extra "middlemen" for referrals when not needed.

For Advanced Cancers

If you have a cancer recurrence, or a tumor has started in a second organ, you should consider yourself advanced.

This will not be so distressing and hard to face if you know that you can still clear it up yourself. Being "in denial" is not all bad. Let it energize you to do two things:

1.) Get the newly discovered cancer-complex out of your water, food, and teeth.
2.) Kill the parasite, Fasciolopsis buski.

Compare yourself to a loaf of bread with its second visible green mold spot. You must snatch this loaf and clean it up immediately, this very minute if you treasure it, and then put it in the freezer. You have no time to lose. You are entered in a race, not of your choosing. The race is between your cancer and your cure. Getting rid of the tumor by whatever means is NOT the answer. How to get rid of polonium and the parasite IS the answer and you can learn how to do this in this book. Of course, you need to see the tumors shrink and disappear, but it needs to be by removing all the radioactivity from your body. This was not discussed in earlier books because I had not yet found the true carcinogen. I had only found the cancer-causing water disinfectant, chlorox bleach that brought it. Cancer is very deceptive. It is seldom visible or painful or diagnosable until it is very late. Of course, it can be found with a Syncrometer® long before that.

To stamp out an advanced cancer completely, you need to remove the cancer-complex from your body and from your teeth. It is now possible to scan the whole body YOURSELF for leftover tumors with the Syncrometer®, not needing an x-ray, MRI or other variety of clinical scan. Supplements are now reduced while "plate-zapping" and "drop-taking" replace them. It is now possible to identify radioactive tooth fillings and extract these teeth exclusively while replacing non-radioactive fillings without extraction.

Again, put up time limits for yourself, when you will do tests and scans. You may be able to find a cooperative therapist to schedule these for you and give interpretations. You may be able to find a Syncrometer® tester who can tell you your status. Best of all, do all the monitoring yourself. Shrinking tumors and lowered cancer markers are easy enough for you to see. But finding and rooting out even the smallest beginning malignancy takes Syncrometer® skills.

In more progressive countries you can schedule tests and scans for yourself. You may need to go there to save your life. Be fair but critical with your results. If they do not give you proof of progress, you need to change something. Improving your compliance is the easiest option you could choose before it is too late. Don't neglect clinical and other alternative options. Review them to choose the wisest path.

With all this realism in one hand and optimism in your other hand you have the best chance to join the ranks of cured advanced cancer cases.

Speed is important. You can jump into action but you must do the program completely. Do not delude yourself that you "did the program" if you left a part out or decided on a different dental path or water solution.

This *2-Week Program* succeeds in 100% of cases when you do it all. In fact, you could realistically succeed with absolute certainty if you did it all. Left out in the past were those so clinically ill they needed a transfusion every week, or needed drainage of effusate every week, and those already in jaundice or kidney failure. **Even these can now be salvaged** with the help of "on the spot" Syncrometer® testing and homeography treatment. It is well suited to emergency care.

You can get extra helpful advice from the earlier books. A therapist, too, will find the technical explanations in the earlier books useful. Where to get items you may want is given in the *Sources* section of this book. Please heed the advice to use only those items listed in these *Sources* because they have been personally tested for quality. In the future such items will be stamped to make it easier to identify them.

You are free to copy pages from my books for yourself or friends (not for commercial purposes). Remember, all the new information was discovered by Syncrometer® and can be verified by yourself, using the *Syncrometer® Science Laboratory Manual*.

CHAPTER 1

THE REAL CAUSE OF CANCER...

has never been known! In this book I will show you the true beginnings of all cancers.

Whether the cancer is in the form of a tumor or single cells, whether it is a sarcoma or carcinoma, whether it is "a very rare variety" or the most common, **each one starts in the same place**, one small region in the **brain**.

This information will make cancer much easier to prevent, to stop, and to cure.

All cancers start in the same organ!

All cancers become malignant along a chain of events. The chain is always the same, except for details. The organ chosen is just a detail.

The cause of all malignancies is a common parasite, the human intestinal **fluke**. Its scientific name is **Fasciolopsis buski**. But it does not act alone. It acts together with 4 or more partners. The first two are **polonium** and **cerium**. These are a radioactive element and a **lanthanide** element. We will learn more about them soon. The participation of the fluke was first described in a book published in 1993. In this book its partners will be revealed. Each is essential to make a cancer and to *keep it growing*.

A fluke is very much like a leech. The adult sticks to one spot where it produces many thousands of eggs inside our bodies. Their attachment causes chronic minor bleeding, which later leads to anemia and pain.

All this was never noticed before because it was not suspected and the eggs do not exit from our intestine. Commercial lab tests for parasitism search for eggs that have exited from the intestine.

You will actually be able to see your adult flukes later, when you succeed in killing them in your intestines, during the *2-Week Cancer-Curing Program*. The disease we call cancer is not caused merely by the adult flukes. That is why fasciolopsiasis does not accompany a cancer case. This is when many adults are present, shedding fertilized eggs into the feces. But sometimes a few adults happen to be in the digestive tract…the esophagus, stomach, or colon. When you kill these, they can be eliminated with the bowel contents, and you have a chance to see them.

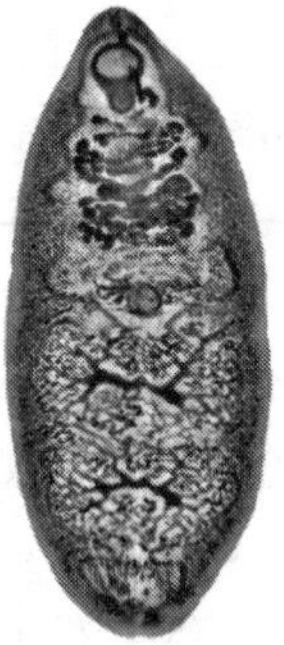

Human intestinal fluke, twice normal size, stretched out and stained (dyed) on a glass microscope slide.

Fig. 2 The cancer parasite

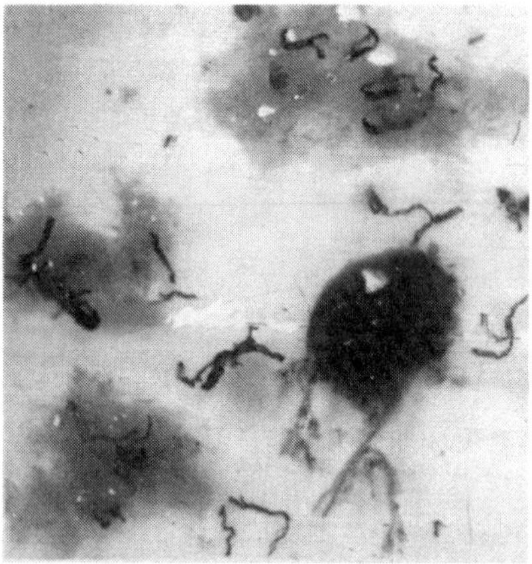

Parasites float when expelled from the bowel. "Black hairy legs" are strings of eggs that hang out when the adult bursts open and deteriorates.

Fig. 3 Five flukes in various stages of decay

You will not be able to see the flukes that are in your tumor or the rest of your body because there is no way for them to be expelled into the toilet. Dead or alive, they are stuck in your tissues. In fact, if they are not promptly removed when you kill them they will cause "side-effects", commonly called "detoxification symptoms".

Tiny primitive animals like flukes go through many phases in their development, somewhat like insects, with their caterpillars and cocoons. These are called **larval stages**. They are not at all like their parents, for example, butterflies or beetles. All fluke stages are too soft and tiny to show up on any scan. But they can be found electronically and then seen physically.

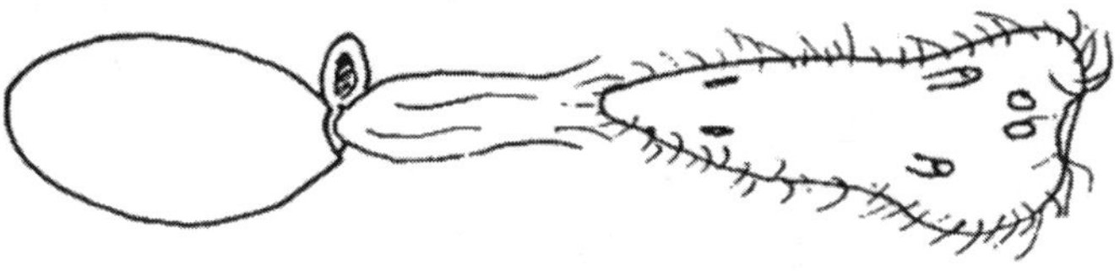

Fig. 4 Miracidia hatching from egg on left

Flukes and fluke stages are in the tissues, not the blood. They have gone unrecognized because only the blood is tested regularly, and the tests are chemical, not physical. Biopsies are prepared by slicing the tissue very thinly. No slice of a parasite stage would ever be recognizable. A biologist could find them, though, by knowing where to search.

Parasites prefer to live packed into your tissues or bunched into stagnant places like vein valves or lymph vessel valves. Other blood rushes along too fast for them and is always patrolled by your immune system. Although a careful search of live blood would show a few of these larval stages, such a search is not a routine part of cancer research or clinical testing. Still, you may actually see adults as you proceed through the *2-Week Program*, sweeping them out as you are doing a liver cleanse.

A liver cleanse is an ancient ritual in which no fat is eaten for a whole day followed by some herbs (now Epsom salts) to relax the bile ducts and a mixture of olive oil and citrus juice later in the evening. This squeezes the bile ducts so a flood of bile is produced. This flood can dislodge and bring out stones that are forming and also parasites.

The presence of Fasciolopsis buski can cause production of a very potent growth stimulant, called **orthophosphotyrosine** or **OPT**. OPT is the hallmark of all our cancers. OPT is made when a radioactive element, polonium, is present along with the lanthanide, cerium, and the DNA of F. buski itself. Even the DNA of bacteria or our own DNA can be attacked by the polonium-cerium partners to produce OPT.

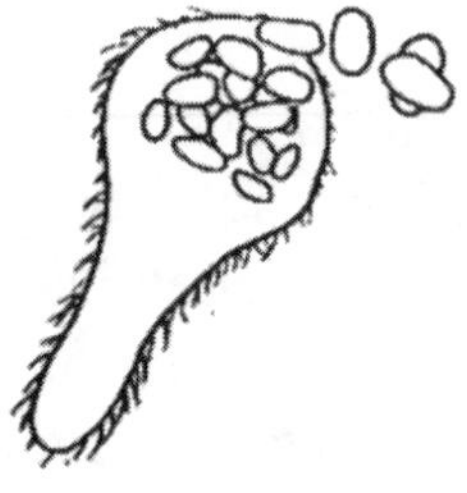

Fig. 5 Miracidia expelling "mother" redia

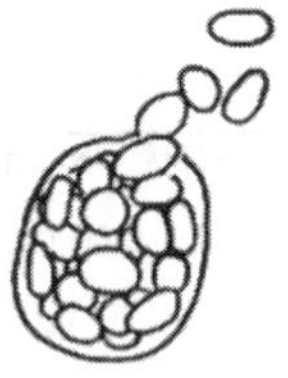

Fig. 6 "Mother" redia bearing "daughter" redia

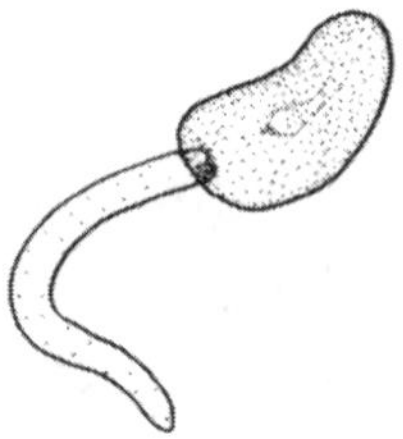

Fig. 7 Cercaria

F. buski's surroundings would normally have both the radioactive element and cerium. We, and all living things, are wading in radioactive elements and lanthanides. Cerium is part of our natural environment, being quite abundant at the same places where the radioactive elements are.

Even parasitism is natural, though excessive parasitism is not. Our bodies begin to kill our parasites as soon as we get them, using powerful body weapons. I will discuss these later. But being trapped in our tissues the dead parasites invite **Clostridium** bacteria. **Isopropyl alcohol** is produced by Clostridium bacteria—those bacteria living in dying flesh and without oxygen. Animal waste is F. buski's normal habitat, namely the colon of animals and people. As soon as any flukes have been killed, Clostridium bacteria travel from the colon to devour their remains; they excrete isopropyl alcohol.

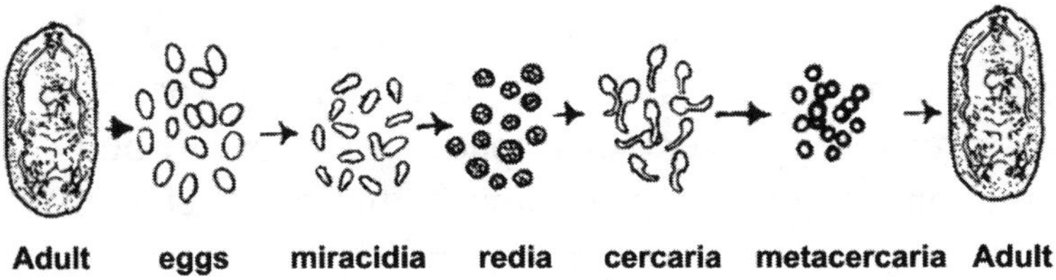

Fig. 8 Life cycle of a fluke

In people, isopropyl alcohol is also provided by a lifestyle that uses it dozens of times each day. It is in our body products and even contaminates our food. So we have two sources of isopropyl alcohol: bacteria and popular products. Isopropyl alcohol is very reactive, chemically, and easily attaches itself to any cerium nearby. Isopropyl alcohol can "hitch a ride" this way with the cerium to the place where they will all act together, our DNA. Logic might tell us that so much polonium, cerium, isopropyl alcohol, Clostridium bacteria and F. buski parasites, in people where much of the population has actual Fasciolopsiasis, should give all these people cancer. People in Asia and other tropical climates should be cancer-ridden. But they are not. The body has learned to make it very difficult for "buski" to make OPT in us…as if to protect us from ever getting cancer! What has gone wrong in the last 100 years? Why do we have a cancer epidemic?

Nature Is On Our Side

Nature is always on our side, protecting us in hundreds of ways. That is why we survived in the past.

In Nature, there are dozens of radioactive elements coming up from the ground if there are uranium phosphate rocks below us. When the uranium atoms break apart, the new pieces formed are radioactive, too, but are different elements now. At the same time the uranium atoms give off radiation. One of the newly created elements is **radon**, a gas. Gases rise and will come to the surface. If your house is located right above some uranium rocks the gas can enter through very tiny spaces and float through your home on the dust. Each new radioactive element will break apart again and again, making more new elements and new kinds of radiation. Radon by itself breaks apart into half a dozen other radioactive elements that we breathe in quite innocently. We do need protection from them and we do get it as we shall see.

Uranium is very reactive with phosphate. That is why they are found together in phosphate rocks. But the elements called lanthanides are very reactive with phosphates too, so they are found at the same places. Many lanthanides are made right there on site as uranium breaks down, again and again. Lanthanides also come up to the surface, riding on dust and gas bubbles. We, living on the surface, are wading in a huge "soup" of radioactive elements and lanthanide elements, mixing and reacting with each other. All the other elements, not radioactive, ride around on dust particles, too, mixing with the others. To make this clearer, see the *Periodic Table of Elements*.

Logic also asks how a huge parasite like Fasciolopsis could get close enough to our DNA to do any harm. After all our genes are safely stowed away inside chromosomes, which are inside the walls of the nucleus.

Periodic table of elements

1 H 1.00797																	2 He 4.00260
3 Li 6.941	4 Be 9.01218											5 B 10.81	6 C 12.01115	7 N 14.0067	8 O 15.9994	9 F 18.99840	10 Ne 20.179
11 Na 22.98977	12 Mg 24.305											13 Al 26.98154	14 Si 28.0861	15 P 30.97376	16 S 32.06	17 Cl 35.453	18 Ar 39.948
19 K 39.098	20 Ca 40.08	21 Sc 44.9559	22 Ti 47.90	23 V 50.9414	24 Cr 51.996	25 Mn 54.9380	26 Fe 55.847	27 Co 58.9332	28 Ni 58.71	29 Cu 63.546	30 Zn 65.38	31 Ga 69.72	32 Ge 72.59	33 As 74.9216	34 Se 78.96	35 Br 79.904	36 Kr 83.80
37 Rb 85.4678	38 Sr 87.62	39 Y 88.9059	40 Zr 91.22	41 Nb 92.9064	42 Mo 95.94	43 Tc 98.9062	44 Ru 101.07	45 Rh 102.9055	46 Pd 106.4	47 Ag 107.868	48 Cd 112.40	49 In 114.82	50 Sn 118.69	51 Sb 121.75	52 Te 127.60	53 I 126.9045	54 Xe 131.30
55 Cs 132.9054	56 Ba 137.34	57 *La 138.9055	72 Hf 178.49	73 Ta 180.9479	74 W 183.85	75 Re 186.2	76 Os 190.2	77 Ir 192.22	78 Pt 195.09	79 Au 196.9665	80 Hg 200.59	81 Tl 204.37	82 Pb 207.19	83 Bi 208.9804	84 Po (210)	85 At (210)	86 Rn (222)
87 Fr (223)	88 Ra 226.0254	89 †Ac (227)	104 (261)	105 (260)	106 (263)												

Lanthanides *	58 Ce 140.12	59 Pr 140.9077	60 Nd 144.24	61 Pm (147)	62 Sm 150.4	63 Eu 151.96	64 Gd 157.25	65 Tb 158.9254	66 Dy 162.50	67 Ho 164.9304	68 Er 167.26	69 Tm 168.9342	70 Yb 173.04	71 Lu 174.97
Actinides †	90 Th 232.0381	91 Pa 231.0359	92 U 238.029	93 Np 237.0482	94 Pu (244)	95 Am (243)	96 Cm (247)	97 Bk (247)	98 Cf (251)	99 Es (254)	100 Fm (257)	101 Md (258)	102 No (255)	103 Lr (256)

Fig. 9 Periodic Table of Elements

Search for the main actors in the cancer story in the chemical (element) table. Find uranium (**U**) in the heaviest set of elements, all radioactive. As uranium breaks apart the pieces are a bit lighter, so are found to the left, for example, thorium (**Th**). Elements at the left side of the table react strongly with elements at the right side. Find the lanthanides, a set of 15, all belonging at the left side, in the same place as lanthanum (**La**). Find cerium (**Ce**), the cancer-making lanthanide. Find promethium (**Pm**), which is the only radioactive lanthanide in Nature. Find radium (**Ra**) to the left of thorium (**Th**), then radon (**Rn**) to the left of radium (**Ra**), then polonium (**Po**) coming from radon's "family". More of radon's family are radioactive bismuth (**Bi**) and lead (**Pb**).

If you test bottled water, any brand, you could find Bi and Pb, suggesting they originated in Rn, and before that Th, and before that U, which started it all. Searching only for U or Rn in public water misses the hazards of drinking radioactive water. I have found every bottle to be radioactive except a few varieties (see *Sources*). Very many bottles had only Th, or Ra, or Bi or Pb, which are radon's "family", and easily get missed when searching for only Rn.

Rn will likely be "spent" while waiting on the supermarket shelves. It breaks apart quite soon, only days, not years. This "time" is called the "half-life". A half-life of 3.8 days means that half of the amount you start with is broken up already in 3.8 days, having changed itself into **polonium**. The radon in a gallon jug of water just shipped from the bottler will be half changed to polonium in 3.8 days. Then another half is changed and another. In a month there would be little Rn left. Except, of course, that more radon is being made from the uranium that got into the jug of water, too. The uranium will "never" be gone, not in a million years (see *The Radon Chain*).

The Radon Chain

Each radioactive element has a "half-life", which is the time for half of it to fall apart (to decay) and give off more radiation.

This table shows the decay chain for Uranium 238, which ends by forming lead that is not radioactive (lead 206, at bottom right).

Isotope	Emits	Half-life	Product
U - 238	alpha	4.5 billion years	Th – 234 Thorium
Th - 234	beta	24.1 days	Pa – 234 Protactinium
Pa - 234	beta	1.17 minutes	U – 234 Uranium
U – 234	alpha	250,000 years	Th – 230 Thorium
Th – 230	alpha	80,000 years	Ra – 226 Radium
Ra – 226	alpha	1,602 years	Rn – 222 Radon
Rn – 222	alpha	3.8 days	Po – 218 Polonium
Po – 218	alpha	3 minutes	Pb – 210 Lead
Pb – 214	beta	26.8 minutes	Bi – 210 Bismuth
Bi – 214	beta	19.7 minutes	Po – 210 Polonium

Isotope	Emits	Half-life	Product
Po – 214	alpha	164 microseconds	Pb – 206 Lead
Pb – 210	beta	21 years	Bi – 210 Bismuth
Bi – 210	beta	5 days	Po – 210 Polonium
Po - 210	alpha	138 days	Pb – 206 Lead

Polonium is regularly "missing" in a water or air sample unless you know how reactive it is and that it might already be combined with phosphate or cerium, or other elements, while you are still searching for the free form.

As humans we have grown up in this cauldron of swirling, reactive elements. It seems though, that Nature has learned to avoid cancer for all its creatures even though the 2 elements that could start it for each of them are all around us, Po and Ce.

A third element, Pm (promethium), is part of the drama, and it is this element that seems to start our cancer protection amidst all the cancer production.

In a cancer victim, Po is attached to Ce, but the Ce is attached to a chemical found in bleach! It is a **cyanide** chemical, added to protect the pipes! The new cyanide is next attached to an **alkylating agent** which appears to be the waste product left by Fasciolopsis buski. It makes alkylating agents, already known for 50 years to cause abundant mutations and cancers. It excretes them because it eats them! The whole body of a cancer patient is full of Po, Ce, the cyanide compound and alkylating agents just as we all are full of nitrogen gas, carbon dioxide and other free molecules from our environment. We all make some alkylating agents, too. They have a rather strong smell, as if mustard and onions plus garlic had been mixed. Our underarm perspiration is always trying to get rid of this "skunk oil" for us. But in cancer patients there are many more ONION, GARLIC and MUSTARD oils because the parasite adds to them. In fact, there are so many right beside the Fasciolopsis stages, that the sweat produced at the skin surface smells like sulfur.

A person without cancer has plenty of Po and Ce, too, because that is our lot on Planet Earth, but these are attached to promethium instead of to cyanides and alkylating agents. The Po is attached to Ce but the Ce is not attached to an ONION, GARLIC or MUSTARD oil coming from a buski parasite. They do not attach to any alkylating agent even though we make a great deal of them by eating onions, garlic and mustard, in the belief they are "good for us". We can sweat them out, but it is a slow process. Often our bodies keep these odors (and the chemicals responsible) for a day or more.

When Po and Ce are attached to Fasciolopsis buski DNA, or to its alkylating agents we see OPT appear quite suddenly.*

My interpretation of this event is that it is produced as a mutation. This has not been proved. However, Po is known as a rather potent mutation causer[13] especially of the large kind where chromosomes are completely broken into pieces. Cerium is known as a "site directing mutagen" (we will discuss this later). And alkylating agents are well known to cause extremely mutilating mutations[14].

Yet Nature has protected us. We cannot get cancer from Nature…although all the ingredients to make OPT are all about us and even within us. Polonium, cerium, and alkylating agents attach to each other in random combinations, yet only <u>one</u> of the many different combinations is <u>ever</u> found in cancer patients and is <u>never</u>

---

* Testers, simulate this situation by placing Po (in bottle-copy form) on left plate. Attach Ce by touching it to Po. Attach buski to Ce. Place OPT on right plate and test for resonance.

[13] Reaney, Patricia, *The Perils of Polonium*, Nov. 2006 www.abc.net

[14] Alberts, Bruce; Johnson, Alexander; Lewis, Julian; Raff, Martin; Roberts, Keith; Walter, Peter, *Molecular Biology of the Cell* – The Preventable Causes of Cancer www.garlandscience.com

found in healthy people. It will originate in only one place as we will see.

To start a cancer requires a very special order between all these partners. That order is not possible in Nature and healthy people...because Pm stands in the way. Pm has already combined with cerium, so the alkylating agents are excluded!

When your biopsy is studied it can easily tell which mutations are probably caused by the polonium. They are the huge "chromosomal aberrations" that cut the DNA right across, leaving large pieces to drift away or stick to other pieces, also cut in this way. But why is it always the same mutations in cases of cancer? Why do they always produce HCG, p53, bcl 2, CEA, CA 125 and many others we have read about over the years? This "site selection" for cancer mutations may be the role of cerium. Site selected mutation by lanthanides was discovered in 1995[15] and possibly earlier.

Fasciolopsis parasites and the radioactive polonium element plus cerium and the ferrocyanide pipe protector, and ONION-like alkylating agents combine to induce OPT, our main cancer marker.

I call this the cancer-complex. The huge cancer-complex produces many mutations besides OPT.

Seeing these chromosome breaks and the extra growth, namely very crowded cells, makes a mass appear malignant to a cytologist who looks at your biopsy. All cancer patients that I analyzed by Syncrometer® and who had already been diagnosed by an oncologist had both OPT and the F. buski fluke stages in the organ with the

[15] Komiyama, Makoto, *Sequence-selective and hydrolytic scission of DNA and RNA by lanthanide complex-oligoDNA hybrids,* J. Biochem., 118, 665-670 (1995) (JB Revies) www.jb.oxfordjournals.org

tumor. There were no exceptions among thousands! That is why OPT is my cancer marker. They also had polonium and cerium stuck together and then linked to F. buski through a ferrocyanide chemical and an alkylating agent. It would seem like a terribly unwieldy cancer-causer. But that will help us to undo it later, as we "cure" it.

It is very easy to stop this early malignancy just by killing this fluke and all its stages as we have done in the past. But now, 12 years later, we can also stop a very advanced malignancy almost as easily. By taking away a single part of the unwieldy cancer-complex we already can stop it. Your tumor cells will stop receiving OPT, their major stimulant. But we can do more. Tumors must have the things they need to grow; otherwise they must stop, regardless of stimulation. Deoxyribonucleic acid (DNA) is one. The stimulation of any radiation, particularly uranium, nearby constantly turns on DNA to make more of itself, but certain ingredients must still be provided. How could the tissues be so deluged in DNA that the Syncrometer® sees they are swamped? It is also being made by the same Clostridium bacteria that devour dead tissue and make isopropyl alcohol.

Clostridium bacteria provide isopropyl alcohol and DNA.

Clostridium produces DNA that is similar to our DNA. DNA flooding is not seen in the presence of other bacteria, like Staphylococcus (staph for short) or Streptococcus (strep for short). Its similarity to our DNA is a unique feature of Clostridium. It allows sharing. Killing all Clostridium colonies will stop providing the tumor with extra DNA to grow on. Meanwhile, the Syncrometer® sees that Clostridium, too, has become a hanger-on of cerium and will get pulled into your chromosomes. When Clostridium reaches the same destination as the rest of the complex it will add to the many mutations being made. Perhaps it will be "excessive DNA of the human kind". Each addition to the cancer-complex adds more and different mutations.

To cure the whole cancer very quickly, we could kill the fluke and its stages, as we did in earlier books. But we could also dislodge the whole cancer-complex. We will be helped by its clumsy construction. We will also be helped by the great water solubility of both polonium and cerium. Simple water could dismantle it and wash it out of you.

If the whole story of cancer causation seems much more complicated now than in the past, we can be consoled when we realize that the complexity makes it more vulnerable.

The whole curing program is much simpler and shorter now than in past programs. Its complexity allows it to be derailed in a single step…swamping.

But we will keep to our *2-Week Program* because there are many more malignancies in your body than your oncologist found. We will be able to find them—but this time without x-rays or ultrasound or any other "scans"—only with "body wipes" that will be tested by Syncrometer®. We will be able to watch as we wash them (our malignancies!) out with hot water.

It is understandable now why an early (first occurrence) cancer could be cured so easily in earlier books. If any one of these clumsy cancer-complex pieces could be removed from the tumor, such as Po or Ce, the cyanide or the alkylating agent, and a *Maintenance Program* kept up for this, no more OPT could be made. It would be removed in hours. Killing the flukes removes the alkylating agents. Stopping the use of chlorox contaminated water stops those alkylating agents coming from automotive greases. Both motor oil and wheel bearing grease have mustard oil alkylating agents. The dinosaurs were probably eating them. Removing all **plastic** and **rubber** would remove the Ce, as we will also see later. All these must be present to develop a cancer.

What was not understandable until recently was why Fasciolopsis was needed at all in this cancer-producing recipe. Surely, the polonium and various alkylating agents could produce enough cancer mutations by themselves, without a parasite. Yet, there is no cancer without the parasite. Evidently, a living force is required too!

One answer came when the Syncrometer® found the popular dye, **methylene blue**, in all chlorox-contaminated water. The dye had attached itself to Fasciolopsis, as a dye could be expected to do: dye something blue. But methylene blue is also an alkylating agent, in this case also dying our DNA. Then why aren't cancer patients blue?

It was known 60 years ago or more that methylene blue is a unique dye, turning colorless, not blue, when a living organism got dyed by it. It is still used for such a purpose—to detect living bacteria in milk, for example. It shows the surgeon where the tissue is alive, not dead. Again, it becomes colorless. Now it was obvious why killing the buski parasite immediately stopped the cancer. A stream of electrons, called reducing power, was coming from buski and was necessary to fuel the cancer-complex at its DNA connections. The real role of F. buski was finally found…as the source of energy to fuel cell division.

Then why not simply focus on killing F. buski?

Because there are so many! And they are given protection by radioactivity. Each parasite stage has its radioactive element attached. When a White Blood Cell attacks, its vitamin C is immediately destroyed. Now it can do nothing, not even attack bacteria and viruses. How radioactivity destroys vitamin C is not known. Why only organic vitamin C (complete with rutin and hesperidin) can win battles against radioactive bacteria and parasites is also not known.

Only removing the radioactivity from the body gives a realistic answer to our baffling parasitism. It will be described in Chapter 16 on Advanced Dentistry.

Summary – Chapter 1

1. The true cause of cancer is not one of the carcinogens listed in Prop 65 in California, or by IARC in its many volumes worldwide. It is not a mutated cell with cancer characteristics.

2. It is a huge chemical complex made of polonium, cerium, iron cyanide in "ferro" form, and MUSTARD, GARLIC and ONION oils in this order. These very odorous oils are called alkylating agents. They can combine with DNA to produce mutations. But the cerium can not be linked to the alkylating agents unless a facilitating substance is present. This will turn out to be potassium ferrocyanide, added to our drinking water as an anticorrosive compound. Adding potassium ferricyanide will not do this. Only chlorox bleach has ferrocyanide. Only ferrocyanide can link the cerium molecule to the ONION chemicals and to F. buski. F. buski gets steered to your DNA by methylene blue, leaving its "living energy" there to somehow turn on the DNA's "magical" reproduction forces.

3. Other items can add themselves to the basic complex at the cerium element attachment. They are isopropyl alcohol, malonic acid, extra DNA, stem cells of any organ, and the tumor nucleus. We will learn about these soon.

4. Each cancer-complex must fit the chromosome at exact points and stick to it tightly. This would satisfy the requirements to make site directed mutations, all those seen over and over in cancer cases.

5. In the earliest book only the Fasciolopsis fluke was given as the true cause of cancer. How it really happened was

still not known. Now, 12 years later, we can see that it is linked to special mutagens that form a large complex I call the cancer-complex.

WANTED DEAD—OR DEADER

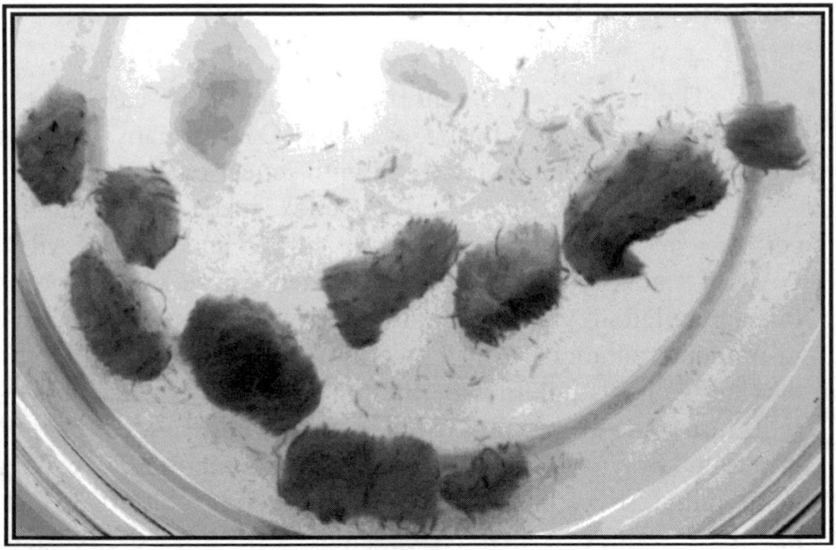

A bowl of proglottids (segments) shows squarish ends as the tapeworm breaks up during the essential oil and suppository treatment. Recipe for elimination is not yet available.

WARNING: DO NOT EXPERIMENT ON YOURSELF to remove tapeworm. The recipes were not complete at time of publishing.

CHAPTER 2

YOUR WATER

At the time *The Cure For All Cancers* was written (1993), it was thought by scientists, myself included, that the malignancy was the entire cancer...that removing it removed the entire cancer and after that, a healthy life could be resumed. Meanwhile, the benign state was considered tolerable and brought a huge sigh of relief. Those were simplistic times. This belief had started the **biopsy** era to distinguish between malignant and benign states. It also brought yet another lucrative arm of treatment that could be carried out in protocol form and in massive numbers of consumers. It separated further the doctor from the doctor's mission, which had always been to cure the patient. Now the doctor did not need to think, ask questions, listen, or wonder, only to carry out a highly skilled technician's task—the **biopsy**. The biopsy, unfortunately, is an invasive procedure, destined to make any wild growth worse, whether skillfully done or not. Any new trauma invites the body to shift into its healing mode, which always consists of new growth to replace the diseased tissue. In the case of cancer the biopsy trauma will be done exactly in that location where there is no growth control. We have all seen the regrowth of tumors along old scars from stomach surgery, breast or thyroid surgery. Growths of any kind, even genital warts seem to favor scar tissue from bladder surgery or episiotomies or even hemorrhoid repair.

If a growth of some kind is not malignant, then what is it? Can it just be given the "watch and see" treatment as was implied by the word "benign"? There would certainly be no justification for surgery, chemotherapy, or radiation treatment of a benign tumor. This stalemate in clinical care seems intolerable now and neglectful to the extreme, knowing its true nature, a suspicious growth. Any cancer suspicion should be challenged with healthful procedures and lifestyle changes, such as I recommend in this book. Yet, they are not even thought about, professionally, as though cancer were not a cause-and-effect disease. There is no precision of course even with biopsies. Finding a chemotherapy that is listed in a catalog to match a biopsy diagnosis can be accurately done, but often does not bring success. Too much is expected of a profession with too little science at its base. Energy medicine using frequency-based detection and treatment could speed this up dramatically. Hopefully, this will soon be remedied with financial investment by society in these new sciences.

In this book the steps are carefully laid out to show how the status of a tumor can be assessed in chemical and physical terms. This will bring treatment into the rational world and into healthy competition with others. Benign tumors have a life of their own both before the malignancy starts and after the malignancy stops. Examples are warts, cysts, fibrocystic masses, polyps, and moles. It even includes extreme obesity. Fat cells become the targeted organ as in cancer.

Wait And See

We all know from our own experience that in the beginning, some kind of growing force gave us a little mass and we lived in fear of this each day. The doctor may have requested a biopsy, but even after that you have not learned why you got it or how you got it or what you really got. And it is certainly not advisable to do nothing, although the doctor wants to reassure you. The "wait and see" approach that is usually recommended seems highly immoral when a whole book of "preventive advice" exists.[16] (See for example, Ralph Moss' book *Cancer Therapy*.) The oncologist should be required to lay one on each patient's report. It could improve that patient's outcome. Whether it does, should also be tested.

We already know what will happen eventually to give us a true malignancy—Fasciolopsis parasites and a host of special chemicals and a polonium-cerium-complex will join the benign tumor.

But what happens between these times? Do all those people who have started a benign tumor or mass reach the point where the tumor becomes malignant?

They do not!

Early tumor-like beginnings that are not visible to the eye are often seen with a Syncrometer® in children when one parent has cancer. Not all of these children go on to develop cancer. Even though the whole family of a cancer patient carries the intestinal fluke parasite and even though the whole family develops early beginnings of tumors, such as moles or polyps, some will get cancer and some will not. Something quite decisive is missing for some of the family members and not for the others to make the difference.

Knowing what makes this difference is very, very important.

Research designed to unravel such a mystery is called epidemiology.

Epidemiology

It was obvious far back to antiquity that the general health and appearance of a person made no difference. The decisive factor whether or not you get cancer was much more subtle.

---

[16] Moss, Ralph W., PhD, *Cancer Therapy*, 1992, 1996

The field of epidemiology grew very strong in the middle of the last century. Different religions, different occupations, different regions of the country, all had different cancer rates. Was it tea and coffee drinking, pork eating, cooking habits, the air, stress levels? Even the heights of chimneys in England were measured, in desperation, to shed light on this mystery.

As promising as all the collected facts and figures looked, nothing could be made of it, nothing could be identified as the deciding factor that leads us to this disease. Yet, the effort was not wasted. Many **carcinogens** (things that could cause cancer) such as **soot** from these chimneys were discovered and were helpful even though they did not lead to solutions. And the failure of every cancer victim's immune power was also discovered.

Immune Power

Immune power was a mysterious concept at first. Researchers could see that animals would not let a transplanted tumor grow in them unless the immune system was first knocked down, by radiation, for example. People who had to have their immune power knocked down to accept an organ transplant got many more cancers than others. Special animals were raised who were missing immune power in order to do cancer research. Special chemicals were developed to destroy immune power at will.

The loss of personal immune power is not visible. You may be a strong, healthy person in the prime of life and yet be losing your immune power. Clinical doctors, researchers and victims of cancer themselves were all aware of this. But the scientific tools available to investigate this were only biochemistry and immunology. These methods are much too slow and much too costly to do such research in a timely way. It would take hundreds of years, if ever, to find the difference between persons who get cancer and those who do not using only these techniques.

Eventually all epidemiology seemed hopeless because everything, even good, nourishing food, seemed to have carcinogens and cause mutations.

> Carcinogens are chemicals that cause cancer and mutagens are chemicals that cause mutations. They overlap a great deal.

Chemicals were studied in bacteria, mice, rabbits, and cancer cell lines, but all rather far removed from our real situation. At the same time chemicals from industry were being dumped into our food and homes in "truckload" amounts, making "good nourishing food" and "fresh air" false concepts. This obscured epidemiological differences. Just as hopes hit bottom, a ray of light shone in.

It was quite by accident that a new technology was born. It held the promise of doing all this difficult and expensive research in a fraction of the time needed before, and for a fraction of the cost. It is the **audio oscillator**.

The device using this technology is called a Syncrometer® (see pages 20 & 21).

The Syncrometer® is momentarily attached to the body with pressure (a probe) to apply a small electrical charge and to note any resistance change. Body resistance changes when a harmful item is passed before the body's open circuit in the form of a single capacitor plate. It could soon verify the close association between getting cancer and losing immunity. It could find precisely what the immune system's defects were. It could find the true causes of these defects. And finally, it could find what the epidemiological factors are that bring these causes to some people and not to others. By 1999 several thousand cancer victims had been studied for toxins in their food, air, water, body products, clothing, and teeth. Which of these were common to all? That was my project.

It all pointed to the water. They were using one kind. No difference though could be seen or tasted or felt in the different waters people were using.

Yet, there was a 100% association between a popular disinfectant in water and cancer. There was also a 100% disassociation between this disinfectant and freedom from cancer.

> The water coming to your kitchen faucet brings the cancer-causing agent.

The same water also has the power to destroy your immune system without you noticing it. Water without this disinfectant has the power to allow recovery.

Proprietary Water Additions

Unfortunately, in spite of our many technical advances, nobody is able to test their own water for those things that are added to it and could be harmful. The additions may even be considered proprietary! Hopefully, this glaring gap in people's freedom to know will be corrected for all in the near future so we can try to prevent future health disasters.

While we were all waiting for our cancer institutes to find any carcinogen hidden in our water, food, and surroundings, it turned out to be the disinfectant itself, the chlorination that was meant to protect us from such dangers and that we had grown to trust. It reminds us of the military trick played in ancient Greece when a wooden horse brought enemy soldiers into the city. After the citizens got accustomed to seeing it inside their city the people overlooked it and in one night were defeated.

The Secret Of Water

There are two kinds of water in the USA and in the world. The world is patterning after the USA in its water processing and delivery. Hopefully, this will be investigated very carefully by all nations trying to sanitize their food and water.

One kind has the cancer-causer, the other kind does not.

Water should be pure and free of bad bacteria; it should bring us minerals, some oxygen, a proper magnetic polarization (to be discussed later) and it should even taste good. The Federal Drug Administration (FDA) and Environmental Protection Agency (EPA) and even the Department of Agriculture have shared the responsibility for good water quality and have done their utmost to keep it so. They could not prevent the universal contamination of our water with hundreds of solvents, metals, pesticides and other chemicals. They could not prevent the tragedy that we now see in an explosion of illnesses beginning in childhood. **We already have a generation of sick children**. There was no reason to suspect the water, which we all, sick or healthy, have come to rely on. It is regularly tested, though not for the correct items.

Gaps In Water Regulation

Nobody recognized the gaps in water vigilance that lie between the last pump house and the residents (see page 67) and between the municipal supplier and the public consumer.

Every inch of the way along the drinkable water trail is regulated, as it should be, but it stops short at your property line. From there to your kitchen sink is your responsibility, namely nobody's.

This is not acceptable in an age of disease like the present. A way must be found to fill this gap.

It is not ordinary water contaminants that make the difference we are searching for. The ordinary ones are present in both waters and consumed by all people and are already being tested. In spite of being undesirable, these do not make the decisive difference between getting cancer or not...although they do for many other diseases.

Adding Aluminum

Water is usually treated with aluminum to help it filter clear of sediment as it is passed through sand beds. It is then disinfected with chlorine gas. This is done in nearly all water treatment plants. Chlorine gas bubbled through water produces assorted harmful and even carcinogenic chemicals, but, again, most people have been drinking such water and do not get cancer. It is not chlorine gas or aluminum that causes cancer.

Adding Chlorine

After the water leaves the treatment plant it is tested for its "free" chlorine level at certain checkpoints, because this level tends to get lower and lower. A certain level needs to be kept up, a few parts per million (ppm) of active chlorine. This is what kills bacteria.

Adding more chlorine gas on a small scale, if the total-chlorine were low, would be prohibitively expensive at these numerous small checkpoints. Chlorine gas is also very dangerous to handle.

Adding Chlorine Bleach

Consequently, technicians have been trained to calculate how much liquid chlorine (bleach) needs to be added at any one checkpoint. This is much less expensive or dangerous. They have been taught which bleach has the EPA registration number and the National Sanitation Foundation (NSF) stamp to legalize its use in drinking water, and where to buy it. It comes in double strength concentration, large bottles, and 4 bottles to a crate, a most unwieldy package! It also comes in larger containers for manufacturer's use and other big consumers. A plastic crate is the only legal way to transport this rather hazardous fluid because it contains 12% chlorine instead of the 6% that we are accustomed to handling. The bottles must always be carried in this crate or returned that way for safety's sake. It is not suited to engineers and workmen who must often speedily repair pipes. It is certainly not convenient for housewives, farmers, or the average citizen.

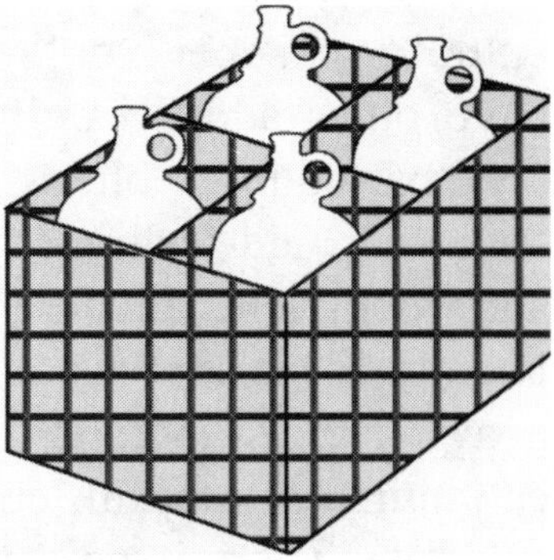

Fig. 10 Crate of bleach bottles

All the detailed requirements for allowing bleach to be added to the public's water were expected to lead to a carefully protected process of adding a food-grade substance to our drinking water. But it did just the opposite.

Bleaches Are Not Equal

Somewhere a myth got started that "bleach is bleach" and any bleach would do. Advertising blurred the difference intentionally. Government memos do not specify the food grade varieties for contact with drinking water. It would justify stopping at the corner store for a bottle of bleach—to fix a water pipe, to pour down a well, to wash tables in a restaurant, to rinse dishes or mixers in a drug manufacturing plant. Before there were many kinds of bleach on the market, perhaps such a myth did little harm. Now that many kinds of bleaches are on the market, it does a great deal of harm. The new bleaches arriving in the supermarkets in the past few decades have changed considerably. Some have "whiteners and brighteners" added, which implies "dyes and metals". The words "ultra", or "super", or "regular" make no difference. Many have other additives. It was already known generations ago that adding "bluing" to your laundry made it appear "whiter". Old-fashioned bluing was a cobalt compound and methylene blue, a heavy metal and a dye. Now laundry bleaches have a huge assortment of dyes, and the heavy metals include barium, lead, lanthanum, nickel, cadmium, chromium, cobalt, ruthenium, and yttrium, for example. There is no set recipe for these, suggesting they are some other industry's wastewater. They were never meant to be drunk, of course, only applied to clothing and bathrooms.

Heavy Metals In Bleaches

The Syncrometer® typically finds about 20 heavy metals in a sample of popular bleach. All have many azo dyes meant for cloth and paper, not food. Most have asbestos and shocking solvents. Shocking, because their PCBs, malonic acid, benzene and isopropyl alcohol are well known to contribute to cancer. Shocking to have motor oil and even wheel bearing grease and a high level of radioactivity. Compare this to the legally designated, NSF grade bleach meant for drinking water (see table on page 62).

Just which brand of bleach is being used can easily be discerned. Bleach varieties only resonate with themselves using the Syncrometer®. So if you test water samples for the presence of local supermarket varieties of bleach, you can tell which one you are inadvertently drinking. You can also find which variety is used in your water filter or softener and on the produce in your supermarket.

Through a simple-minded error of using chlorox laundry bleach instead of NSF grade bleach, your water can receive the stamp of cancer.

Azo Dyes In Drinking Water

Modern bleaches contain extremely toxic dyes. Being used for laundry, we could not expect these to be safe, edible dyes. The Syncrometer® detects those already banned 50 years ago in food. Some are legally allowed. The Syncrometer® always finds Fast Garnet, Fast Green, Fast Red, Fast Red Violet, Fast Blue, Dimethylaminoazobenzene (DAB, or butter yellow), Sudan Black, in fact, the entire list on page 645.

Unknowns In The Drinking Water

I do not know the source of the dyes, asbestos nor heavy metal ingredients shown in the table on page 62. I do not know the source of the malonic acid, motor oil or wheel bearing grease. I do not know the source of the isopropyl alcohol or even the potassium ferrocyanide. The polonium, cerium, and promethium could be expected in any large body of water. They are everywhere in the air.

The water with laundry bleach disinfectant does not look different from healthful water. It is clear and sparkling, tastes good, and meets all the requirements of the water regulators. The requirements do not include tests for the ingredients I

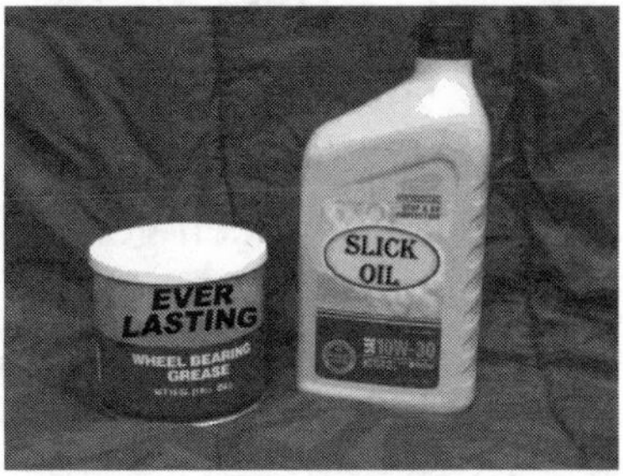

Regular wheel bearing grease and motor oil are in your drinking water from addition of chlorox laundry bleach.

Fig. 11 Common wheel bearing grease & motor oil

found. Such non-NSF bleach also appears to be allowed in water filters although water in contact with a filter is meant to be drunk!

Maybe the activated carbon (filter) makers believe the carbon will filter itself when in use. It does not. It contaminates all the water passing through it, instead. Was this not tested?

Water Softeners Contaminate

Maybe the water softener manufacturers believe that their softener salts will obediently keep to one side of the kitchen faucets and that nobody will use the hot water faucet to cook with, or make instant tea. But they do. And softener salts do not keep to one side. They contaminate both sides, in fact, all the water pipes. It is tempting to justify this belief on the basis that the crossing over of chemicals from the "hot" faucet to the cold faucet must be very small. Indeed it "must". But if we were dealing with plutonium or are dealing with polonium we should certainly apply a much more stringent standard than ever before! These are some of our most toxic elements.

Project of 1999

My project in 1999 became "which one of the ingredients in laundry bleached drinking water made the difference between getting cancer or not in all cases?"

I had already found the PCBs, benzene, asbestos, set of azo dyes, set of heavy metals, malonic acid, isopropyl alcohol, motor oil and wheel bearing grease to distinguish the 2 bleaches. But not one of those was present in 100% of cancer cases. Those that were a part of sets or in the form of compounds seemed unreachable in their vast numbers and many were unavailable as test standards.

24 Common Solvents

Nevertheless, I tested each of a set of 24 common solvents, about 40 more metals, 14 lanthanide elements, and a few radioactive elements (radon, uranium, americium, thorium, and radium). None of these were 100% associated with cancerous tumors. None was present in the water sample of each cancer patient. The task looked infinite, requiring more time than might be available for me (age 72).

Amateur Radio To The Rescue

The clue came by accident. A fellow amateur radio operator had used his old military Geiger counter and found a higher level of radioactivity than normal "background". He had tested the skin surface of his wife who had just been diagnosed with lung cancer. He implored me to revisit such a study with a similar Geiger counter he had loaned me a number of years earlier. My first data looked surprisingly high in radioactivity. Could it be? The Geiger counter is not meant for a skin study. Most of the radioactivity would get missed! Then why were his wife's readings higher, especially over the bones in special "hot spots"? I immediately tested 2 lung cancer cases myself. The readings seemed exceptionally high, but it would take much too long to reach figures that were statistically significant. I invested in an automatic counter with timer. Meanwhile my colleague's measurements had to stop when his wife, Julie, died. From diagnosis to death was a scant month. The tragedy was unspeakable. His mourning turned into action and spurred mine.

A New Geiger Mueller Counter

With my new counter and samples of water, food, even the very walls of a house, potting soil, softener salts, potassium supplements, fertilizers, the picture soon became clearer. We are not suffering from average spreading of radioactivity from postwar bomb testing. We are suffering from surprising indiscretions, right now. Our chlorinated water, grapes, strawberries, tomatoes, citrus fruit and raisins are much higher in radioactivity than the background! Our dental supplies including caps, composite, anesthetics are much higher and will become permanently attached to the inside of the body as they solidify. The amalgam itself, and porcelain, or veneers are much higher, too! How could we put the toxins we fear most, such as spread of contamination along with nuclear capability, right in our mouths?

Moreover, our 2 kinds of drinking water had 2 kinds of radioactivity.

Background Radioactivity

There is radioactivity all around us…from outer space, from underground, from our houses, even from ourselves. It all adds up to an average amount. So when you wish to measure the radioactivity in some potting soil you must know what is "normal" for that spot first and then subtract it from the gross count. It is called "background".

The radon-family, often called "daughters", was often present in the saliva of a cancer case, but not always. In fact, polonium, the most suspect, could not be studied for lack of a pure sample. Two lanthanides were present much too often, cerium in cancer victims and promethium in healthy people. These results brought more questions than answers.

Sampling The Environment

People came to my assistance. I was given a set of 15 tobacco varieties and a one-foot stack of computer printouts on the subject of radioactivity and cancer. I still had several cigarettes from past smokers—cancer patients.

I was sent various IARC journals, samples of fertilizer, softener salts and dozens of bleaches. The search was on in earnest. **What was the true carcinogen in the laundry bleach water?** Was it the same as appeared to be raising the radioactivity level of any average cancer case?

"Maybe Po" In Tobacco?

A year later, with only a few metals left to study—radioactive ones, not available for purchase, I made a single test sample out of the tobacco set. I called it "Maybe Po" to study a new lung cancer case that had just arrived. I found a match! But the match was not simply to Maybe Po. It was to Maybe PoCe and to Maybe PoCe-ferrocyanide. There was no free Po or Ce. Soon these same chemical complexes were found in every cancer patient, whether they had ever smoked or not. In fact, it was in their kitchen water supply, though often not in the outside garden hose water. It was in all the most popular bleaches, but not in NSF bleaches.

Pure Polonium Passes All Tests

Eventually, I obtained very small samples of rather pure radioactive elements (within legal limits). They included promethium as well as polonium. Fortunately my "Maybe polonium" did possess the true element and a year's data was saved.

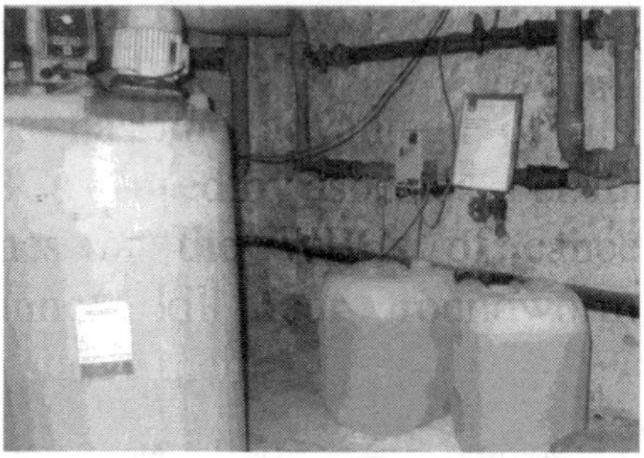

Fig. 12 Water additives are inconspicuous

The difference between cancer-causing waters and NSF water is polonium, in a complex with cerium (a lanthanide), followed by potassium ferr<u>o</u>cyanide instead of the NSF PoCe-potassium ferricyanide. This time there were no exceptions. Every cancer case had the ferro chemical. Others had the ferri variety. Was the bleach company putting in the wrong chemical to prevent scaling and save the water pipes?

"Scaling" refers to the deposit that settles on the inside of a water pipe, making it pass less water. Chemicals can be added to reduce this. Of course, you drink the chemicals along with the "loosened" "scale".

Chemicals In Bleach **Undiluted bleaches tested by Syncrometer®**

The two iron compounds and polarizations are not toxins.
An asterisk means the level detected was exceptionally high.

Toxin	popular laundry bleach	NSF grade bleach	Toxin	popular laundry bleach	NSF grade bleach
acetone S	Neg	Neg	molybdenum	Pos	Neg
alpha radiation♦	Pos	Neg	motor oil S	*Pos	Neg
aluminum	Neg	Neg	neodymium L	Pos	Neg
antimony	Pos	Neg	methylene blue	Pos	Neg
arsenic	*Pos	Neg	nickel	*Pos	Neg
asbestos	*Pos		niobium	Neg	Neg
azo dyes	Pos	Neg	north polarization	Neg	Pos
barium	*Pos	Neg	palladium	Pos	Neg
benzene S	Pos	Neg	PCB S	Pos	Neg
beryllium	Neg	Neg	platinum	Neg	Neg
bismuth	Neg	Neg	polonium R	Pos	Neg
boron	Pos	Neg	praseodymium L	Neg	Neg
bromine, gas	Neg	Neg	Promethium R	Pos	Neg
cadmium	Pos	Neg	rhenium	Pos	Neg
cerium L	Pos	Neg	rhodium	Neg	Neg
cesium	Neg	Neg	rubidium	Neg	nt
chromium III &VI	Pos	Neg	ruthenium	Neg	Neg
cobalt	Pos	Neg	samarium L	Neg	Neg
copper	Pos	Neg	scandium L	Neg	Neg
dodecane S	*Pos	Neg	selenium	Neg	Neg
dysprosium L	Pos	Neg	silicic acid	Neg	Neg
europium L	Pos	Neg	silicon	Pos	Neg

♦ preliminary data

Fe2O3*, ferrite	Pos	Neg	silver	Neg	Neg
Fe3O4, magnetite	Neg	Pos	south polarization	Pos	Neg
ferricyanide	Neg	Pos	strontium	Pos	Neg
ferrocyanide	Pos	Neg	tantalum	*Pos	Neg
formaldehyde S	Neg	Neg	tin	Neg	Neg
gadoliniumL	Pos	Neg	tellurium	Neg	Neg
germanium	Neg	Neg	terbium L	Neg	Neg
gold	Neg	Neg	thallium	Neg	Neg
holmium L	Pos	Neg	thulium L	Neg	Neg
indium	Pos	Neg	toluene S	Pos	Neg
iridium	Neg	Neg	tungsten	*Pos	Neg
isopropyl alcohol S	Neg	Neg	uranium R	Pos	Neg
lanthanum L	Pos	Neg	vanadium	Pos	Neg
lead	Neg	Neg	wheel bearing grease	Pos	Neg
lithium	Neg	Neg	xylenes S	Pos	Neg
lutetium L	Neg	Neg	ytterbium	Neg	Neg
manganese	Neg	Neg	yttrium	Neg	Neg
mercury	Neg	Neg	zinc	Neg	Neg
methanol S	Neg	Neg	zirconium	Neg	Neg
nt = not tested	**L = lanthanide**		**S = solvent**	**R = radioactive**	

Fig. 13 Toxins in bleach

Maybe it does little harm to rub the polonium-cerium-ferrocyanide bleach against your skin after doing the laundry. But the Syncrometer® sees the cancer-complex being absorbed by the skin and passing right through to a deeper organ. I suspect it causes our skin cancers, as well as metastases. Skin cancer is so common now that it equals all other cancers combined. It is not even counted in the statistics regularly given for cancer. Skin cancer is blamed on the sun! Added to your drinking water, the following dozen toxins do incredible harm: **PCBs, benzene, asbestos, a heavy metal panel, azo dye set, isopropyl alcohol, malonic acid, wheel bearing grease, motor oil, dissolved plastic** and **rubber, iron cyanides,**

♦ preliminary data

methylene blue. Children suffer greatly from such water, getting kidney disease, lowered immunity and poor appetite.

> The bleach variety in your kitchen water makes the difference between those who get cancer and those who do not.

Legitimate food-grade bleach, the kind stamped with the NSF mark and given a registration number has none of these dozen toxins (categories), nor the cancer-complexes. But it does have radioactivity—no doubt from the buffers used to manufacture it, which are mainly phosphates. It does have the disease complex: PoCe-potassium ferricyanide. This combines with other parasites if MUSTARD oil is present. This is how we get our non-cancer diseases.

All the cancer patients seen in the last 7 years, including many not seen but merely tested, had these same dozen toxins and potassium ferrocyanide together with popular **chlorox laundry bleach** in their drinking water. The same set was seen in their saliva, lymph, organs, and tumors. This comes to a very large number of patients, well over a thousand. Not a single cancer case was missing this set in their bodies. But a few patients had the evidence only in their tumors or lymph, not saliva. These persons had recently moved to a new home and luckily found good water so the body was already detoxifying itself.

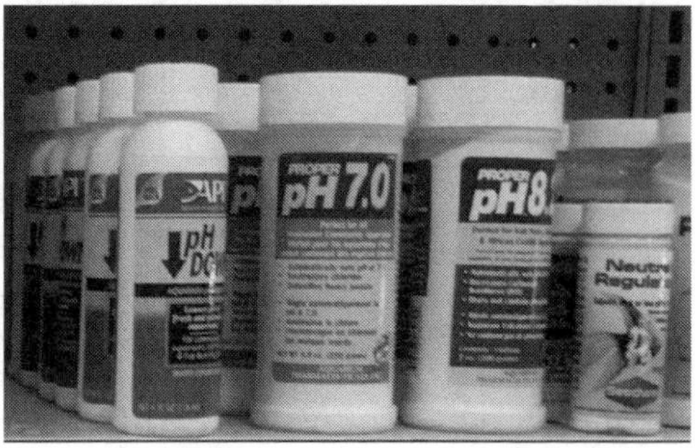

Buffers keep the acid-base balance regulated. Test yours with a Geiger counter if in dry form.

Fig. 14 Buffers may be radioactive

European Laundry Bleach

Cancer victims in Europe showed a different brand of laundry bleach I have named *European laundry bleach.* This is particularly high in polonium, azo dyes, motor oil, wheel bearing grease and malonic acid, but with less PCBs and benzene. The manufacturing plant given for it was American. Cancer victims in Central America, India, UK, and all HIV victims in Africa showed the same chlorox bleach brands as in the USA. Victims in Mexico showed a Mexican brand of bleach with the USA brand as an ingredient. African laundry bleach was particularly high in benzene.

There were no exceptions among cancer patients, making this a compelling statistic. Of course, family members of cancer victims may not have cancer yet although they are using the same water. Their risk is much higher than others but maybe they will move away before it happens. Now it is understandable how a parent with cancer could raise a family where only some children get cancer. They all moved to different residences. It only takes a few weeks to lower the level of all these toxins in your body if you are still healthy. Your body is still capable of detoxifying itself and excreting the complex. But if cancer has already developed, it is too late.

You already have the cancer-complex stuck in your DNA and its genes. One organ connects to the cancer-complex. The complex will hold tight like the intertwined branches of a thorn bush. One of your organs will start to produce cancer mutations over and over until the complex is removed, if ever.

You must quickly clean up your water supply and your contaminated house and separate the cancer-complex from this organ. Each patient seen by us was asked to obtain water samples from friends and relatives until clean kitchen water was found where they could stay till their homes were ready for them.

Testing The Outside Water

Four out of five of the patients were already getting NSF rated bleach in their own water! This was obvious by testing the outside faucet water. It did not have the polonium-cerium-ferro-complex and did have an NSF bleach. What went wrong for this patient? How could the kitchen and entire house be so contaminated if the municipal water did not bring it?

Almost everyone had attached a filter. Many kinds of filters were used. The filters all contained the cancer-complex along with a multitude of other toxins. We tested very many (hundreds). As the safe water from the municipality passed through the filter it got contaminated with the cancer-causing bleach that was used to "sanitize" the filter and the die was cast upon the family.

The same thing happened when a softener salt was added. So far, none that I have tested in all these (15) years has had NSF bleach disinfection. It always had polonium-cerium-ferro-complex. It did not stay on the hot water side of the sink. All water sometimes refluxes. In a single pass the pipes are contaminated.

Genetic Diseases

All persons with serious diseases and genetic diseases, besides cancer and HIV or AIDS had such filters or a water softener attached to their water pipes at one time. Often, none was visible, though. It had been done by a previous resident. The water heater had become contaminated in many cases. It only takes one small filter attached to one small pipe in a distant room to contaminate the whole house with polonium. When the house touches you, with its floors, carpets, chairs, bedding, and dishes, your skin immediately absorbs it, as it would poison ivy.

The Last Pump House

Sometimes the cancer-complex comes directly from the city. As thorough and demanding as our agencies have been with water regulations, the control has not extended to the end-of-the-line. Which grade bleach to use for periodically cleaning the small tank where bleach and water are premixed before pumping it to the large tank, which oil and grease to use for the pumps themselves and which kinds of pumps to use are not specified. Which bleach to use when repairing water pipes is not specified. Nor is it specified when giving cautionary advice about cutlery, kitchen counters and sinks for restaurants. Nor is it specified for filters and water softeners attached to water pipes. And which bleach to use for manufacturing activated carbon that regularly touches your food and water in the form of filters is not specified. It is human nature to reach for the quickest, easiest source, and cheapest brands. We must not trust any company regardless of its good intentions. They mean no harm, certainly, but drinking water must be guardable to the very last detail of its delivery path. It should be guarded even beyond the agency's present day jurisdiction. Good to the last drop must be literally interpreted. The record of procedure must be provable in detail with a log, dated and signed, as for any manufacturing business.

Water filters of all types should have their disinfectant specified. They should be tested for radioactivity, at least polonium and uranium.

Water softeners should have their disinfectant specified. They should be tested for radioactivity, although this can be done by any individual using a handheld Geiger Mueller counter (see *Sources*).

The public drinking water should not have added radioactivity. The uranium in the source water may be far less than suspected and only removal of wrong bleach and buffering agents be needed!

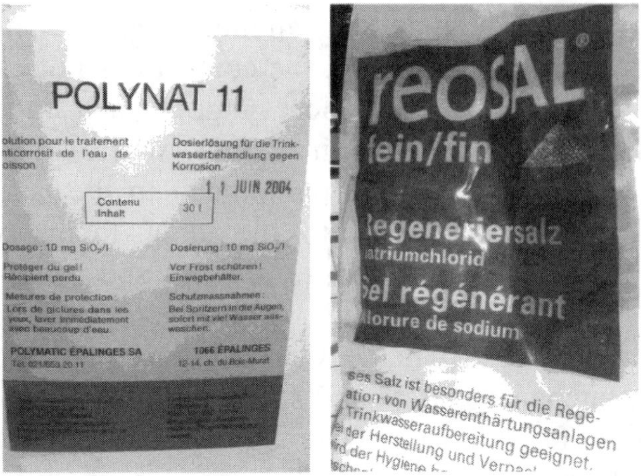

Popular water conditioners combine softening and boiler and pipe protection, especially in hotels, restaurants and public buildings.

Fig. 15 Polynat II and Reosal, side by side, in every big building's basement.

The average citizen could be made much healthier by disallowing radioactivity to be added to water. Don't believe the assurances given on your water department's annual statement when it blames the radioactivity on "natural rock formation". Water departments are kind, deserving people, concerned about our environment and our water quality. They would be eager to find less radioactive water additives or a way to avoid them altogether. Perhaps they need help to change old metal pipes to HDPE pipes that have much less scale formation and less metal corrosion to prevent.

The gap in quality control between the end of the water departments' service line and your kitchen sink should be filled. Independent labs could be found or created, to test for the dozen toxin categories that now exist. The polonium, cerium, potassium ferrocyanide tests, and tests for motor oil, which brings the alkylating agents, should get special attention, to stop the exploding cancer statistics.

Your first and most important task is to find out if your municipality is sending you the correct bleach in your water. There is no such test in existence now. There is still no way you can do this without using a Syncrometer®. Chances are good that the city is bleaching correctly, but chance is not satisfactory. You may be able to find a Syncrometer® tester on the Internet. Send the tester a cold water sample from your outside faucets as well as the kitchen.

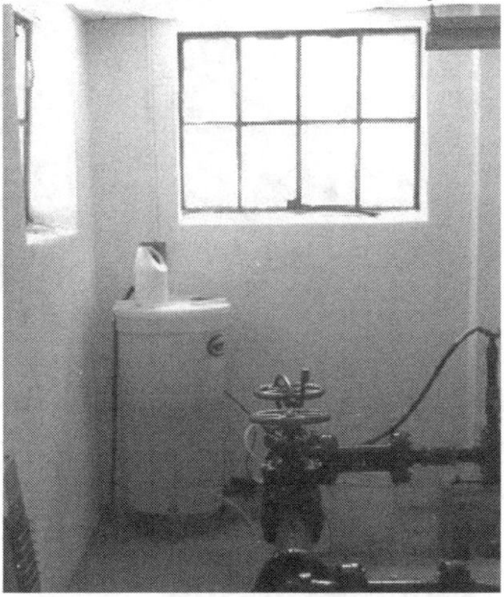

Bleach is first added to a small tank of water (in the corner), using pump at center front to make a premix.

Fig. 16 A water department pump house

Interested Agencies?

Of course the FDA, EPA and Department of Agriculture who are in charge of disinfectants and sterilization methods cannot be expected to accept results obtained with a Syncrometer®. The Syncrometer® is not an FDA-approved device nor will it be for some time to come. Automation of the device must come first. The interest of our agencies would help us arrive at this. It should be known that polonium already has a cancer-causing reputation (see the Internet for a fairly large body of scientific literature). Agencies as well as individuals can send water to a radiochemistry lab for testing (see *Sources*).

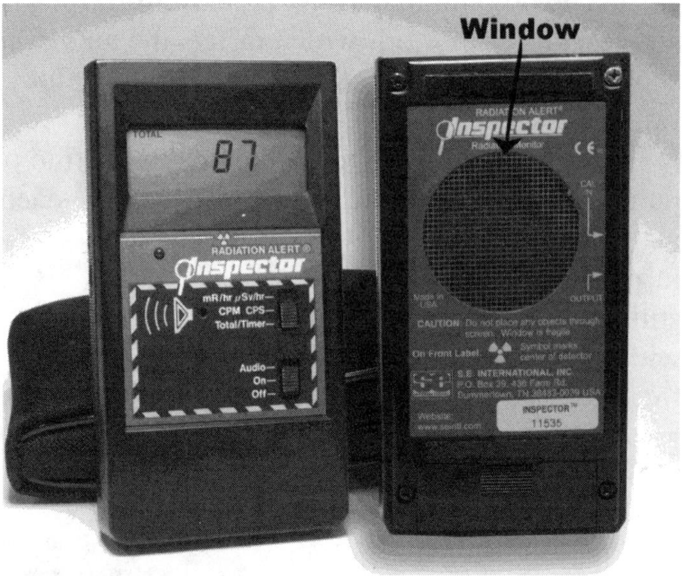

Fig. 17 Geiger Mueller counter with timer and counter

Alpha, Beta And Gamma Radiation Tests

Regular analytical laboratory tests are approved and could be used by anybody to validate the Syncrometer® results. I have already done this, finding the BTEX* analysis, heavy metal panels, and "gross alpha, beta and gamma" tests to be the most reproducible and least expensive. I recommend these tests for anyone who gets cancer, or wishes to prevent it and wants to confirm the extraordinary carcinogens and solvents in their own drinking water. See the list of laboratories on page 646. Remember that what you find will probably not be the water department's responsibility. All the more enlightening this will be.

* BTEX stands for benzene, toluene, ethylbenzene, xylenes, a solvent panel.

Testing for PCBs by labs is more expensive and much less reliable than for benzene. Often no results are seen by a lab because of the tendency for grease to stick to the sides of the container. PCBs are greasy. They came with the motor oil and grease in the bleach. Just pouring out the water sample into the labs' own containers or sucking up a portion of it leaves these toxins behind! They miss being tested, especially when plastic bottles have been used in sampling. Grease sticks to the container the way it sticks to a dishpan if no soap is used. Grease holds the oil soluble metals and benzene so they regularly get missed, too.

If you wish to send a sample to a radiochemistry laboratory, ask for Gross alpha radiation, not just polonium and uranium, since the half-life of polonium is only 138 days, meaning it will soon be half gone. It could have disintegrated to an undetectable amount by the time the test is done. Be sure to listen to the lab's advice.

Dry materials like your softener salts, charcoal, fertilizer, drywall can be sent to radiochemistry labs. Test for gross alpha and beta, as well as total gamma, the 3 main radiation types. Try to identify the culprits chemically. It is not expensive (see *Sources*).

Radioactive liquids require special testing methods, so fruit and water cannot be tested this way. Foods like strawberries and oranges should be dried and then crumbled to a powder, and poured onto a very thin (1 mil) plastic sheet over the window of the Geiger counter. The citrus fruit should be peeled and the peels dried. Be very careful not to get any radioactive powder or dust into your counter. Do all this with a dust mask on. You will not be able to get it out of the counter and it will raise the background radiation level. Be sure to buy one with automatic counting and timing (see *Sources*).

Asbestos and azo dyes cannot be tested at all because no commercial labs have been found that can do this. Even research labs can only detect asbestos spears above a certain (10 micron) length. Most asbestos in water is shorter than this and gets missed. When a pollutant gets missed, it ruins the epidemiological study. Even the short asbestos spears are easily found by Syncrometer®. The smaller ones are the most harmful because they can be eaten whole by your white blood cells. The number of longer spears that are legally allowed is 7 million per quart!

Of course, if you know you have a water filter or softener attached anywhere, the most reasonable assumption is that the cancer-complex is coming from these since they are liberally disinfected with chlorox laundry bleach. The newer they are the more bleach they diffuse, but quantity is not meaningful when an amount the size of a dot can start a cancer as for Po.

If you could remove all filters, distillers (because they have filters attached) and softeners, then wash all the pipes (see page 77) with very hot water you could wash them clean. You should replace the water heater, and then attach a special prewashed, back-flushing, whole house filter that is able to trap the whole polonium-cerium-ferrocyanide-alkylating agent-complex (see water filter in *Sources*), not just Po or Ce.

The charcoal used for the filter should be of plant origin (coconut shell) and be specially boiled. It should have no methylene blue dye. The effluent (wash water), when the filter is self-cleaning (backwashing), will be extremely radioactive. It should have a safe exit down a sewer pipe. This is not good for the environment and eventually a sure killer for the biosphere, but it is not safer to be consumed by you. The backwashing interval can be set to suit your needs. It will be based on family size, about 5 to 6 days. Be sure to get the same prewashed charcoal for a refill in a year or two. Most important is protecting your family from any contact with the filtered, concentrated, radioactivity that is to be drained down the sewer.

Hungry Water

Distilled water or filtered water is very hungry water! It has no minerals in it. It will try harder to pull the metals from the pipes. If you have copper pipes it will pull copper and lead (from solder joints) from the pipes much more than before. Position the filter so this can't happen. Change at least the pipes to the kitchen, hot and cold, to PVC (or the new POLYETHYLENE PIPE) as well as the pipe to the water heater. Best is to change all your pipes to PVC at the same time. It is very inexpensive and therefore fought by the plumbing industry.

Another Ray Of Hope

Recently, NSF bleaches have reached the supermarkets (see *Sources*) not just the pool stores. You can now start to clean up your home, the dishwasher, furniture, walls and carpets with easy to find and to pour varieties with the same strength as you are accustomed to. Remember to remove your own filters and softeners first. You cannot clean up anything that you are contaminating at the same time. Don't "use up" Po-containing supplies before starting safe ones. Detergents and many other house cleaning supplies should be carefully chosen (see *Sources*) to avoid the cancer-complex.

True Cancer Prevention

No case of cancer in a series of well over a thousand in a 7-year period was without the presence of **chlorox** laundry bleach in their tumors and their kitchen water. We looked further. All of our failures, patients who later died and had sent us a water sample beforehand, had moved back home to bad water. It was done innocently, since they believed the water had been cleaned somehow. And all patients who returned to the clinic because their cancer had returned while at home had been using bad water again. Still further, all follow-up patients who were doing well at home had switched to NSF bleached water, rainwater in a cistern or well water, unchlorinated. The picture is clear. How could you get cancer unless you had cancer-complex polluted water? It is true that our planet is steeped in polonium from underground sources such as uranium rocks. We are also steeped in cerium but they never arrange themselves into the cancer-causing-complex. This is artificially done during manufacture of chlorox bleach and spread over the entire world to add to the safe clean water! The probability of getting cancer without such water seems to be less than one in a thousand (assuming I did only a thousand tests).

A cancer that has already started is in a different position. The tumor is alive and obeys the rules of biology. One rule is that every molecule replaces itself in time called the turnover rate. Po will replace itself as long as it is available nearby from the Po or radon in air, water, food or your own tooth fillings! Rn produces Po as one of its daughters (see page 38). The other ingredients of the cancer-complex can do the same. But if F. buski is killed it can no longer turn over or produce alkylating agents. Cancer must stop abruptly.

Is It A Cure?

The first step in curing your cancer, if the chlorox bleach is coming from your water department, is to flee from it. You can't change the water department but you can get away from it. Move without delay. Your water is equivalent to smoking cigarettes continually. Without this, there will be no chance of curing your cancer or preventing its return. A clinical or alternative treatment may give you quick success, at first, as any band-aid would to a wound, but not a permanent cure…only remission. Moving your residence will give you many other advantages, too, getting you away from pets, air pollutants, and contaminated furniture at the same time. Unless you move, cancer would always come back because the cause would still be arriving in your body! The same elements, giving you the same mutations make it inevitable.

Find a Syncrometer® tester on the Internet. Send samples of your outside water (to the garden hose) to be tested. Do it 2 or 3 times to avoid all mistakes. If all have chlorox send samples from the nearest gas stations. They would have city water that was not softened or filtered to help you find a good water zone. Remove all filters, even the small one going to your refrigerator. Do not keep a bathroom filter or any filter that is not tested for chlorox bleach. Expect to find about 95% chlorox bleach filters or other water devices in your collection.

Take Off Filters And Softeners

Of course, when you move it must be to a location where the kitchen water arrives correctly bleached. Your friends and family may also have put filters and softeners on their pipes and contaminated their pipes and house. Test first. When you change to radiation-free water, precancerous growths and very early tumors often clear themselves. But if you have already been diagnosed with cancer, you must do more. Only taking the cancer-complex out of your body can cure you.

Carrying "Good" Water Does Not Work

Finding a new way of distilling your water or treating it in some new "purifying" way does not work. We might imagine that carrying in clean water for drinking and cooking purposes would work. These methods do not. All patients got a cancer recurrence after trying one of these "shortcuts". At first, their health merely declined. Then they got cancer again. It is not possible to live in a PoCe-ferrocyanide contaminated house and be protected from cancer.

Moving Is Best

Guard your first success, whether you got it using natural means or by the usual clinical means. You cannot change the water department's policies or manufacturers' habits. After finding good water in another water district, move immediately. Be certain there is nothing attached to the water pipes. Do not attach anything yourself! The new water you will drink exchanges with all your body's water in 2 days! This is much faster than the rate for food. Don't delay this because it is the most significant and fast-acting part of the cure. Besides using it internally we will use it externally to wash away the water soluble part of the cancer-complex. In 2 weeks you can be rid of the polonium-cerium-ferro-complexes and have no more malignancy. The time required is shorter if your washing efforts are more intense and dental clean up is included.

What guarantee do you have that the water you switch to will stay good? None! But habits get ingrained for responsible or irresponsible behavior. Over a 7-year period I have only seen three switches in water bleaching policy by water departments.

How can you get your outside (city) water tested for laundry bleach? If you can't find a Syncrometer® tester learn it yourself. Share results with other testers. They will benefit, too. If you don't have confidence in the results, attend classes. A friendly water department employee might even help personally to set things straight.

And if you find that your city water is good, immediately remove every attachment to your water system. Filters of any kind, softeners of any kind, distillers of any kind were well intended; nobody knew the hazard. Pass 3 tankfuls of very hot water from your water heater through all your pipes, or replace them along with the water heater. (This time use PVC pipes.) Remember to wash the cold pipes, too, using a garden hose attached to the bottom of the heater to reach all your cold pipes. If the water heater is contaminated buy a new one.

The New Water Heater...

...should be a gas, glass-lined heater, not electric. The hot water samples tested recently from electric heaters have every imaginable heavy metal, even tungsten, vanadium, titanium, palladium! The electrodes stick boldly into the water without a housing or separation from the water to be used in food! This is very toxic to kidneys. The gas heated water is protected from such gross contamination.

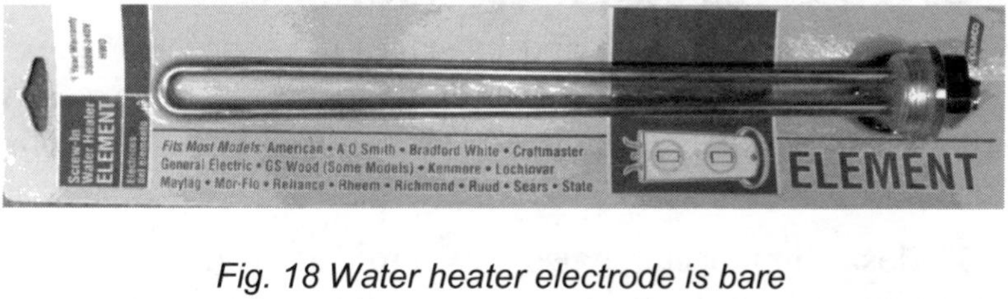

Fig. 18 Water heater electrode is bare

As soon as your water is changed and the house washed with new safe bleach and new safe detergent, you can start the program. It will not work otherwise. If there are carpets or furniture not washed, cover them with a plastic sheet till they are. Send carpet wipes for testing to a Syncrometer® tester.

Summary — Chapter 2

1. Every tumor has a beginning, middle, and end period.

2. Between beginning and end we see the tumor growing and accumulating many things that would normally be excreted or eliminated. This is due to large-scale destruction of the immune system and blockage of the kidneys.

3. Malignancy is caused by the arrival of the human intestinal fluke. It acts with a polonium-cerium-ferrocyanide and alkylating agent-complex to cause site-specified mutations. The main one is assumed to be orthophosphotyrosine, OPT. The large amount of OPT in the tumor zone shows us intense stimulation of the enzymes that attach a phosphate group to tyrosine groups in proteins. Cell division, called **mitosis**, is accelerated explosively.

> Specific pollutants are responsible for additional cancer mutations: PCBs, isopropyl alcohol, benzene, asbestos, malonic acid, wheel bearing grease and motor oil, certain heavy metals, azo dyes, polonium, cerium, ferrocyanide, methylene blue dye, bromine, and fluorine. They attach themselves to the cancer-complex at various locations.

4. By killing this fluke and its stages the cancer-complex is broken up and the mutations are stopped. The excessive production of OPT is stopped, as well as HCG and other "markers".

5. Clostridium bacteria also play a role early in every cancer. By killing Clostridium bacteria and stopping personal use of isopropyl alcohol, excessive amounts of DNA and HCG disappear.

6. By switching to a clean water source we stop the intake of the real carcinogen and the accumulation of a dozen or so extreme toxins, including ferrocyanide. Each of these must next be eliminated from the body to regain immunity and health. This is done in the *2-Week Program*.

7. A tumor must be constantly fed the cancer-complex ingredients. Otherwise it loses its malignancy and shrinks.

8. By removing the polonium and uranium replacement sources, usually air, food and tooth fillings, each cancer stops, while the tumor remains. This is part 1 of the cure. It is the most important part. Your body will feel relief from pain and fatigue.

Three things must still happen to shrink the tumors that are left behind. They must be able to digest themselves, be digested by your digestive enzymes and be eaten by your white blood cells. These three steps can be monitored with the Syncrometer® to be sure they are happening. Nothing must be left out. It includes clearing the radioactivity out of the teeth...a dental challenge for the alternative dentist (see Chapter 16). Benign growth can continue as long as there is any uranium left in the dental supplies used for a tooth repair. It is seen in people with left over amalgam in their mouths in the form of tattoos and scattered bits hidden inside the gums and old cavities. It originated with the uranium contamination of amalgam and porcelain and the use of chlorox bleach to disinfect dental supplies.

The *2-Week Program* eliminates all phases of cancer. Rescue is still possible even when the body is emaciated and coma not far away.

Let us go back to the beginning now and see how easy it would be to prevent a tumor from ever starting.

WANTED DEAD—OR DEADER

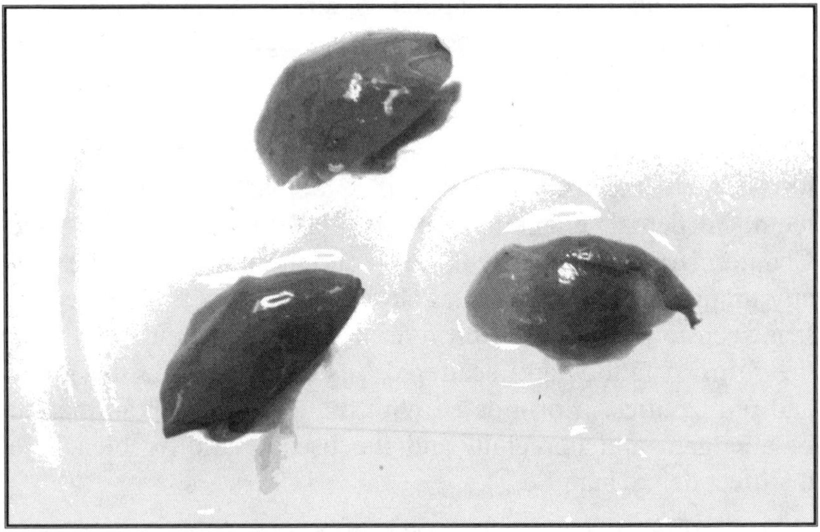

Three dehydrated adult F. buski's fled from the bile ducts during a prolonged liver cleanse, using 3 or 4 doses of Epsom salts, only 1 Tbsp. each, the morning after, 2 hours apart.

CHAPTER 3

STARTING A TUMOR

This is how every tumor starts whether it becomes malignant or not.

Step 1

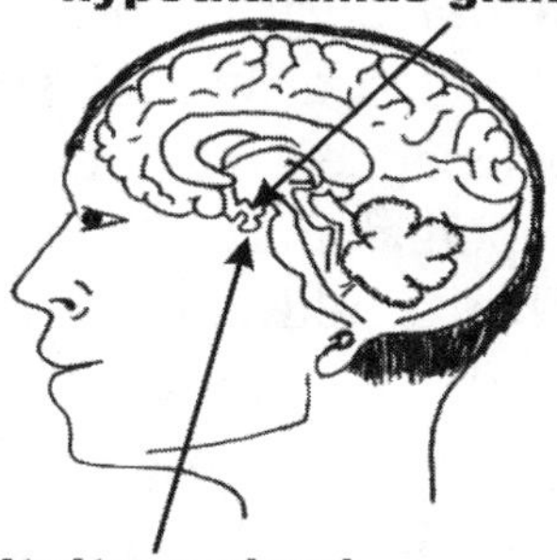

Fig. 19 Master glands in the brain

Far away from the real tumor, in one small corner of the brain where the hypothalamus gland is located, a quiet explosion takes place. Tiny bits and pieces fly away from it. Cells of the hypothalamus land in the blood, in the lymph, and in the cerebrospinal fluid that bathes the brain. They float beside the red blood cells, white blood cells, and platelets, wherever they are, quite undisturbed.

We might think these cells should die, separated this far from their parent organ, but they do not. Nor do white blood cells eat them. White blood cells, being your immune system, should somehow eliminate them. They are acting like diseased cells. But your white blood cells have been trained to protect, never to eat, or even attack, cells that belong to your very own body. If they were dead they would be quickly eaten up, but these are not. Are they exempt because they are still alive? Will they never die? Are they doing any harm?

Step 2

Not far away, in a small part of the pituitary gland, another tissue explosion is taking place. The pituitary is just a tiny marble hanging down from the hypothalamus in the floor of the brain. This is just above the roof of your mouth near your throat. The pituitary explosion is independent of the hypothalamus explosion. They could happen before or after each other.

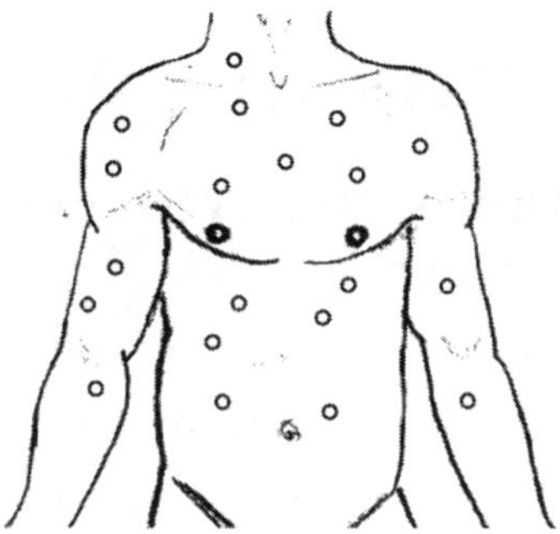

Fig. 20 Our body fluids distribute the tiny bits of hypothalamus

Now two organs are doing this very strange thing—coming apart, letting bits of themselves come loose, to float away in the body's fluids. How long will the tiny bits live? No white blood cells will eat them unless they are dead. To kill them, **complement** has to arrive.

Complement C_3

An arm of our immune system is called **complement**. There are many actors in this arm, called C_1, C_2, C_3 and so on. Each contributes to the daily chores. They round up bacteria, get them into a vulnerable position and pierce them with their daggers. We must remember that bacteria are a thousand times bigger than complement molecules. This achievement is spectacular.

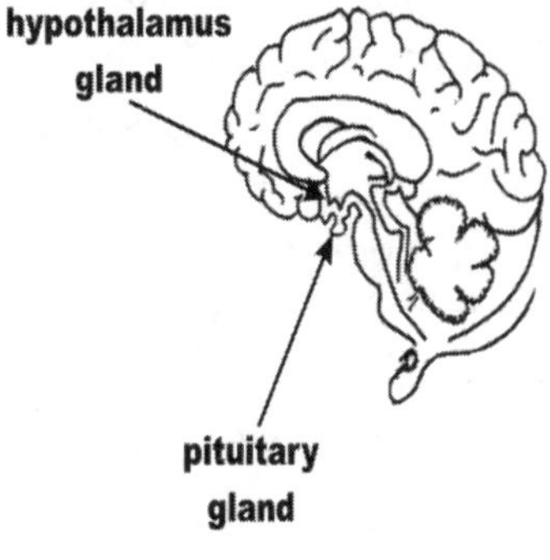

Fig. 21 The pituitary gland hangs below the hypothalamus

The job of dispatching the runaway hypothalamus and

pituitary cells is, evidently, the complement's. The Syncrometer® sees C_3 attached to these cells at first.

All the runaway cells get caught by complement C_3 and pierced. Now the white blood cells will be able to attack and eat them.

Soon the blood, lymph, and brain fluid are all cleared of wandering hypothalamus and pituitary cells.

> Remember, the Syncrometer® is the audio oscillator, a detection device that lets us identify our own tissues, parasites, or chemicals **very accurately** inside ourselves. We can eavesdrop on events happening, wherever they are happening. Opportunities for discovery are almost endless. Details on how to build one and use one are given in the *Syncrometer® Science Laboratory Manual* by this author. Nobody is too old to learn to use this powerful scientific tool. It promises health as nothing could before it.

But then another flood of runaway cells arrives, and another, as if hailstorm after hailstorm had loosened them and set them free. It can be difficult for complement C_3 molecules to keep up with their skewering task. Once these molecules have pierced their prey, they can't be used again. They remind us of bees who have used their stingers. The C_3 molecules get devoured by the white blood cells along with the speared cells. The body must make more C_3. Perhaps it is expected to make 10 times more than normal and keep this up day after day.

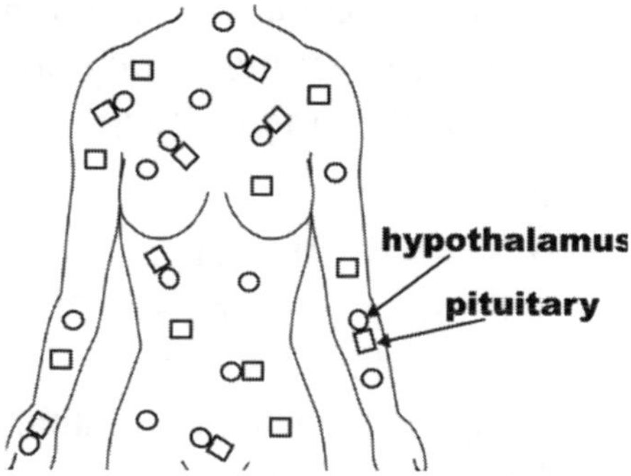

Fig. 22 Diagram of single cells & duplexes afloat in the body's fluids

Soon your body can't keep up with the big demand for complement C_3. Then both kinds of brain cells float side by side. Will they communicate with each other? They normally do, when they are in their own glands in the brain.

Hypothalamus And Pituitary Cells Join

Maybe they often bump into each other as they float. Maybe they normally attract each other. Maybe they are just sticky. Suddenly the Syncrometer® sees tiny duplexes, part hypothalamus and part pituitary. They fused!

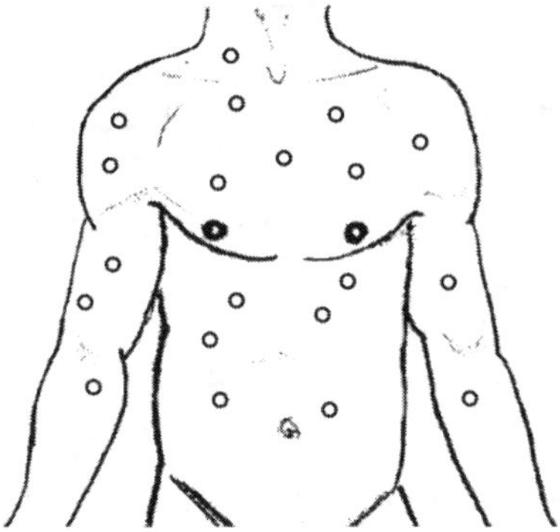

Fig. 23 Now both hypothalamus & pituitary gland bits are afloat

Now duplexes as well as single cells are circulating. Undaunted, complement now attacks the duplexes too, trying to take them all out of the circulation as well as the single cells. There is more demand for C_3.

Step 3

Just above the navel and a tiny bit to the right is the "head" of the pancreas. From here it stretches around to your left side. The same sinister force is beginning to act. A tissue erosion begins. Pancreas cells begin to float free in the body fluids.

Suddenly, a "snowball" forms. The duplexes that were formed before now stick and fuse to the new loose pancreas cells to make triplets. They are in this order: the pancreas cells stick to the pituitary, not to the hypothalamus portion. Complement tries again to kill all triplets as well as duplexes and single cells.

Finally, there is no more complement. Single cells of all three organs, their duplexes and their triplets, fill the body fluids. The Syncrometer® finds them in the saliva, blood, **lymph** and **cerebrospinal fluid**.

Lymph is the fluid that is not in your arteries or veins; it is around your organs, bathing them and taking care of their daily needs. Part of the space around organs is called the "**matrix**" since it has more than just fluid. Close to our cells there is a meshwork of fibers lashed about the cells and each other like ropes and anchors to keep everything securely in place.

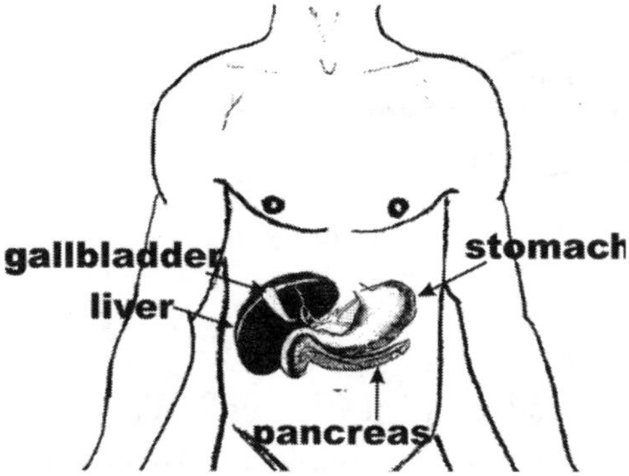

Fig. 24 The pancreas will contribute the third tissue

Cerebrospinal fluid is a lymph for the brain, bathing it and taking care of its daily needs. It reaches down the center of the spinal cord. Then it flows out and back up to reach the brain again, round and round.

The renegade tissue bits float through organ after organ by means of our arteries and veins, lymph and cerebrospinal fluid (CSF). They travel much slower through the lymph and matrix meshwork as they get near our cells. Do they pose a danger to our cells? Without complement to help, the white blood cells now

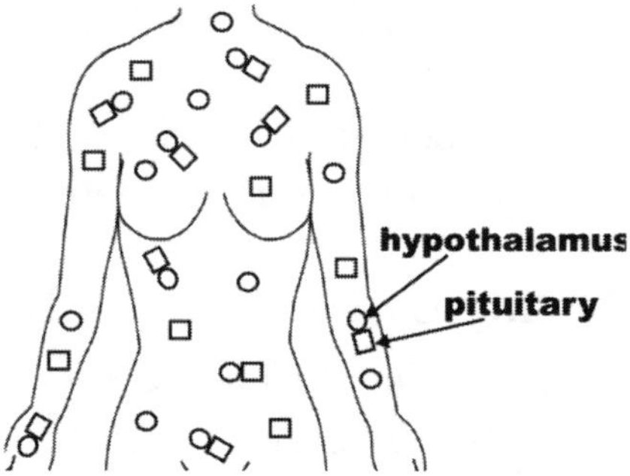

Fig. 25 Single cells, duplexes & triplets everywhere

resort to other tactics to kill them. Nitric oxide is used as a chemical weapon. It is present whenever complement C_3 has run out. But all these tactics are "too little and too late". They do not control the tide of tissue bits awash in the body.

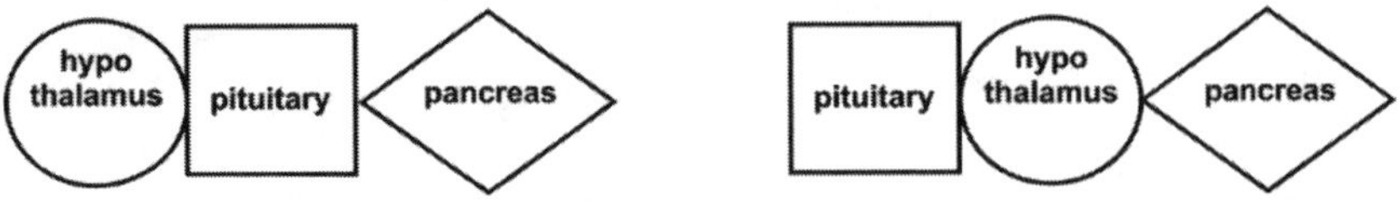

Fig. 26 This is the triplet.......................Not this...

Why did it happen? Was it caused by radioactivity, by parasites, by bacteria, by viruses? How did it happen? What will happen next? Was it due to inflammation? Why were these organs inflamed? Why were there no symptoms?

It reminds us of cows who have their most common disease, **mastitis**.

Cow's milk always has udder (breast) cells in it. When **mastitis** (udder infection) strikes her she has many more loosened cells. A device is used to measure this "somatic cell count". The mastitis is usually caused by Staphylococcus bacteria. Is this a clue? Have we missed finding some common bacteria that loosen our cells?

Destiny Of The Hypothalamus Renegades

It appears to be the job of our pepsin, made by the stomach to digest the free cells coming from the hypothalamus. The stem cell factor gets removed and the remainder gets reduced to an indigestible bit identical to PRIONS. Is this the true origin of the deadly prion? A cancer patient's tumor swarms with prions. Could cows and people prevent brain diseases with added pepsin?

Finding A Home

Sooner or later, a fourth organ will follow the trend and begin its micro-explosion. Unless we know what is causing these, we cannot stop them. We will study this soon.

Now, cells of a fourth organ are let go to join all the others in the circulating body fluids. Whether it is the prostate, breast, or another organ, new loose cells are being added to those already afloat and traveling.

The fourth organ has a difference from the other three. It is making glue. Sticky substances are being made along with fine threads, called **fibronectin**, **laminin**, and **cadherin E**. These glues ooze like sticky mucous. They could form a trap.

As the tiny triplet finds itself floating through this organ, the glue slows it down. The triplet suddenly sticks to the fourth organ. They fuse. A quadruplet is made!

The fourth organ has triplets stuck to it all around. They will never let go. Many new "quads" are already swimming away like the triplets did before. But many stay stuck right there in the sticky matrix of the fourth organ. This fourth organ will make the "primary tumor". The triplet only gets attached to an organ with excessive fibronectin and laminin threads and with cadherin E, the glue.

But why was so much glue produced? It is, after all, normal to have some—and normal to have some laminin and fibronectin. It only happens when totally different, quite independent parasites are living nearby. Wherever these parasites exist, all these are overproduced. It is probably for their own purposes—not to get washed away easily. But the triplet gets caught in it, like a moth in a spider web, and then fuses itself to the fourth organ cells. Or do mutations play a role making excess glue when certain other parasites are present? This has not been studied yet.

It (the triplet) will provide the growing point of the tumor, so I call it the **tumor nucleus**.

The parasites are common Fasciola and Ascaris, not others! Fasciola and Ascaris parasites increase, too, as the immune system is destroyed by chlorox bleach. It is part of the increased parasitism always seen with immunity destruction.

Fasciola is another fluke, fairly easily killed, like Fasciolopsis. Ascaris is a roundworm, harder to kill, it seems, than flukes. And the gluey trap substances, fibronectin, laminin, and cadherin E can be digested. Our ordinary digestive enzymes produced by the stomach and pancreas can digest them in days. We will do this, but why did our digestive organs not do this automatically? We will see later.

The Primary Tumor

When you or your doctor find your first tumor it is called the "primary tumor".

If the tumor is in the breast, there will be a tumor nucleus of hypothalamus, pituitary and pancreas—fused to breast cells. Every tumor so far searched (hundreds upon hundreds) has the same nucleus. And the order is always the same: hypothalamus, pituitary, pancreas, followed by the organ that develops the primary tumor.

Even non-tumorous cancers like the leukemias or eosinophilia or thrombocytosis, have the same tumor nucleus in the bone marrow or lymph nodes or spleen. These cancers remain dispersed instead of forming solid masses. Even masses that form away from an organ, like Hodgkin's and non-Hodgkin's have the same tumor nucleus, but this time attached to lymph node cells that have gotten themselves wrapped up by a filaria parasite here. The growing force for each is the same tumor nucleus.

Soon there will be a genuine tiny tumor wherever the tumor nucleus has fused with the organ cells. They cluster together, making it look like "one cell started it all". But the tumor nuclei are numerous.

After this the tumor begins to accumulate things and grow. Now immunity destruction by chlorox bleach will play a more visible role. And several new actors will join this tragic drama.

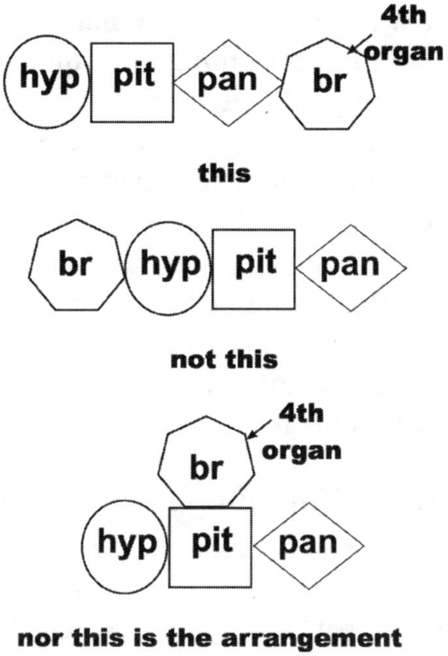

hyp = hypothalamus; pit = pituitary; pan = pancreas; br = breast

Fig. 27 The primary tumor forms

Would it not be an easy matter to prevent the first step from ever happening? Because there is an orderly sequence in this snowballing behavior, couldn't we prevent any one of these steps and already achieve our goal? There will not be just one way to prevent cancer, but at least a dozen ways. It will be possible to stamp out this disease to completion—for our pets, and for domestic animals, too. To accomplish this we must know what causes all these events.

Back At The Hypothalamus…

an extraordinary chemical has accumulated. Whenever it is loosening its cells and letting them go free into the circulation this chemical appears. It is absent when there are no cells being shed. All cancer patients have such an accumulation and it is the same chemical for each person.

The chemical is **chlorogenic acid**, a well-known plant compound! It is considered an **antigen** (or **allergen**) by "ecological allergy" specialists. It is known by botanists to be a common "intermediate" in plant growth, often taking part in the forming of fruits and vegetables. It is there naturally, although how plants grow and ripen must surely affect the compounds produced in them. How foods are cooked could also affect this chemical. Research is badly needed.

A search of the ordinary foods people eat showed chlorogenic acid to be present in some of our popular foods. Certain less common foods contain it, too. We should certainly avoid foods containing chlorogenic acid. Here is the list:

Foods Containing Chlorogenic Acid

- potatoes, except sweet potatoes
- cow's milk and all dairy products, except goat milk
- peppers of all kinds, except jalapeño seeds
- unripe fruits of many kinds,
- watermelon, except grown in Mexico
- coffee and regular tea

For potatoes very thorough cooking destroys chlorogenic acid, but frying does not. This agrees with Dr. Charles Ivy's[17] results of 50 years ago that fried food is carcinogenic in some way. He was the world's most renowned gastroenterologist, a researcher at the University of Chicago.

---

[17] Lane, A., Blickenstaff, D., and A.C. Ivy, *The Carcinogenicity of Fat "Browned" by Heating*, Cancer, v. 3, 1950, pp. 1044-51

Dairy products and beverages are not normally cooked, but this could change.

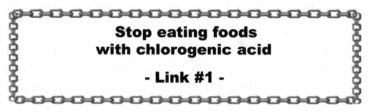

Stop eating foods with chlorogenic acid

- Link #1 -

Because there is a chain of events—only one chain—that leads to cancer could we not pluck out one link to stop it all? It has not been tried on a large scale but is so tantalizing a thought that I will list the links as I find them.

The food list for chlorogenic acid is not perfectly complete, but avoiding these already gives excellent results. In five days no more hypothalamus single cells can be found in the body. The erosion has stopped. What could be easier?

Back At The Pituitary…

another extraordinary chemical has accumulated. The pituitary gland is the "downstairs" neighbor of the hypothalamus gland. The chemical is called **phloridzin** (or phlorizin), again, a plant substance. It, too, is a "phenolic" substance, belonging to the list of food antigens or allergens. Food allergists have studied it, too. In fact, it has even been found to be associated with cancer in the past, rather often, about 80% of the time![18]

Phloridzin has been studied in another connection for nearly 100 years. It could give rabbits instant diabetes if they were given a small dose. The diabetes was permanent. It was a popular way to do research on diabetes in the 1940s and 50s. It was not suspected that

[18] Ber, A. MD, FRCP, *Neutralization of phenolic food compounds in a holistic general practice* J. Orthomolecular Psychiatry, 1983 4th quarter p. 283

phloridzin was actually a cause of our own diabetes, even though phloridzin could be obtained from apples, a popular human food! Eating too much sugar was suspected, instead.

The Syncrometer® detects phloridzin accumulation in the pancreas of every diabetic. It is right at the tiny islands of tissue called "islets of Langerhans", where insulin is made.

Banting and Best[19], the discoverers of insulin in the 1920s, saved many lives of diabetics. It was not a cure but a replacement. They could not have guessed that basic research would stop after their departure so that doctors are still without a true cure for diabetes. The connection to phloridzin in foods, and later the arrival of a parasite, the pancreatic fluke and the solvent, wood alcohol, would have excited them greatly.

So for two reasons we should not be eating phloridzin in our food. It is part of cancer development and it leads to diabetes.

Foods Containing Phloridzin

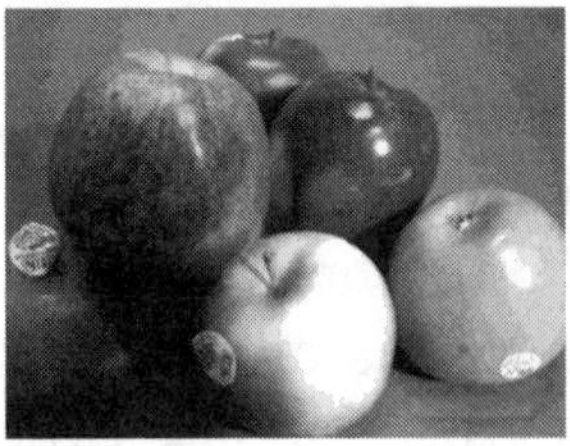

Fig. 28 Pick your fruit carefully

- apples, *EXCEPT* Red Delicious and Golden Delicious, both very ripe
- pork, ham and derivatives
- soy products including oil
- unripe fruits of many kinds
- bananas with any tinge of green at the ends
- cauliflower, kohlrabi, dark green zucchini (all raw)
- cashews
- amaranth, millet (uncooked)

[19] Banting MB, F.G. and Best BA, C.H. *The internal secretion of the pancreas* The Journal of Laboratory and Clinical Medicine, Vol. VII 1922

We must avoid phloridzin in our foods to stop fragmenting the pituitary gland in the brain (and protect the islets of Langerhans in the pancreas).

After avoiding all foods on the phloridzin list for five days, we again find no single cells or fragments of the pituitary gland in the blood or lymph. Success is swift. Neither duplexes nor triplets can be found. We have stopped the formation of tumor nuclei as we had hoped.

Stop eating foods with phloridzin

- Link #2 -

Back At The Pancreas...

still another chemical is responsible for its micro explosion. It is **gallic acid**, another phenolic substance coming from food. All cancer patients have an accumulation in their pancreas.

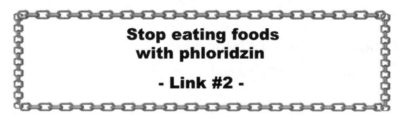

Its presence on all our grains in the USA makes it the most pervasive of the three food antigens. It is not native to the grains, though. We place it there by spraying our grains with it (!) for its antioxidant, anti-mold, (preservative) action. We put it in the oils on supermarket shelves for the same preservative effect. Only a few foods have it naturally. Many milk varieties, many chickens, and most eggs in the USA have it. Others don't, like eggs from Mexico. I am guessing this depends on the feed used. It explains why cow's milk has it while goat milk does not (goats shun processed feed such as "rations" and "supplements"). It could explain why chickens are so full of tumors; they are primarily grain eaters. And perhaps why other **alternative therapists** have taken chicken and eggs off the cancer patients' diet. One therapist, a bacteriologist, Virginia Livingston M.D. founded an institute based on the concept that the cancer "bug" came from chickens (and eggs).[20] We will see more evidence for this, later.

Gallic acid, too, has been studied by allergists. It causes many allergic symptoms, especially muscle spasms and very painful cramps, but it does not cause pain in the pancreas and its role in cancer development was not suspected.

Foods Containing Gallic Acid

- grains of all kinds, treated for longer shelf life with antioxidant preservatives
- oils of all kinds, treated to prevent rancidity (antioxidant)
- flour, enriched and bleached
- chickens fed supplementary rations and their eggs
- cows milk and dairy products
- most maple syrup

How to grow and handle foods so they do not have these three food allergens will hopefully become one of our Agriculture Department's high priorities. How to avoid eating them will be our highest priority.

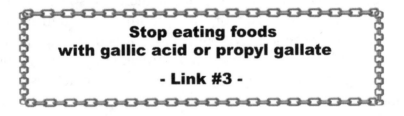

Stop eating foods with gallic acid or propyl gallate

- Link #3 -

Foods tested by Syncrometer® for these three food antigens are listed in the *Food Table* on page 97. Foods

[20] Livingston-Wheeler, MD, Virginia and Addeo, Edmond G., *The Conquest of Cancer, Vaccines and Diet,* New York, F. Watts, 1984, Chicago, Advanced Century Pub. Co. 1978

with other antigens are also listed. We will soon see what role they play.

After your tumors are gone you may use certain tips and "loopholes" to regain some of these foods but not sooner. By then you will have acquired some new tastes and will be able to diversify your food better than before.

Food Table

Use this table to identify which foods are safe for you to eat. Find the food you are interested in, for example, almonds. They are *Positive* (*P*) for acetaldehyde, meaning they <u>do</u> contain it. Another example is avocados. They are *Negative* (*N*) for all food phenolics tested, meaning they do <u>not</u> contain them. Foods that are *P*/*N* means they can be either.

Foods do not always give consistent results. Ripeness, handling methods, and growing methods can make a difference to the phenolic content of food. Test yours to be certain*.

Sometimes I find a food that acts as an allergen, but I have not identified the substance involved. Those foods are shown in capital letters, for example, CORN.

PIT stands for phenylisothiocyanate, a food phenolic.

The three columns that are shaded are the three that cause the tumor nucleus to form. They are always a top priority.

Thallium is a popular pesticide in foreign countries. Unfortunately, they can expect leg pain, nervous system diseases, and birth defects now. (See *Dangerous Properties of Industrial Materials* 7th ed. by N. Irving Sax and Richard J. Lewis Sr., Van Nostrand Reinhold, N.Y. 1989.) Thallium has been banned in USA, even for rodents.

---

*Syncrometer® testers, please accumulate your findings with as much detail as possible. It will be a timeless treasure.

TRY is free tryptophane, an amino acid. NGF is nerve growth factor. Mo is molybdenum.

D-mannitol is a sugar isomer (form) that appears after heating to high temperatures. It changes only a bond or two in its molecular structure, but that is enough to make it harmful.

All honey and corn products can have air pollutants: beryllium, strontium, vanadium, and chromium in metal form. Now that artificial "beeswax" frames are used, disinfected with chlorox bleach, we can soon expect radioactive honey and sickly bees. Test commercial honey for gold, too, an upcoming serious toxin that leads to new, modern diseases.

Food Table

FOOD PHENOLIC ALLERGENS / FOOD OILS

N = Negative P = Positive N/P = both Negative&Positive FOOD ITEM	Apiol	ASA(aspirin)	Asparagine	Acetaldehyd	Caffeic acid	D-Carnitine	Cinnamic	Chlorogenic	Coumarin	Gallic acid	Limonene	Malvin	Menadione	PIT*	Phenylalanin	Phloridzin	Quercitin	SHRIMP	ONION	Tyramine	Umbelliferon	Linoleic oil	Linolenic oil	Lauric acid oil	Myristic oil	Oleic acid oil	Palmitic oil
agave, syrup	N	N	N	N	P		P	N	N	N	N	N	N	N	N	N	N	N	N	N	N	both gone if boiled					
	has fructose, which is changed to mannitol by boiling																										
alfalfa sprouts	N							N		N						N			N								
almond	N			P				N		N						N			N		have mandelonitrile						
aloe vera								N		N						N			P								
amaranth	N							N		N						P			N			gone if cooked					
anise seed	N				N		N	N	N	N		N		N	N	N		N	N	N							
apple, Golden & Red Delicious	N	N	N	N	N	N	N	N	N	N	N	N	N	N	N	N	N	N	N	N	N	phloridzin present if unripe; sodium pyruvate in red peel					
	Granny Smith has caffeic. Golden Delicious has myristic.																										
apple, others	N									N		N				P			N		phloridzin gone if cooked						
apricot, raw, very ripe	N	N	N	N	N	N	N	N	N	N	N	N	N	N	N	N	N	N	N	N	N	no naringenin, NGF; has myristic					
arrowroot flour	N	N	N	N	N	N	N	N	N	N	N	N	N	N	N	N	N	N	N	N	N	no naringenin, NGF, mannitol					
artichoke	N							N	N	N						N			N			cooked					
asparagus	N		P					N		N						N			P			cooked					

N = Negative P = Positive N/P = both Negative&Positive FOOD ITEM	Apiol	ASA(aspirin)	Asparagine	Acetaldehyd	Caffeic acid	D-Carnitine	Cinnamic	Chlorogenic	Coumarin	Gallic acid	Limonene	Malvin	Menadione	PIT*	Phenylalanin	Phloridzin	Quercitin	SHRIMP	ONION	Tyramine	Umbelliferon	Linoleic oil	Linolenic oil	Lauric acid oil	Myristic oil	Oleic acid oil	Palmitic oil
avocado	N	N	N	N	N	N	N	N	N	N	N	N	N	N	N	N	N	N	N	N	N	N	P	N	P	N	N
banana	N	N	N	N	N	N	N	N	N	N	N	N	N	N	N	P	N	N	N	P	black center has Bacillus cereus; test for thallium						
banana, frozen	N							N		N						N			N	N	freezing removes phloridzin, tyramine, and Bacillus cereus						
banana, small	N	N	N	N	N	N	N	N	N	N	N	N	N	N	N	N	N	N	N	N	has no Bacillus cereus						
barley, cooked	N	N	N	N	N	N	N	N	N	N	N	N	N	N	N	N	N	N	N	N	has manganese metal						
barley, raw	N	N	N	N	N	N	N	N	N	N	N	N	N	N	N	N	N	N	N	N	has organic manganese, rutin, hesperidin						
basil, fresh	N	N	N	N	N	N	N	N	N	N	N										has piperine						
bay leaf	N	N	N	N	N	N	N	N	N	N	N	N	N	N	N	N	N		N	N	N						
beans, green	N	P		N				N		N						N			N			cooked					
beans, pinto, lima, cooked	N	N	N	N	N	N	N	N	N	N	N	N	N	N	N	N	N	N	P	N	N	ONION gone if slow cooked twice					
	All develop ONION if cooked at high temperature																										
bee pollen	N	N	N	N	N	N	N	N	N	N	N	N	N	N	N	N	N	N	N	N	N	has naringenin and phenol in US varieties* *Mexican sources have neither					
beef, cooked	N							N		N						N			N			P	P	has F. buski, gold			
beef, range fed	N	N	N	N	N	N	N	N	N	N	N	N	N	N	N	N	N	N	N	N	N	N	N	has F. buski, no oils			
buffalo	N	N	N	N	N	N	N	N	N	N	N	N	N	N	N	N	N	N	N	N	N	N	N	N	N	N	N
beet greens	N	N	N	N	N	N	N	N	N	N	N	N	N	N	N	N	N	N	N	N	N	has no mannitol					

N = Negative P = Positive N/P = both Negative&Positive FOOD ITEM	Apiol	ASA(aspirin)	Asparagine	Acetaldehyd	Caffeic acid	D-Carnitine	Cinnamic	Chlorogenic	Coumarin	Gallic acid	Limonene	Malvin	Menadione	PIT*	Phenylalanin	Phloridzin	Quercitin	SHRIMP	ONION	Tyramine	Umbelliferon	Linoleic oil	Linolenic oil	Lauric acid oil	Myristic oil	Oleic acid oil	Palmitic oil
beet, raw	N	N	N	N	N	N	N	N	N	N	N	N	N	N	N	N	N	N	N	N	N						
beet, cooked	N	N	N	N	N	N	N	N	N	N	P	N	N	N	N	N	N	N	N	N	N						has NGF, mannitol
bok choy, raw	N	N	N	N	N	N	N	N	N	N	N	N	P	N	N	N	N	N	N	N							gone if very fresh
boneset herb	N	N	N	N	N	N	N	N	N	N	N	N	N	N	N	N	N	N	N	N	N						no naringenin, NGF
Brazil nuts	N			P				N		N						N							P				
bread, bakery					N		N	N	N	P		N			N	N		N		N							has gold & mannitol
bread, (Mex) bolillo	N	N	N	N	N	N	N	N	N	N	N	N	N	N	N	N	N	N	N	N	N						no mannitol, bromine or live yeast
bread, supermarket	N							N		P			P			N			P								has mannitol, bromine, gold & live yeast
bread, health food store	P							N		P			P			N			P								has live yeast
bread, machine, or homemade	N							N		N						N			N								no live yeast or gallic acid
broccoli	N	N	N	N	P	N	N	N	N	N	N	N	N	P	N	N	N	N	N	N	N						gone if cooked
Brussels sprout	N							N		N				P		N			N								cooked
buckwheat	N	N	N	N	N		N	N	N	N	N	N	P	N	N	N	N	N	N		N						cooked
burdock root	N	N	N	N	N	N	N	N	N	N	N	N	N	N	N	N	N	N	N	N	N						no naringenin, NGF
butter, organic	N	N	N	N	N		N	N	N	N	N	N	P	N	N	N	N	N	N		N						has HGH
butter	P							P		P						P			P								

N = Negative P = Positive N/P = both Negative&Positive FOOD ITEM	Apiol	ASA(aspirin)	Asparagine	Acetaldehyd	Caffeic acid	D-Carnitine	Cinnamic	Chlorogenic	Coumarin	Gallic acid	Limonene	Malvin	Menadione	PIT*	Phenylalanin	Phloridzin	Quercitin	SHRIMP	ONION	Tyramine	Umbelliferon	Linoleic oil	Linolenic oil	Lauric acid oil	Myristic oil	Oleic acid oil	Palmitic oil
buttermilk	N							P								N			P								
cabbage, raw	N	N	N	N	N	N	N	N	N	N	N	N	N	P	N	N	N	N	N	N							PIT gone if cooked
cactus, raw	N	N	N	N	N	N	N	N	N	N	N	N	N	N	N	N	N	N	N	N	N						has ASA if cooked, has hesperidin
cantaloupe	N	N		N	N		N	N	N	N	N	N	N	N		N	P	N	N	N	N						no MELON allergen
cardamom					N		N	N	N	N		N		N	N	N		N	N	N							
carrots, raw	N				N		N	N	N	N		N		N	N	N		P		N	P						no umbelli if peeled
cashew, raw	N		N	P				N		N						P			N								no phlor if roasted
cauliflower														P		P											both gone if cooked
celery	N	N	N	N	N	N	N	N	N	N	N	N	N	N	N	N	N	N	N	N	N						
chard, Swiss	N	N	N	N	N	N	N	N	N	N	N	N	N	N	N	N	N	N	N	N	N						has no mannitol
cheese, cottage, other	P							P		P					P	P	P										most cheeses have Bacillus cereus, pituitary, hypothalamus, vasopressin, HGH, TSH, FSH
cheese, goat	N							P		N					P	N/P											
cheese, organic	N							P		P						N			N								
cherimoya								N	N	N						N											have phloridzin if unripe
cherries, Bing, ripe, black	N	N	N	N	N		N	N	N	N	N	N	N	N	N	N	N	N	N								have chlorogenic and phloridzin if only red
cherries, red	N							P		P						N			N								

N = Negative P = Positive N/P = both Negative&Positive FOOD ITEM	Apiol	ASA(aspirin)	Asparagine	Acetaldehyd	Caffeic acid	D-Carnitine	Cinnamic	Chlorogenic	Coumarin	Gallic acid	Limonene	Malvin	Menadione	PIT*	Phenylalanin	Phloridzin	Quercitin	SHRIMP	ONION	Tyramine	Umbelliferon	Linoleic oil	Linolenic oil	Lauric acid oil	Myristic oil	Oleic acid oil	Palmitic oil
cherries, yellow	N							N		N						N			N								
chicken, cooked	N	N	P	N	N	P	N	N	N	N/P	P	P/N	N	N	N	N	N	N	N	N	N	has lauric acid, MYC oncovirus, limonene, E. recurvatum fluke					
	range fed has no gallic, MYC, SV40, malvin, but has limonene																										
cilantro, fresh	N	N		N	N		N	N	N	N	N	N	N	N	N	N	N	N	P	N	N						
cinnamon	N	N	N	N	N	N	P	N	N	N	N	N	N	N	N	N	N	N	N	N	N	N	N	N	P	N	N
clover, red	N							N	P	N						N			N								
cloves, whole	N	N	N	N	N	N	N	N	N	N	N	N	N	N	N	N	N	N	N	N	N	N	N	N	N	N	N
coconut	N	N	N	N	N	N	N	N	N	N	N	N	N	N	N	N	N	N	N	N	N	P	P	P	P	P	P
collards	N							N		N				P		N			N			gone if cooked					
comfrey leaf or root, dried								N	N	N						N			N								
corn	N	N	N	N	N		N	N	N	N	N	N	N	N	N	N	N	N	N	N	N						
	All corn varieties and products: in husk, cooked, popped, organic have incorporated major air pollutants: strontium, beryllium, chromium, vanadium																										
coriander	N							N		N						N			N								
cranberries	N	N	N	N	N		N	N	N	N	N	N	N	N	N	N	N	N	N		N	have hippuric acid					
whipping cream, heavy:								N/														has lactose and galacturonic acid					

N = Negative P = Positive N/P = both Negative&Positive FOOD ITEM	Apiol	ASA(aspirin)	Asparagine	Acetaldehyd	Caffeic acid	D-Carnitine	Cinnamic	Chlorogenic	Coumarin	Gallic acid	Limonene	Malvin	Menadione	PIT*	Phenylalanin	Phloridzin	Quercitin	SHRIMP	ONION	Tyramine	Umbelliferon	Linoleic oil	Linolenic oil	Lauric acid oil	Myristic oil	Oleic acid oil	Palmitic oil
• supermarket			P		N		N	**P**		**P**		N	P	N	P	**N**		N		P		no lactose, or piperine					
• org, kosher	N	N	N	N	N		N	**N**	N	**N**	N	N	P	N	N	**N**	N	N	N	N	N						
• Lala (Mex)	N	N	N	N	N	N	N	**N**	N	**N**	N	N	N	N	N	**N**	N	N	N	N	N						
cucumbers	N	N	N	N	N	N	N	**N**	N	**N**	N	N	N	N	N		P	N	N	N	N						
cumquat, raw	N	N	N	N	N	N	N	**N**	N	**N**	N	N	N	N	N	**N**	N	N	N	N	N	has no naringenin					
dates, dried	N							**N**		**N**						**N**			have acetic acid, hippuric acid								
dextrose	N	N	N	N				**N**	N	**N**		N				**N**			N	has CORN (air) pollutants							
eggs USA, raw or cooked	N	N	N	N	N	N	N	**N**	N	**P**	N	P	N	N	N	**N**	N	N	N	N	N	P					
	Hypothalamus and pituitary cells as well as SV40 and MYC oncoviruses are present in most USA, raw or cooked eggs, but they can be destroyed with HCL, 3 drops each. All eggs have hippuric acid.																										
eggs (Mex)	N have hippuric acid							**N**		**N**		N				**N**			N		have no hypothalamus, pituitary, SV40, MYC						
eggplant	N				N		N	**N**	N	**N**		N		N	N	**N**	N	N		N			P	cooked			
epazote	N	N	N	N	N	N	N	**N**	N	**N**	N	N	N	N	N	**N**	N	N	N	N	N	soup flavoring					
eucalyptus	N	N	N	N	N	N	N	**N**	N	**N**	N	N	N	N	N	**N**	N	N	N	N	N	all parts					
fennel, seed	N	N	N	N	N	N	N	**N**	N	**N**	N	N	N	N	N	**N**	N	N	N	N	leaves have ONION						
fenugreek	N	N	N	N	N	N	N	**N**	N	**N**	N	N	N	N	N	**N**	N	N	N	N	N						
fig, raw, dried	N							**N**		**N**						**N**		N	N	has acetic acid							
fish, fresh or canned	N							**N**		**N**						**N**		P	N	has Fast Garnet, Fast Red, Fast Red Violet dyes							

N = Negative P = Positive N/P = both Negative&Positive FOOD ITEM	Apiol	ASA(aspirin)	Asparagine	Acetaldehyd	Caffeic acid	D-Carnitine	Cinnamic	Chlorogenic	Coumarin	Gallic acid	Limonene	Malvin	Menadione	PIT*	Phenylalanin	Phloridzin	Quercitin	SHRIMP	ONION	Tyramine	Umbelliferon	Linoleic oil	Linolenic oil	Lauric acid oil	Myristic oil	Oleic acid oil	Palmitic oil
flax seed, oil	N	N						P	N	P						N			P				P				
flour, wheat	N	N	N	N	N		N	N	N	N	N	N	P	N	N	N	N	N	N	N		no bromine or gallic if unbleached					
flour, white	N				N		N	N	N	P		N	N	N	N	N	N	N		N							
flour, rye	N	N	N	N	N	N	N	N	N	N	N	N	N	N	N	N	N	N	N	N	N	has no menadione					
garbanzo beans, cooked	N	N	N	N	N	N	N	N	N	N	N	N	N	N	N	N	N	N	N/P	N	N	develops ONION at high temperature					
ginger	N	N	N	N	N	N	N	N	N	N	N	N	N	N	N	N	N	N	N	N	N	has hippuric acid and D-malic if unpeeled, no limonene in capsules					
garlic, raw	N							N	N	N						N		N	P			has alkylators					
grapes, red, blue	N	N	N	N	N	N	N	N	N	N	N	P	N	N	N	N	N	N	N	N	N	no benzoic, citric acid or fructose; have radioactivity					
grapes, green	N	N	N	P	N	N	N	N	N	N	N	N	N	N	N	N	N	N	N	N	N						
grapefruit					P			N		N	N					N				caffeic gone if tree ripened							
grape seed oil	N	N			N		N	P	N	P	P	P	N			N	N										
grain, Kamut								P		N						P											
guayaba		P		N	N		N	N		N	P	N	N	N		N	N			N	cooking removes both						
gum, chewing	P						P	N		N		P				N			P				has mannitol				
hamburger					N		N	N	N	N		N		N	N	N		N		N			has pyrrole				

N = Negative P = Positive N/P = both Negative&Positive FOOD ITEM	Apiol	ASA(aspirin)	Asparagine	Acetaldehyd	Caffeic acid	D-Carnitine	Cinnamic	Chlorogenic	Coumarin	Gallic acid	Limonene	Malvin	Menadione	PIT*	Phenylalanin	Phloridzin	Quercitin	SHRIMP	ONION	Tyramine	Umbelliferon	Linoleic oil	Linolenic oil	Lauric acid oil	Myristic oil	Oleic acid oil	Palmitic oil
honey	N							**N**	P	**N**						**N**			N	has fructose, L-DOPA, does not have mannitol							
	All honey has incorporated air pollutants: strontium, beryllium, chromium, vanadium; test also for gold.																										
horseradish	N	N	N	N	N	N	N	**N**	N	**N**	N	N	N	N	N	**N**	N	N		N	N						
hydrangea root	N	N	N	N	N	N	N	**N**	N	**N**	N	N	N	N	N	**N**	N	N	N	N	N	N	N	N	P	N	N
Jalapeño seed								**P**		**P**	P			N		**P**			P			all gone if ripe					
Jamaica flower								**P**		**P**						**P**			P		popular Mexican drink						
jicama, raw	N	N	N	N	N		N	**N**	N	**N**	P	N	N	N	N	**N**	N	N	N	N	N						
kipper snacks	N									**N**						**N**			P		has pyrrole, NGF						
kiwi	N	N	N	N	N	N	N	**N**	N	**N**	N	N	N	N	N	**N**	P	N	N		has no mannitol						
kohlrabi herb								**N**	N	**N**						**N**		N		kills SV40, tumor nucleus							
kohlrabi, raw								**N**	N	**N**						**P**		N									
lard																**N**						N	N	P	N	N	N
lamb	N	N	N	N	N	N	N	**N**	N	**N**	N	N	N	N	N	**N**	N	N	N	N	N	N	N	N	N	N	N
leeks, raw								**N**	N	**N**						**N**			P								
lecithin, soy	P															**P**											
lemons	N	N	N	N	N	N	N	**N**	N	**N**	P	N	N	N	N	**N**	N	N	N	N	N	have citric acid					
lentils, cooked	N	N	N	N	N	N	N	**N**	N	**N**	N	N	N	N	N	**N**	N	N	P	gone if slow cooked, has rutin							

N = Negative P = Positive N/P = both Negative&Positive FOOD ITEM	Apiol	ASA(aspirin)	Asparagine	Acetaldehyd	Caffeic acid	D-Carnitine	Cinnamic	Chlorogenic	Coumarin	Gallic acid	Limonene	Malvin	Menadione	PIT*	Phenylalanin	Phloridzin	Quercitin	SHRIMP	ONION	Tyramine	Umbelliferon	Linoleic oil	Linolenic oil	Lauric acid oil	Myristic oil	Oleic acid oil	Palmitic oil
lettuce, iceberg	N	N	N	N	N	N	N	**N**	N	**N**	P/N	N	N	N	N	**N**	N	N	N	N	has menadione if wilted						
licorice root																							has ruthenium				
limes, all					P		P																				
mango	N							**P**		**P**		P				**P**			N								
margarine	P							**P**		**P**					P	**P**		P	P								
maple syrup	N	P/N			N		N	**N**	N	**N/P**		N			N	**N**	P	N		N				has mannitol			
melon	N							**N**		**N**	P					**N**	P		N			has MELON antigen					
- honeydew	N	N		N	N		N	**N**	N	**N**	N	N	N	N		**N**	P	N		N	N						
milk, goat,(ultra pasteurized)	N	N		N	N		N	**N**	N	**N**	N	N	N	N	N	**N**	N	N	N	N	N	no HGH,TRY, casein, piperine, or free cells					
milk, goat	N	P						**N**		**N**						**N**			N		N	has mannitol, TRY					
milk, cow, all kinds	N							**P**		**N/P**					P	**N**			N	P	has hypothalamus, pituitary cells, TRY						
mint, fresh	N	N	N	N	N		N	**N**	N	**N**	N	N	N	N	N	**N**	N	N	N	N	N		no naringenin				
mustard seed	N							**N**		**N**				P		**N**			N								
nectarines	N	N	N	N	N		N	**N**	N	**N**	N	N	N	N	N	**N**	N	N	N		N						
nutmeg	N	N	N	N	N	N	N	**N**	N	**N**	N	N	N	N	N	**N**	N	N	N	N	N	N	N		P		
nuts, Hazel	N	N	N	N	N	N	N	**N**	N	**N**	N	N	N	N	N	**N**	N	N	N	N	N	N	N	N	N	N	N

N = Negative P = Positive N/P = both Negative&Positive FOOD ITEM	Apiol	ASA(aspirin)	Asparagine	Acetaldehyd	Caffeic acid	D-Carnitine	Cinnamic	Chlorogenic	Coumarin	Gallic acid	Limonene	Malvin	Menadione	PIT*	Phenylalanin	Phloridzin	Quercitin	SHRIMP	ONION	Tyramine	Umbelliferon	Linoleic oil	Linolenic oil	Lauric acid oil	Myristic oil	Oleic acid oil	Palmitic oil
oats, cooked, raw	N							N	N	N			P			N	P		N		has manganese metal						
oil, almond	N			P				N		N						N			N								
oil, canola	P							N		P						P			P								
oil, corn	P							P		P						P			P								
oil, cottonseed	P									P																	
oil, olive	P antigens gone if pure							P		P						P			N								
oil, peanut, pure	N							N		N						N			N/P			all these oils had malonic and maleic acids, whether "pure" or not. Only two Mexican olive oils did not (Olibaja, Carbonell).					
oil, safflower	N							N		N						N			N								
oil, sesame	N/P							N/P		N/P						N/P			N								
oil, soy, pure	P															P											
oil, sunflower	N							N		N						N			N								
oil, vegetable	P									P																	
okra, cooked	N	N	N	N	N	N	N	N	N	N	N	N	N	N	N	N	N	N	N	N	N						
olive leaf, dried	N							N		N						N			N								
olives, black	P							P		P						P			P			all absent if fresh					
ONION, raw								N	N	N						N		N	P		ONION gone if cooked						

N = Negative P = Positive N/P = both Negative&Positive FOOD ITEM	Apiol	ASA(aspirin)	Asparagine	Acetaldehyd	Caffeic acid	D-Carnitine	Cinnamic	Chlorogenic	Coumarin	Gallic acid	Limonene	Malvin	Menadione	PIT*	Phenylalanin	Phloridzin	Quercitin	SHRIMP	ONION	Tyramine	Umbelliferon	Linoleic oil	Linolenic oil	Lauric acid oil	Myristic oil	Oleic acid oil	Palmitic oil
oranges, supermarket	N	N	N	N	P	N	N	N	N	N	N	N	N	N		N	N	N	N	N	N	have naringenin					
	caffeic not present in homegrown oranges; Mandarin & tangerine have no naringenin, have rutin and hesperidin																										
oregano, dried	N	N	N	N	N	N	N	N	N	N	N	N	N	N	N	N	N	N	N	N							
papaya, ripe	N	N	N	N	N	N	N	N	N	N	N	N	N	N	N	N	P	N	N	N	N	no naringenin					
parsley, raw	N	N	N	N	N	N	N	N	P/N	N	N	N	P	N	N	N	N	N	N		N	both gone if boiled, no D-malic					
pasta	N	N	N	N	N		N	N	N	N	N	N	N	N	N	N	N	N	N		N						
peaches, ripe	N	N	N	N	N	N	N	N	N	N	N	N	N	N	N	N	N	N	N	N	no naringenin, NGF						
peas, green, split, yellow	N	N	N	N	N	N	N	N/P	N	N/P	N	N	N	P		N/P	N	N	N	have ONION after cooking, have Cu, Co, Cr, V, Ge, Se if roasted							
peanuts, raw in shell	N	N	N	N	N	N	N	N	N	N	N	N	N	N	N	N	N	N	N	N	have ONION if roasted, have linolenic						
peanut butter, old fashioned					N		N	N	N	N		N		N	N	N		N	P	N/P	smooth ground has nickel and chromium						
pears, ripe	N	N	N	N	N	N	N	N	N	N	N	N	N	N	N	N	N	N	N	N	have limonene if cooked						
pecans	N		N	P				N		N						N			N				P				
peppermint	N	N	N	N	N	N	N	N	N	N	N	N	N	N	N	N	N	N	N	N							
peppers, all	N							P		N						N			N		gone if cooked						
pineapple	N	N					N	N	N	N	P	N	N	N	N	N			N		raw or cooked						

N = Negative P = Positive N/P = both Negative&Positive FOOD ITEM	Apiol	ASA(aspirin)	Asparagine	Acetaldehyd	Caffeic acid	D-Carnitine	Cinnamic	Chlorogenic	Coumarin	Gallic acid	Limonene	Malvin	Menadione	PIT*	Phenylalanin	Phloridzin	Quercitin	SHRIMP	ONION	Tyramine	Umbelliferon	Linoleic oil	Linolenic oil	Lauric acid oil	Myristic oil	Oleic acid oil	Palmitic oil
plantain, fried	N	N	N	N	N	N	N	N	N	N	N	N	N	N	N	P	N	N	N	P	N	both gone if ripe					
plums, black	N	N	N	N	N	N	N	N	N	N	N	N	N	N	N	N	N	N	N	N	have phlor if under ripe						
pomegranate								N	N	N					N	N	P	N	N								
potatoes, well cooked, baked	N							N		N						N			N	test for malonic acid							
potatoes, fried	N							P		N						P			N								
potato starch	N	N	N	N	N	N	N	N	N	N	N	N	N	N	N	N	N	N	N	no piperine, NGF							
potato, sweet, or yam	N	N	N	N	N	N	N	N	N	N	N	N	N	N	N	N	P	N	N	N	N	has mandelonitrile, test for malonic, apiol					
potato chips	P							P		P						P			P								
pumpkin	N							N		N						N	P			not in seeds, gone if cooked							
pumpkin seed	N	N	N	N	N	N	N	N	N	N	N	N	N	N	N	N	N	N	N	N	N	has Mo if roasted					
quassia herb	N							P								P											
radish, red	N	N	N	N	N	N	N	N	N	N	N	N	N	P	N	N	N	N	N	N	N	no naringenin, NGF					
radish, white																		P	SHRIMP gone if cooked								
raisins, all	N	N	N	N	N	N	N	N	N	N	N	P	N	N	N	N	N	N	N	N	N	have mannitol					
raspberries								N	N	N						N		N									
rice, USA, cooked	N	N	N	N	N	N	N	N	P	N	N	N	P	N	N	N	N	N	N	N	N	Mexican varieties have no coumarin					
rose hips capsule																	N										

N = Negative P = Positive N/P = both Negative&Positive FOOD ITEM	Apiol	ASA(aspirin)	Asparagine	Acetaldehyd	Caffeic acid	D-Carnitine	Cinnamic	Chlorogenic	Coumarin	Gallic acid	Limonene	Malvin	Menadione	PIT*	Phenylalanin	Phloridzin	Quercitin	SHRIMP	ONION	Tyramine	Umbelliferon	Linoleic oil	Linolenic oil	Lauric acid oil	Myristic oil	Oleic acid oil	Palmitic oil
rosemary	N	N			N		N	**N**		**N**	N	N		N	N	**N**	N	N	N	N							
sage, dried	N	N	N	N	N	N	N	**P**	N	**N**	N	N	N	N	N	**N**	N	N	N	N	N	gone if cooked					
salmon, fresh canned	N							**N**		**N**						**N**		N	N			test for dyes, SHRIMP					
sardines, oil	P							**N**		**N**						**N**		P	N			have NGF					
sardines, water	N							**N**		**N**						**N**		P	N			have NGF					
seafood, fish, shrimp, crab	N							**N**		**N**						**N**		P	N		no SHRIMP in first 6 hours after catch						
sesame seed	N				N		N	**N**	N	**N**						**N**	N		N	N			P				
soybeans	P							**N**		**N**						**N**			N		all soy products have apiol						
soy beverage	P							**P**		**P**						**P**			P								
spinach, raw	N							**N**		**N**						**N**			N		has oxalate, use little						
squash, all	N	N	N	N	N	N	N	**N**	N	**N**	N	N	N	N	N	**N**	P	N	N	N	gone if cooked; no naringenin, NGF, mannitol						
Stevia, herb	N	N	N	N	N	N	N	**N**	N	**N**	N	N	N	N	N	**N**	N	N	N	N	N						
strawberries, org., supermkt	N				P		P	**N**		**N/P**		P				**P/N**			N		supermarket variety has radioactivity						
sugar, icing	N	N	N	N				**N**	N	**N**		N				**N**			N	has fructose, CORN, mannitol							
sugar, org. USA	N							**N**		**N**						**N**				has mannitol; test for CORN							
sugar (MEX)	N	N		N	N		N	**N**	N	**N**	N	N	N	N		**N**	N			N	N	test for CORN					

N = Negative P = Positive N/P = both Negative&Positive FOOD ITEM	Apiol	ASA(aspirin)	Asparagine	Acetaldehyd	Caffeic acid	D-Carnitine	Cinnamic	Chlorogenic	Coumarin	Gallic acid	Limonene	Malvin	Menadione	PIT*	Phenylalanin	Phloridzin	Quercitin	SHRIMP	ONION	Tyramine	Umbelliferon	Linoleic oil	Linolenic oil	Lauric acid oil	Myristic oil	Oleic acid oil	Palmitic oil
	zulka azuca estandar and azucar estandar (CALIMAX) dark have no mannitol																										
sunflower seed	N	N	N	N	N	N	N	**N**	N	**N**	N	N	N	N	N	**N**	N	N	N	N	N	N	P	N	N	raw	
tahini, organic	N							**N**		**N**						**N**			N				P				
tapioca, cooked	N	N	N	N	N	N	N	**N**	N	**N**	N	N	N	N	N	**N**	N	N	N	N	has PIT if undercooked						
tea, regular		P			P			**P**		**P**		N				**P**											
thyme																				has piperine (causes knee pain)							
thyme, dried	N	N	N	N	N	N	N	**N**	N	**N**	N	N	N	N	N	**N**	N	N	N	N	P						
tomatoes, raw or cooked	Roma has no malvin							**N**	N		N/P	P				**N/P**		N		malvin gone if cooked 5 min.							
tomato, cherry	N	N	N	N	N	N	N	**N**	N	**N**	N	N	N	N	N	**N**	N	N	N	N	N	N	malvin if blemished				
tuna, canned	N							**N**		**N**						**N**		P	N				in water				
tuna, canned	P							**N**		**N**						**N**		P	N				in oil			P	
tuna (kosher), Albacore, Tongol, Skipjack, canned in water has no SHRIMP																											
turkey, free range, organic	N	N	N	N	N	N	N	**N**	N	**N**	P	N	N	N	N	**N**	N	N	N	N	N	N	has no hippuric				
turkey, regular						P																P					
turmeric, pwd	N	N	N	N	N	N	N	**N**	N	**N**	N	N	N	N	N	**N**	N	N	N	N	N				N		
uva ursi, pwd	N	N	N	N	N	N	N	**N**	N	**N**	N	N	N	N	N	**N**	N	N	N	N	N	N	N	N	N	N	N
vanilla	N							**N**	P	**N**						**N**			N								
walnuts	N		N	P				**N**		**N**						**N**			N				P				

N = Negative P = Positive N/P = both Negative&Positive FOOD ITEM	Apiol	ASA(aspirin)	Asparagine	Acetaldehyd	Caffeic acid	D-Carnitine	Cinnamic	Chlorogenic	Coumarin	Gallic acid	Limonene	Malvin	Menadione	PIT*	Phenylalanin	Phloridzin	Quercitin	SHRIMP	ONION	Tyramine	Umbelliferon	Linoleic oil	Linolenic oil	Lauric acid oil	Myristic oil	Oleic acid oil	Palmitic oil
walnut, Black, hull tincture	N	N	N	N	N	N	N	**N**	N	**N**	N	N	N	N	N	**N**	N	N	N	N	N				N		
watercress	N							**N**		**N**						**N**			N		tablets have coumarin						
watermelon				P																							
wheat, sprouts	N							**N**		**P**			N			**N**			N								
wheat germ	N	N	N	N	N	N	N	**N**	N	**N**	N	N	P	N	N	**N**	N	N	N	N	N	gone if nitrogen packed					
wheat, cooked	N	N	N	N	N		N	**N**	N	**N**	N	N	P	N	N	**N**	N	N	N		N						
wild rice	N	N	N	N	N	N	N	**N**	N	**N**	N	N	N	N	N	**N**	N	N	N	N	has no hippuric, gluten, has vitamin E						
wormwood																	P										
yam, raw		P																			gone if cooked						
yogurt, all varieties	P				N/P		N/P	**P/N**		**P/N**		P		P/N	P	**P/N**		N/P		P		has mannitol					
zucchini	N	N	N	N	N	N	N	**N**	N	**N**	N	N	N	N	N	**N**	N	N	N	N	N	cooked					

*bee hives in US are supplied with commercial wax comb contaminated with benzene, which could be oxidized to phenol by the bees

**lauric oil comes from coconut and animals fed coconut

Allergens Destroyed by Ozonation (ozonate 10 minutes; then close container and wait another 10 minutes to complete the action; see page 548).

- casein
- CHEESE
- estradiol
- estriol
- estrone
- PIT
- quercitin

Note the 3 estrogens, which should be inappropriate food for young children in any large quantity.

Allergens Destroyed by Boiling (keep up a rolling boil for 5 minutes; add liquid to thick foods like beans or porridge to help it boil; microwaving is not satisfactory).

- caffeic acid
- chlorogenic acid
- gallic acid
- menadione
- ONION, raw
- phloridzin
- quercitin
- SHRIMP
- umbelliferone
- PIT

Special Attractions

Food antigens can be especially attracted to certain organs, just as bacteria or medicines are. Such attractions are called **tropisms**. We have many examples. For instance, herbs expected to help the eye or throat should have a tropism for these organs, to be truly useful. Bacteria with tropisms are, for example, tuberculosis for the lungs, and Staphylococcus aureus for the skin and breast. The three allergenic food substances are specifically attracted to the three eroding organs. Is the erosion causing or caused by the allergies? Research is badly needed.

Chlorogenic acid has a tropism for the hypothalamus. When a tiny bit of potato is chewed, raw or fried, we can detect chlorogenic acid in the hypothalamus in <u>seconds</u>, before it could have reached the liver!

Even when free hypothalamus cells have already settled in a different organ, where they are living as part of the tumor nucleus, chlorogenic acid is immediately there from a food.

When a tiny bit of the wrong apple is nibbled, phloridzin goes immediately to the pituitary gland. In less than a minute it can be detected in free pituitary cells passing through some organ. And a tropism exists for the islets of Langerhans too; it is the same substance, phloridzin! We could stop all diabetes. In fact, this cancer cure routinely cures diabetes, too.

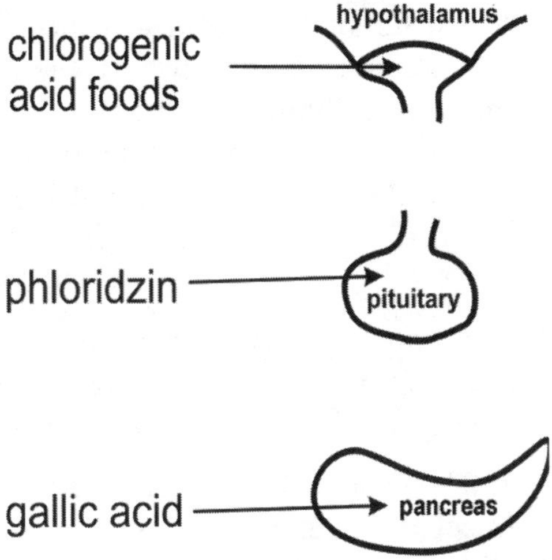

Fig. 29 Food antigens go to specific organs

Gallic acid has a tropism for the pancreas, not the islets of Langerhans where your insulin is made. It is there in three seconds after putting a bit of gallic acid-containing food in your mouth. Again, it arrives before it could have reached the liver where detoxification would occur.

The tropisms of chlorogenic acid, phloridzin, and gallic acid are the same for all of us, whether or not we have cancer or allergies or other illnesses or are completely well. What matters for our health is how long it stays in the target organ. It depends on parasitism, as we will see.

Summary — Chapter 3

1. All tumors that lead to cancer start with a tiny string of cells that come from 3 organs: the hypothalamus and pituitary glands in the brain and the pancreas just under the stomach. They stick together in a certain order, not randomly. This is the tumor nucleus. A cancer patient is teeming with tumor nuclei. The pancreas cells, not the others, are infected with the SV40 virus.

2. A cancer patient is also teeming with parts of the unique cancer-complex that will attach itself to the DNA in an organ destined to form the primary tumor.

3. The cancer-complex, as well as the tumor nucleus, attach themselves to this organ, specifically at the cerium element. Preliminary evidence shows that stem cells are chosen as contact points for both the tumor nucleus and the cancer-complex.

4. The cancer patient-to-be runs out of complement C3 molecules, so prevention of a growing tumor will be impossible.

5. All 3 organs that contribute to the tumor nucleus are inflamed—they make prostaglandin E2 (PGE2).

6. The processes leading to a cancerous tumor form a chain, so any scheme that pulls out a link would also prevent cancer. Omitting one or two foods that belong to the chain of events seems like an easy way to prevent any cancer.

7. The 3 organs that start the tumor nucleus each have an allergy to a particular food substance called a food phenolic. The *Food Table* on page 95 lists the allergens brought by many foods.

CHAPTER 4

WE ALL HAVE PARASITES

Humans, like other animals, have always had parasites, both outside and inside our bodies. It is easy to see in animals when you dissect a frog or fish in a college classroom. You would be taught that every organ has its parasite. Some are **flukes**, some are **roundworms**, some are **tapeworms**. Most parasites belong to one of these 3 groups.

Flukes are like little leeches, stuck in one spot, just feeding and making eggs. The animal that is parasitized with the adult fluke is the **primary host**. The animal with the larvae is the **secondary host**, often a snail. Inside the snail the larvae go through their developmental stages. This suits the parasites' need to, somehow, hitchhike from animal to animal till it can reach its primary host again. This has changed since immunity has dropped. The Syncrometer® finds that instead of requiring a single, specific snail, many snails can be used as the secondary host. Shortcuts can be taken by the parasite because the vigilance of the immune system is gone.

People go through infancy, childhood, teenage, and adulthood, to reproduce and arrive at infancy again. All with the same purpose: to survive and thrive. Our parasites survive with us, but how they will thrive depends on our health. They do not thrive when we are healthy. It is the less healthy animal that is the most parasitized in Nature.

In times of plentiful, nourishing food and clean water for animals, parasites do not take them over. But if food is scarce, and the water source is crowded with other animals, their general health declines and parasites thrive instead. Poor health and parasitism go hand in hand.

The roundworms look a lot like earthworms without feet, or means of travel. A roundworm just wiggles and molts its skin off a number of times to grow till it is an adult. Our common roundworms are **Ascaris**, **Strongyloides** and **filaria** (long, thin filaments) like **heartworms**. Cats have learned to spit up their Ascaris by eating grass. Puppies, too, are taught to eat "dog grass" to entangle their stomach Ascaris and spit them up. But people, with all their intelligence, seem to be doing nothing to keep their parasitism in check.

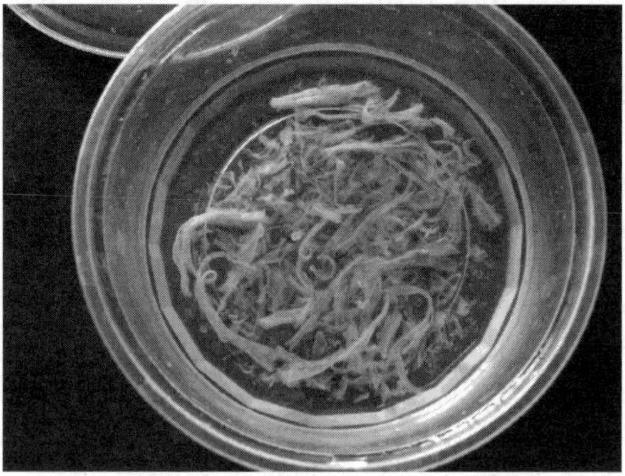

Fig. 30 Bowl of Ascaris from cancer patient

The Syncrometer® shows that we all, from early childhood, harbor Ascaris eggs and larvae, the young hatchlings that go through molts. These tiny wormlets, too small to see, give us seizures, eczema, the common cold, and our childhood diseases.

Parasites even live in other parasites. They have their own bacteria and viruses. The bacteria themselves have viruses. And at least one bacterium, common Salmonella, has Flu virus.

Ascaris brings us **Chicken Pox** and **mumps**, **Herpes 1** and **2**, **Coxsackie viruses**, and **Adenovirus** (the common cold). It brings us **Mycobacterium avium** that causes night sweats. We didn't notice these connections in the past because these diseases are commonplace and the parasites so tiny and quiet.

It takes a special astuteness to be suspicious of commonplace things. Ancient and primitive societies had special astuteness. Why did the Hebrew nation ban pork in the diet? Did they notice that herdsmen of swine often had epilepsy, skin disease and other health problems?

Modern American citizens have some astuteness, too, having recognized that smoking cigarettes often leads to lung cancer.

Strongyloides bring us **migraine** headaches and maybe our addictions as well as the very beginning of all tumors, as we saw in Chapter 3. Which problem they bring depends on where they colonize and what we, the host, are eating.

The filaria are as thin as a single filament of silk, but very long so they can make a tangle of themselves and trap other cells. Dirofilaria is the common heartworm of dogs. It is a major contributor to all heart disease. Since our lives are ended in heart disease more than any other way, heartworm should really have our greatest attention. So far, the Syncrometer® has found it not just in the heart, but everywhere we have fluids. Our eyes even have tiny threads of filaria suspended in their fluids. The chest with its lymph fluids around the lungs has heartworm bits. The belly with its **peritoneal** fluid has its short bits. If any of these short pieces of Dirofilaria manage to escape both the immune system and your digestive enzymes so that it can grow long, it produces a snarl. Such a snarl is the starting point for **Hodgkin's Lymphoma, but non-Hodgkin's abdominal tumor masses** grow with Oncocerca, another filaria. Heartworms have gained ground in us by growing longer, even inside the bowel, so their clear glass-like threads make loops in the bowel contents, easy to recognize.

Onchocerca has gained ground, too. Its stages hide in our vein valves, giving us blue **varicose veins**. It gives us small hard nodules under the skin.

For animals it is the availability of clean food and water that decides if they are heavily parasitized and short-lived.

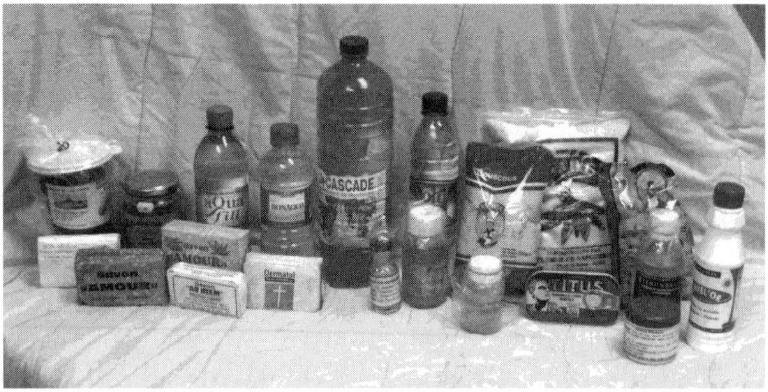

The local water quality decides the food and product quality for that region. Two out of all these African products did not have PCBs, benzene, azo dyes, heavy metals, motor oil, wheel bearing grease, and polonium, all from the chlorox bleach disinfectant used. They were the imported jam and pasta. At extreme right is a bottle of chlorox bleach, meant to be added to food, a direct form of a radioactive immune depressant.

Fig. 31 African products bring immunity depressors

For humans it is also the food and water that decides our health and whether we are heavily parasitized and destined to a life of low energy and lots of medicine.

> For humans, unclean food and water has brought immunodepression, so parasites can increase.

Water has brought these critical immune system depressants: PCBs, benzene, asbestos, azo dyes, heavy metals, motor oil and radioactive elements. Food has brought the same depressants, through food processing that uses the same polluted water to accomplish it all.

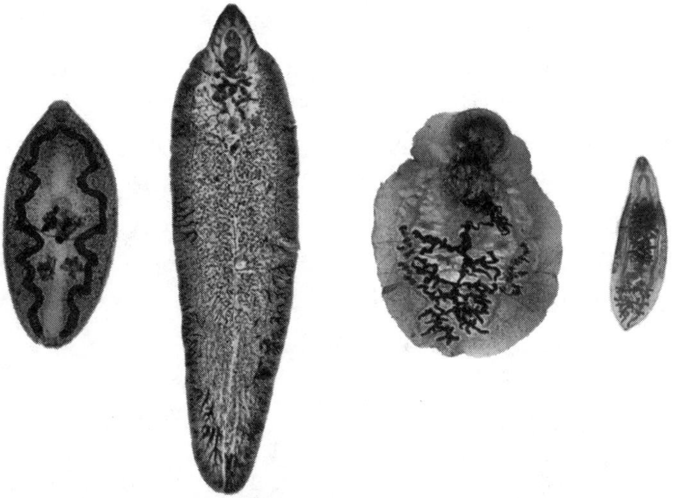

L to R: lung fluke (enlargement 6 times, 6X); sheep liver fluke (3X); pancreatic fluke (5X, causes diabetes, nucleates our cancerous tumors and brings SV40 virus); and human liver fluke (5X).

Fig. 32 Four common flukes on microscope slides

As a result humans now have four very common flukes, besides Fasciolopsis: the sheep liver fluke, the lung fluke, the pancreatic fluke and human liver fluke. Don't believe that the sheep liver fluke is for sheep alone. Hosts can be substituted when immunity is down so that we can become the "accidental" or "incidental" host, already known for decades. Less common parasites are becoming more frequent, too, such as Gastrothylax, which brings us Cystic Fibrosis, Down's

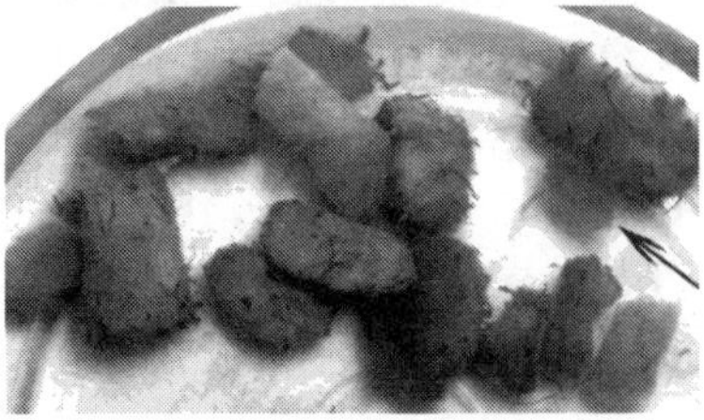

A bowl of F. buski without "hairy legs" can be caught during a liver cleanse if the Gary Technique (see page 184) is used to collect them. Arrow points to lone Fasciola.

Fig. 33 Intact F. buski

Syndrome and Polycystic Kidney Disease, 3 genetic diseases. Echinostoma revolutum, the parasite for all wheelchair cases and Echinoporyphium recurvatum one of our diabetes parasites (besides pancreatic fluke) have gained ground, too. You may see any of these now while you are killing parasites with a vigorous program that induces a brief diarrhea. Get a strong flashlight and keep plastic cups and utensils in the bathroom, as well as Lugol's iodine, so you can see your own parasites safely and identify them.

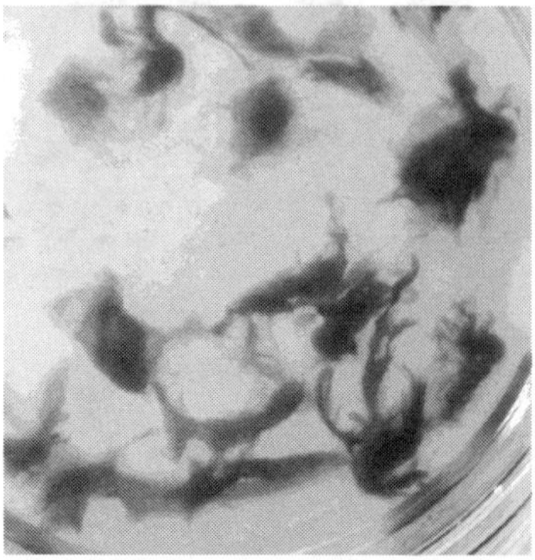

Wispy connections between individuals are easy to spot during a liver cleanse.

Fig. 34 Acanthocephala

The parasite-killing recipe given in earlier books is by far the best to kill flukes. It is a combination of Black Walnut Hulls (still green), wormwood leaves and cloves, very freshly ground. A slow, easy to manage pace is given in earlier books to help those who must be cautious about new treatments. If you are inexperienced with herbs, you should try a very small dose first and work up to the really effective doses.

Herbs are our greatest gift on this planet! They do not have just one active ingredient that kills a parasite or kills bacteria or viruses. Each herb has many active ingredients. The concept of extracting one principle compound, and making its "sister" chemical (analogs, derivatives) is mistaken and unwise. An active ingredient, such as l-ascorbic acid, for example, has its "sisters" right with it in Nature! Potency of an herb does not depend so much on the amount of active ingredient you eat. Potency is increased much more by eating all the natural "sister" compounds, which means, the herb intact. Rose hips have much more potency than l-ascorbic acid in my experience. The Syncrometer® shows that several nuts or a few rose hips can accomplish as much as germanium capsules or pure vitamin C.

For this reason and because herbs belong to you, being your own true treasure, I have chosen herbs wherever possible to deparasitize yourself, kill bacteria and viruses, and maintain your health in a regular way. This is besides electronic and "starvation" ways I will discuss later.

Parasites In The Hypothalamus

In a healthy person chlorogenic acid goes straight to the hypothalamus after eating it. But in five minutes, at most 20 minutes, it is gone. It has been detoxified, digested, or removed.

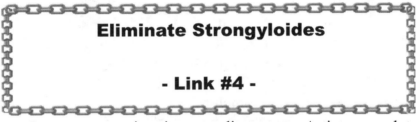

Eliminate Strongyloides

- Link #4 -

In a cancer patient it never disappears. A tiny wormlet is present, microscopically small. It is Strongyloides stercalis. This wormlet belongs to the **roundworm** family, not the flukes, nor the tapeworms. Its larval stages have **molts**. Molting brings special molting chemicals. Perhaps it is one of these that interferes with the removal of chlorogenic acid from

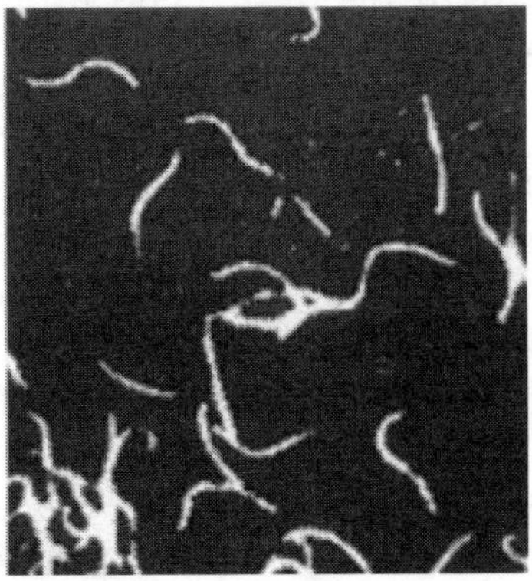

Fig. 35 Strongyloides drawn from a microscope slide, too small to see

the hypothalamus. Maybe this wormlet needs this food antigen to molt or accomplish other purposes. The worm is never there unless chlorogenic acid is there.

How we humans can allow our very brains to be consumed by common worms shows how little control we have. We must do better in our effort to survive as a species. They are easily killed by levamisole (see page 157).

Parasites In The Pituitary

Phloridzin, too, goes directly to the brain, lodging in the pituitary gland even in healthy persons. But it is there only for minutes. Then it has already moved on.

In a cancer patient it is always there. This irritating allergen is present constantly—yet only if the common human liver fluke is there. Somehow this parasite prevents the removal of phloridzin or, again, perhaps it needs it. The human liver fluke is a small parasite, less than ¼ inch long even when it is stretched flat. Its scientific name is Clonorchis sinensis.

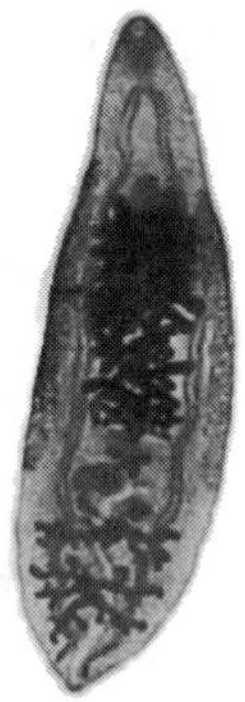

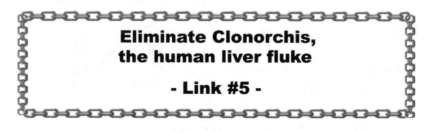

Stretched to ¼ inch on a microscope slide and stained with dyes, its organs are clearly visible.

Fig. 36 Clonorchis, the human liver fluke

Eliminate Clonorchis, the human liver fluke

- Link #5 -

Human Liver Flukes And Cancer

Human liver flukes are very common, and like Strongyloides, they become more plentiful as we age. It is not surprising that they play a role in cancer. In fact, scientists in Asian countries have often proclaimed their theories that this fluke actually is the chief cause of cancer, at least, liver cancer. After a traditional liver cleanse you may see dozens of these in the toilet bowl, but having shrunk to $^1/_8$ inch to $^1/_{16}$ inch in length, they go unnoticed. Use the method on page 181 to find, identify and store yours. The association between this fluke and liver cancer has been studied for decades.[21] The fact that it plays a role in every cancer would be more obscure, without the technology of the Syncrometer®.

The smallest piece of apple, a wedge the size of a penny, brings phloridzin to the pituitary gland in the brain, and some to every other bit of pituitary in the body, such as bits traveling in the blood and lymph. It only persists, though, if Clonorchis is present.

Parasites In The Pancreas

The food allergen, gallic acid, has accumulated in the pancreas in cancer patients. Again, there is an associated parasite; this time it is the pancreatic fluke, with the scientific name, *Eurytrema pancreaticum*. This is the same parasite that brings us diabetes. It is very common,

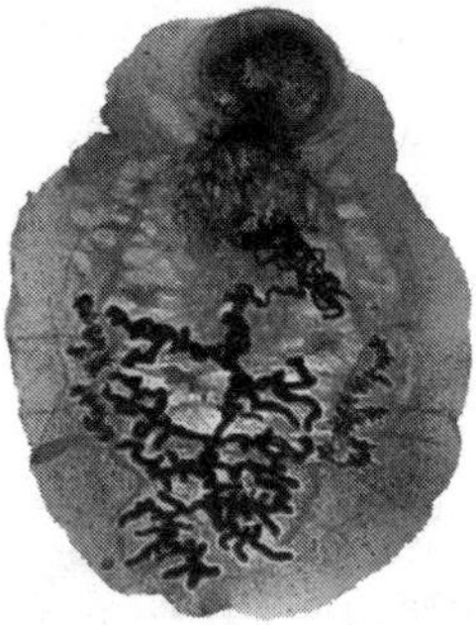

2 red dots near top and a third smaller one midway along one side identifies it.

Fig. 37 Eurytrema, the pancreatic fluke photographed from a slide

[21] *Infection With Liver Flukes* (IARC) Summary & Evaluation, Vol. 61, 1994; (p.121) Last updated 08/26/1997

probably due to our consumption of non-sterile dairy products. Cow's milk and cheese always have eggs and larval stages of the pancreatic fluke. Its essential role in the initiation of cancer could not have been guessed because milk drinking and cancer seem quite far apart. Without Eurytrema, gallic acid does not accumulate; in fact, it is gone in minutes! Nor does the pancreas begin its micro-explosion.

Eliminate Eurytrema, the pancreatic fluke

- Link #6 -

3 Parasites, 3 Allergens and 3 Target Organs

All three parasites must be present to make the three food allergens pile up at the three organs involved in starting a tumor. Without them no sticky "snowball" could form to become the tumor nucleus.

Not only should we avoid the foods with these allergens, we should kill the parasites responsible for it all. We will have 3 more links to perfect prevention of cancer.

Allergies

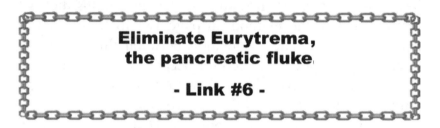

We are all damaged by eating foods we are allergic to and we all respond the same way. Our organs fight back when they get certain substances by making **prostaglandin E2** (PGE2). It is not made immediately—not the first few times we eat it. It is made later, when a south pole force has arrived at that organ. It arrives with **nickel** and **radioactivity**. No matter which food allergen is causing your never-ending symptoms, the organ cells respond by making the same compound, PGE2, after nickel or radioactivity reach it.

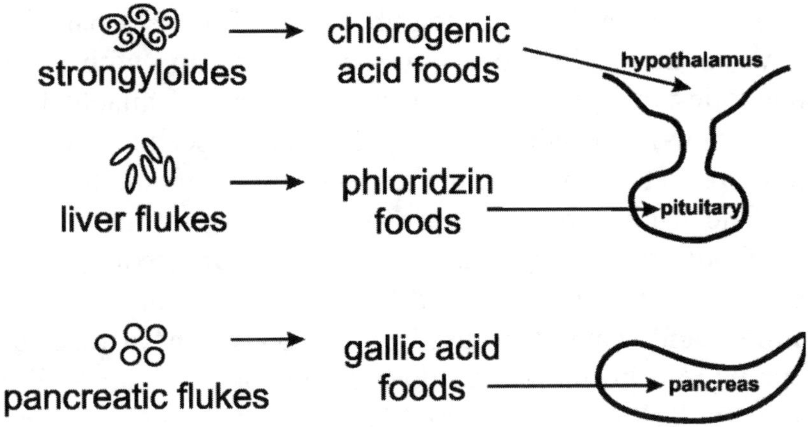

Fig. 38 Three events start the tumor nucleus

The Allergy Explosion

When Fasciolopsis buski arrives in the tumor zone it produces a growth stimulant, orthophosphotyrosine (OPT). It does this by becoming part of the large cancer-complex that makes so many mutations seen in cancer patients. A bacterium, *Bacillus cereus*, constantly streams from this fluke, its own personal host. These bacteria produce **d-tyramine**, a special **amine** that can turn nearby substances from l-form to d-form, like itself. Amines are made from amino acids by the body's chemistry. Northerly zones have changed to southerly zones where the d-forms are made.

l-tyramine is a normal amine, formed from the amino acids, l-tyrosine, and l-phenyl alanine. l-tyrosine will make your l-thyroxine, your normal thyroid hormone. Your metabolism always uses l-forms but Bacillus cereus makes d-forms of tyramine. You can think of l- and d-forms as the left and right glove of a pair. Your body only uses "left gloves" saving itself half of all the materials and enzymes and genes it would otherwise need.

Yet how could the d-form be contagious? All the l-amino acids in the near neighborhood of a buski parasite have soon switched to d-forms! By interacting with other phenolic-type amino acids (those with a OH attached to their rings) to establish an equilibrium, it seems possible to perpetuate d-forms in the presence of south pole forces.

The d-form process spreads from d-tyramine to the neighboring phenolics making d-thyroxine, d-phenylalanine, d-tyrosine, d-histidine, and more. The d-amino acids cannot be used by the body. The d-form of our thyroid hormone can do nothing for our bodies. We are now lacking this essential hormone. It is an emergency for the tissue. This should get immediate attention and it will. PGE2 will be made.

The change in amino acid structure from l- to d- alerts the tissue to call in the allergy-fighting mechanism. But the situation is made much worse when food after food that we eat has many d-forms of amino acids and d-forms of phenolics. They stimulate more PGE2 because the body considers them allergens, too. We should not eat them. I believe it is the similarity between phenolic food allergens and our phenolic amino acids that allows this "creeping allergy" of l-forms to d-forms to extend to our foods. We should eat only the freshest of food that has l-forms exclusively. We should carefully avoid aged food, regardless of its chemical preservation, to avoid getting more d-forms. The F. buski fluke is acting as a catalyst for this allergy explosion; it is bringing in these special bacteria. This is the forerunner of metastasis. Once more F. buski plays a role in cancer…metastasis.

The allergy explosion fills us up with inflammations from PGE2. The inflammations open the doorways of our cells to bacteria and viruses. Now we get sick. Pain bacteria, bloating and gas bacteria, cough-mycoplasmas, sweats-mycobacteria, diarrhea bacteria...all these make the cancer patient miserable. We must stop the allergy process by killing more F. buski. To stop the allergy immediately we must stop eating the responsible phenolics, our allergens.

A Mild Scurvy

After PGE2 is made the cells no longer seem to stick together properly. They let go of each other. Maybe (and this is only a theory) they are forced to spill their enzymes, like **collagenase**.

Collagenase digests collagen. Without collagen cells would loosen their hold on neighbor-cells and set themselves free to roam.

To make collagen requires vitamin C. But vitamin C is also required by our white blood cells, precisely to get rid of radioactivity. It becomes a vicious cycle that leads to less and less vitamin C. Radioactivity from chlorine bleach uses up our vitamin C. All chlorine bleaches contain radioactivity from the manufacturing process that uses phosphate buffers to protect the pipes. In this way a chronic mild vitamin C deficiency leads to a low level scurvy that weakens our tissues. When we can't make or repair our collagen promptly tissues come apart.

Inflammation

Inflammation goes hand in hand with PGE2. Both are made by our tissues. Inflammation lets the doorways into our cells stand wide open. You can see this when the electrical resistance of the tissue has gone far down, using various "electro medicine" devices. We can see it with a Syncrometer® when we get a "*Positive*" result. The cells' doorways are open and current is increased.

Although the details of our allergies are not worked out yet, I can see there are only 2 causes for all of them: nickel and radioactivity (besides the food itself). We know we must avoid our allergies or they get worse. And if we do avoid them, sometimes they go away. If we stop getting nickel and radioactivity into our bodies they always go away. A few days of avoiding the food allergy at the same time as removing nickel and radioactivity clears them up. This will be an extra benefit of doing this *2-Week Program*.

Allergies make PGE2.

Parasitism Increasing

We can see that parasitism has been increasing in humans, although nobody is keeping a count or identifying varieties that I am aware of. So important a subject certainly deserves a department of scientists, not affiliated with medical personnel.

It would be wise to protect ourselves—and all of society—by exterminating our parasites constantly with anti-parasite herbs and the traditional practice of herbal "cleaning" of the liver and kidneys. (See earlier books by this author for many details.) They are inexpensive and well tolerated, a practice that was relied on in primitive societies. We should hurry to revive such priceless knowledge.

It would be wise for society to stop using radioactivity in chlorine bleach manufacture, in fertilizers, in water softener salts, and, most importantly, in dental supplies. It would be wise for you to own a Geiger Mueller counter (see *Sources*) to test some of these items yourself.

It should be possible to prevent all newly starting cancers and be free of this risk in society, by stopping the spread of polonium-cerium-ferrocyanide-alkylating agent "complexes" in drinking water. It is a societal responsibility. But you can do it for yourself without waiting.

Choose food and prepare it so it is consistently free of any one of the three tumor starting chemicals. This is another way to protect yourself. You may soon belong to the first cancer-free society that people have ever known.

Cancers that have already started and even progressed to an advanced stage need more than prevention, understandably. But the first step to be taken here, too, is to stop making any more tumor nuclei. In five days the effect of your new diet can be easily seen with a Syncrometer®. The tumor nuclei are gone from blood and lymph.

Prevention Of All Cancers In 5 Days

There will be no single cells, no duplexes, nor triplet combinations of the three glands to be seen anywhere, except inside tumors after 5 days on this diet. You do not need to kill or destroy the tumor nuclei. Although there are special herbs and substances that can do this (6 fresh seed recipe for example), your body will catch up with these chores by itself, now that no more tumor nuclei are being made.

> Prevention of diseases, not cure, or treatment, should be society's foremost goal.

Although I do not know how phenolic food allergens bring about organ erosions except through a PGE2 effect, and I do not know how a parasite can interfere with the allergen's removal, and I do not know how nickel and radioactivity cause allergies, I do know it can all be stopped in 5 days. Preventing cancer; like preventing malaria or a forest fire is very easy, and much more powerful than curing it.

Curing All Cancers

Once the tumor nucleus fuses itself to one of your organs and the complete polonium-cerium-ferrocyanide-ONION-GARLIC-MUSTARD alkylator has attached itself to your tumor nucleus DNA, and Fasciolopsis DNA, a cancer is attacking you. The complex has landed on your DNA and the mutant chemicals are being produced. First is OPT. You have a malignancy now and are forced to keep on producing the family of cancer compounds and markers. But you will not know it until it is discovered much later by yourself or your doctor. By then it is large enough to appear dense on an x-ray or scan. Your immediate goal then will be to kill Fasciolopsis buski because this parasite brings the ONION- GARLIC- and MUSTARD-compounds and it's DNA. After removing it the cancer-complex is no longer complete. But you should at once stop making tumor nuclei, too. This way you will stop making new tumors first, and then reverse the malignancy by breaking up the cancer-complex.

Fortunately, flukes are quite easy to kill. The first cancer book, *The Cure For All Cancers*, was devoted to getting rid of them and if you succeeded you would be cured quite quickly. But if you did not succeed, your cancer would become advanced and require the more intensive *21-Day Program* from the second book, *The Cure For All Advanced Cancers*.

If you succeeded this time, you would again be cured. This time you would need to be much more vigilant afterwards to prevent a recurrence.

But if important steps were left out, a recurrence would be inevitable, and the terminal state would not be far away.

The *2-Week Program* in this book can prevent a recurrence, prevent metastases, and cure even the terminal state.

This time round you will find yourself again overrun by Fasciolopsis buski parasite stages, but this time many more bleach toxins have accumulated to play a role, and to make you feel sick as well. The dyes and malonic acid have caused effusions. Benzene has caused bleeding and pain. Polonium located in your tooth crowns, bridges, and fillings has had time to find a route to each buski parasite attached to a tumor. Root canals have filled your body with cerium and more chlorox bleach.

In addition, you will be taken over, almost completely by Salmonella, E. coli, Clostridium, *and their* viruses, Yeast and sometimes *prions*.

This time round you might have all the conditions that are typical of advanced cancer and success will depend on eliminating them quickly. There can be no omissions.

In this book you will learn for the first time that F. buski can be "starved" as a killing tactic. The starvation principle can be applied to other parasites, too, even our oncoviruses and bacteria. We will learn for the first time that our laundry bleach toxins can be washed out from our skin to break up the cancer-complexes underneath. New mouthwashing procedures can even clear part of the gum tissue that is still saturated with mercury, radioactive residue and metals.

Summary — Chapter 4

1. We have a dozen common parasites in USA and can learn to recognize them, using photos, and eliminate them.

2. Three parasites cause the beginning of all tumors, which is the tumor nucleus: Strongyloides, Clonorchis, Eurytrema.

3. Allergies to a certain food substance (food phenolic) makes a specific organ inflamed and produce PGE2 (prostaglandin E2).

4. Allergy in all circumstances is due to radioactivity in the organ, nickel in the organ, or continued use of the allergic food.

5. Parasitism increases as immunity decreases.

6. Parasitism increases as radioactivity increases.

7. Only organs that are making PGE2, that is, are allergic to something you are eating get chosen to become cancerous. These organs are full of radioactivity as we already knew from the polonium discovery.

CHAPTER 5

KILLING PARASITES

Individual parasites are very very fragile. Any little change in temperature, or salt concentration, or interruption of their own vitamin supply removes them immediately. In fact, Barlow, the early researcher who had a grant to study Fasciolopsiasis in China in the mid 1920's, could not keep them alive by feeding and culturing them in any way at all. But he did not get done with his research in time for his departure date and he wished to continue his research at home in the USA. He resorted to swallowing them (counting them carefully first) and retrieving them after he arrived home (researchers can be very dedicated to the betterment of society and the search for truth). Then why are they so hard to eradicate? We still do not know their weaknesses and exact requirements. We can see that they carry a tiny chip of radioactivity on themselves; this seems to protect them and to destroy our immunity instead. It can be a chip of free polonium or polonium-bromide or polonium-fluoride or a particle of uranium with polonium attached to it.

Our white blood cells refuse to attack our invaders when tiny radioactive particles are sticking to them. We must remove our radioactivity. We are wallowing in radioactivity besides the immunity destroyers both from laundry bleach. At the same time we are wallowing in pet excretions, domestic animal excretions and our own excretions without even recognizing them! Our food is tainted with all of them. The very name "E. coli" shows us its origin! Chronic infection with intestinal bacteria, such as Salmonella and E. coli, should not be tolerated in an age of running water, splendid plumbing fixtures and the microscope.

Visit a pet shop and a feed store. Notice the shelves are full of medicines for parasites. Notice the refrigerators are full of antibiotics and further medicines for parasites. They are to be given repeatedly, because the situation does not improve for them. Parasitism does not go away without deeper intervention than medicine. Our animals and pets have become immune depressed with us by drinking the same chlorox bleach in their water. Our health and their health are intertwined. We must care for their health in order to care for ours. See *Curing Cancer in Pets* page 487.

As you learn how to regain your immunity, and how to cure your own cancer as well as your family's cancers, you will see what needs to be done for animals and the rest of society.

> To prevent our cancers we must prevent immune depression from radioactivity in our animals besides ourselves. This will prevent parasitism for both of us.

Now your immediate task is to kill your <u>own</u> parasites—and your <u>own</u> bacteria—at the same time as regaining your immunity. The more advanced your cancer is, the more varieties you have. They are contributing to your illness, even if not directly to your cancer. Killing many will not be harder than killing a few, but we will need to be mindful of detox-illness.

The parasites to conquer are:

- Ascaris lumbricoides
- Ascaris megalocephala
- Dirofilaria, dog heartworm
- Malaria
- Fasciola
- Human liver fluke
- Onchocerca
- Pancreatic fluke

- Fasciolopsis buski
- Echinoporyphium recurvatum
- Paragonimus
- Strongyloides
- Macracanthorhynchus
- Acanthocephala

The bacteria to conquer are:
- Clostridium varieties
- Salmonella varieties
- Staphylococcus aureus
- Bacillus cereus
- Streptococcus G, S. pneumoniae, and S. pyogenes
- Shigella varieties
- E. coli

Extra invaders to conquer are:
- yeast, the bread and alcohol-making kind
- prions

The viruses to conquer are:
- Mumps
- MYC (oncovirus)
- RAS (oncovirus)
- JUN (oncovirus)
- FOS (oncovirus)
- SV40 (oncovirus)
- NEU (oncovirus)
- SRC (oncovirus)
- EBV (Epstein Barre virus)
- CMV (Cytomegalovirus)
- Hepatitis B virus
- Hepatitis C virus
- Adenovirus
- Influenza A and B and recently avian variety

Starving Our Parasites

Just as people need vitamins with their food, parasites need quite specific things, too. Monarch butterflies need milkweed plants for their larvae (caterpillars). Other butterflies need cabbage for their larvae. How fortunate it was to discover that Fasciolopsis needs **ONIONS**. They seem to require them. When their ONION stores are digested away with huge amounts of digestive enzymes the larvae leave. In a few days half of the larvae are gone. Strict avoidance of any food with raw onion-like substances that are also in garlic and mustard gets rid of them. A small deposit of **ONION** will still be seen stored inside tumors and at the organ that has the most attraction for **ONION**, which is the medulla (plus 1 pF). This is at the base of the brain, apparently in the crevice between the medulla and base of the cerebellum on the right side. ONIONS seem to have a tropism for the medulla, and F. buski follows. If the ONION stash is at the left side of the medulla, F. buski will be seen there. If it is on the right side, F. buski will be seen there. But health problems come to the opposite side of the body. Cancer in the right breast, right lung or right kidney means F. buski and its ONION stash are at the left side of the medulla. The role of the medulla is not yet clear.

It is most important to starve F. buski, but other parasites can be starved, too.

These are the essential foods for the 3 parasites that start the tumor nucleus:

3 Essential Foods

- for pancreatic fluke – gallic acid and lemons
- for Strongyloides – potatoes
- for human liver fluke – oats

Even viruses have special food requirements that we must eat for them if they are to survive in us. Food oils are required for nearly all so far studied.

The Syncrometer® finds many foods, in fact, parts of every meal, distributed in tiny deposits in cancer patients and even in their urine. Oils in particular are common. They may be essential in the human diet, but it seems the patients were eating much more than could be digested. Certainly, the patient should catch up on digestion of oil before eating more. Going off all food oils, as well as potatoes, lemons, oats, and gallic acid preservative would give us the fastest way to pull these parasite links out of the chain leading to cancer. At the same time our virus infections would be greatly reduced. In the future you will be able to eat small amounts of those that can be completely digested, especially with help from digestive enzymes. These food factors will not be available then, for viruses or parasites to reestablish themselves.

Starving parasites has one huge advantage over killing them directly; you do not get dead parasites that need to be disposed of. In other words, you do not get detoxification-illness. It seems the parasites simply leave.

Starving parasites is surprisingly quick. They seem to know in 2 days that their food supply is dwindling. In less than a week, I have estimated half the parasites are gone. And in 2 weeks they are essentially gone—but not completely. After 2 weeks you could begin to experiment with one small serving per week to see if they return.

How could you know if parasites or viruses had returned? Direct stool observation is the most reliable, using techniques that have been learned by parasitologists over many years (see page 181). Getting a symptom back is the most reliable for viruses. Of course, you should never return to using gallic acid.

Parasites have fought back, over time, by giving each of their larval stages a <u>different</u> essential food. It is much more difficult for people, the hosts, to manage such diets. That is why we must also <u>kill</u> them. Fortunately, for us, fluke metacercaria also require a <u>special</u> <u>trigger</u> to hatch and when these are known we will have yet another way to eliminate them.

After you have starved your parasites for 2 or 3 weeks, their numbers will be far down. Then eating a small serving of one of these foods does not build up their numbers immediately. Keeping to once a week would not let their population grow. This does not include the ONION family. That should be off limits forever. Not only onions, but garlic and mustard should not be considered people-food. They all turn into alkylating agents after you and your buski's digest them. Alkylating agents do not belong in our diet. They are strong mutagens.

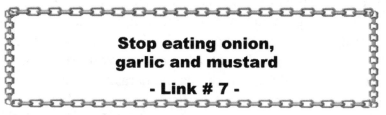

Stop eating onion, garlic and mustard

- Link # 7 -

Preventing parasitism should be the way of the future rather than killing parasites directly. This means we should preserve our immune power. Radioactivity has the greatest immune-lowering impact. We should stop the intrusion of radioactivity into our lives. Radioactive elements and lanthanide elements come up from the earth side by side. We should not settle in those regions that produce these in large quantity. We should measure the background radioactivity in any house we are considering to buy. We should not distribute radioactive elements in the form of fertilizer, home building materials and in the public water supply. It is not too late to turn the human fate around, but first more people must cure themselves of cancer (and other diseases) to understand the real challenge to our existence. Radioactivity and lanthanides must come under our control. We will soon see why.

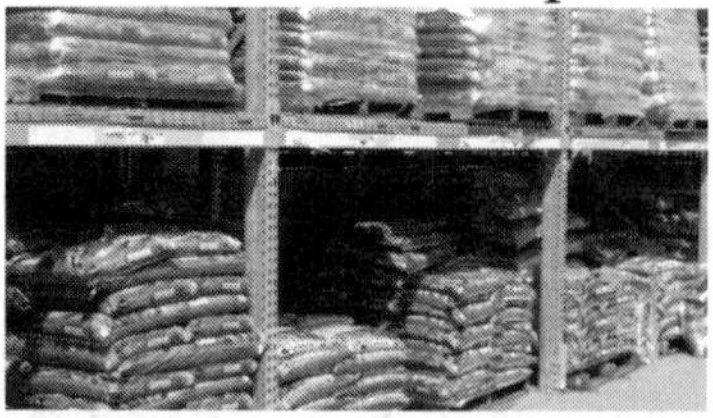

Fig. 39 Test your fertilizer with a Geiger counter in the store

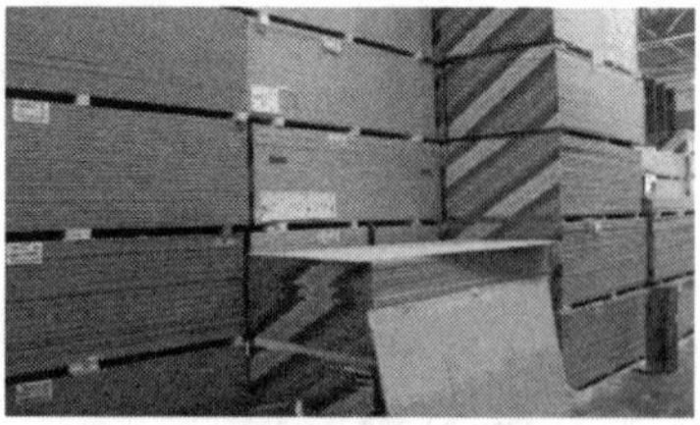

Fig. 40 Test your drywall materials and kitchen counter for radioactivity with a Geiger Mueller counter

Preventing parasitism is already beyond your personal reach. You now need to kill them as fast as you can. But it will do no good if it cannot be lasting. Nobody can do such an intensive parasite-killing program daily. And it will be quite difficult if killing them makes you sicker than not killing them. In other words, you need to get your immunity back and protect yourself from the after effects of killing parasites before you should actually kill them.

Stop eating oats regularly

- Link # 8 -

That is why the *2-Week Program* draws a line between the first part of the program, (taken for 5 or 6 days) and the second part where we actually kill our parasites.

In the first part of the program you will get your immunity back by stopping the contaminated kitchen water, cleaning the contaminated house, and changing food and body products. It is the removal of many things in your lifestyle that will bring back your immune power, not taking boosters or enhancers. We must stand in wonder at the great power of your immune system, the white blood cells (WBCs), swimming alongside your RBCs and platelets in your blood and tissues, like chaperones everywhere, to keep you clean and healthy.

You can get started now, ahead of time, to remove all the attachments ever made to your water system. Or plunk yourself into a different house that doesn't have them and where the water has been tested free of chlorox bleach with a Syncrometer®.

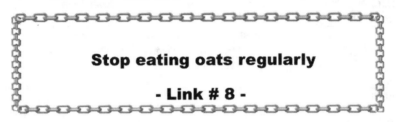

Table Of Parasite Essential Foods

Parasite	Food Required	Killed by
Ascaris lumbricoides, pet roundworm	quercitin (squash & pumpkin, undercooked)	BQ* drops, levamisole, cysteine
Ascaris megalocephala, pet roundworm	D-carnitine (meat of domestic animals, not free-range, organic)	RZ** drops, levamisole, cysteine
Clonorchis sinensis, human liver fluke	oats, cooked or raw	BWT***
Dirofilaria, dog heartworm	lactose (milk sugar) chromium	levamisole
Echinoporyphium recurvatum	Cinnamic acid, hippuric acid, (dairy, eggs), vitamin D3, copper, vanadium	glyoxal in form of homeographic drops; pomegranate (seeds and peel)
Echinostoma revolutum (neurological diseases)	zein, sorghum (CORN), acetaldehyde (nuts)	glyoxylic acid in form of homeographic drops
Eurytrema pancreaticum, pancreatic fluke	LEMON & lauric acid (food oil), gallic acid preservative	BWT
Fasciolopsis buski, human intestinal fluke	raw ONION (allyl sulfide, diallyl sulfide, allyl methyl sulfide, & other ONION-like substances in the lily family)	BWT, 6 fresh seeds, zapping. MSM removes alkylating agents & leftover ONION
Fasciola	WHEAT (gluten, gliadin); metacercaria require lauric acid food oil	
Gastrothylax (causes polycystic kidney disease, Down's Syndrome, cystic fibrosis	Cinnamic acid (cinnamon)	
Macracanthorhynchus	BEEF, BANANA, BUTTER, RICE	removal of gold
Onchocerca, filaria roundworm	CORN, MANNITOL (sugar), linolenic oil, vitamin D3	Decaris (levamisole) vinegar
Paragonimus, lung fluke	LEMON	BWT

* benzoquinone, homeographic copy
** RZ, rhodizonic acid, homeographic copy
*** BWT (green) Black Walnut, Wormwood, Cloves combination

Parasite	Food Required	Killed by
Plasmodium falciparum, vivax, malariae (malaria)	different stages need iron disulfide, wheat, lemon, melanin, plantain, ASA, pyrrole, others	avoidance of benzene and allergens (honey, ASA, limonene) (potatoes in HIV/AIDS)
Strongyloides, roundworm	potatoes, raw or cooked, linolenic acid (food oil)	levamisole
By not eating their required food, you can starve the parasites.		

Fig. 41 Parasites' essential foods

In the first part of the program you will also help your kidneys pour themselves clean many more times a day than before by drinking many herbal teas. We will also use special supporting kidney "drops", but you could use the *Kidney Cleanse* from earlier books instead if you are not advanced. It is an herbal recipe that removes several kidney blocks listed here.

- the methyl malonate block
- the heavy metal block
- the gold block
- the azo dye block
- the asbestos block
- the radioactivity block
- the wheel bearing grease and motor oil block
- the plastic and rubber block

The first 7 blocks came from the chlorox bleach contaminants, but the plastic and rubber comes from many more sources. All the water in existence, all your food, all your clothing and your products are contaminated with rubber and plastic of many kinds. As plastic and rubber replace the whole world's wood and metal we fill up more and more with our gaskets, O-rings, washers and valves. As fabric gets fused with rubber in clothing there is no way of escaping the **cerium** that flows from them. Yet, there are parts of plastic and rubber that cannot be excreted by our bodies. Eventually, they form a blockage of the kidneys. Black, white and green rubber, as well as plastic, fills our kidneys, coming from the hoses and pipes that transport our processed food, dairy products, and even bread. That is why, in our *2-Week Program*, we switch to well water, pumped ourselves, and bake our own bread with a bread machine. Our own choices can easily be tested with a Syncrometer® and changed if they do seep. We do not need to be perfect—only successful in unblocking our kidneys so swellings disappear, effusions stay away and health returns. It is miraculous that herbs exist able to do such technical tasks, and that they were already known to help kidneys thousands of years ago.

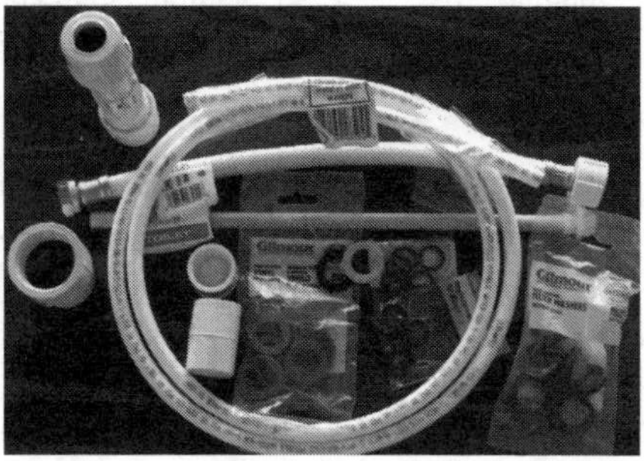

Avoid flexible hose and all rubber

Fig. 42 Hose and plumbing parts block our kidneys

Also in the first part of the program we will use 3 supplements that feed your immune system. All the "immune boosters" in the marketplace cannot substitute for these. WBCs need organic selenium to remove automotive grease and motor oil, among others. They need organic germanium to remove chlorinated chemicals like bleach, even the "good" variety. Chlorine does not belong in the living body and must be constantly removed. Your body considers it so important that chlorine is even excreted in the night. Our WBCs also need organic vitamin C for many tasks, but mainly to remove radioactivity in some mysterious way.

The Organic Part Of Vitamin C

In nature, vitamin C comes with 2 partners, **rutin** and **hesperidin**. It is these that tackle radioactivity. To get the help of manufactured vitamin C, you should add these organic parts. They are also needed for malonic acid detoxification.

Currants and even raisins have them, but do not heat them nor add liquid. Just freeze and eat.

There are, of course, synthetically made germanium, selenium and more vitamin C varieties. They would certainly help if they could be found without chlorox disinfectant or heavy metal contamination or their own radioactivity. But all these are regularly used in their manufacture. All supplements require disinfection, and although these may be very "pure", the bleach always remains as a residue. Even "good" NSF bleach has radioactivity, precisely the item we are trying to remove. Search for varieties that have no chlorine disinfectant at all.

Radioactivity keeps tumors growing.

This makes it inefficient to use synthetic vitamin C when it has been chlorinated. It adds to the radioactivity burden. Fairly often a supplement can be found that has a different disinfectant, not chlorine.

From the very first day that you start to feed your WBCs with their 3 supplements, you can see them getting to work. Truckload after truckload of toxins gets taken to the kidney WBCs, without getting stuck in the kidneys themselves. Soon you will be able to detoxify your whole body without clogging your kidneys or liver. You can understand why helping the kidneys is in the first part of the cure. From here all the toxins go to the bladder…and out. It will be important not to get the parts of the program reversed. The order is important to prevent ankle swelling, loading the liver with toxins, or even sending them to your lymph nodes so they must enlarge. All mistakes are fixable, but you should be in charge yourself to help prevent them. If you must slow down at any point, stop killing parasites until you have caught up again with feeding your WBCs.

Taking protective supplements comes next. Why do you need protection?

It is because your WBCs are suddenly able to work again and your body often decides on its own to kill parasites instead of only removing toxins. That will bring detox-illness because dead parasites release bacteria.

We must hurry to prepare properly for killing parasites so you can avoid detox-illness.

Detoxification-Illness

As soon as you kill an F. buski fluke the common Flu virus and several varieties of Salmonella bacteria jump away…and into you! Before killing a fluke the Syncrometer® can not hear any Salmonella frequency emissions. Immediately after killing buski's, within minutes, one or more varieties of Salmonella can be heard, at exactly the same place where the fluke was but no longer is. And soon after this, Flu viruses appear at the same spot. The F. buski flukes, although quietly causing your cancer, were not making you feel physically unwell. But Flu viruses and Salmonella bacteria do make you feel unwell, very unwell if you don't have remedies. This explains how you can feel sicker from killing the parasites than leaving them be. We must expect and prevent as much Flu and Salmonella illness as possible.

Detox-syndrome, or detox-symptoms have been known a very long time. Sometimes it was given a special name and sometimes it was given a moralistic interpretation like "No pain, no gain" and "It has to get worse before it gets better". But the Syncrometer® could see what it really was, merely escapees from newly killed parasites. In fact, the same escapees always come from particular parasites. Flu and Salmonella always come from F. buski. Salmonella alone, a different variety, comes from killing Fasciola. A particular Clostridium comes from killing the human liver fluke. And the common cold, Adenovirus, jumps out of Ascaris larvae when they are killed. This subject needs much more study…the more so, because detox-symptoms are the real deterrent to killing parasites on a large scale in our pets and animal friends besides ourselves.

Most extremely ill patients, just arrived from a hospital or from hospice care, have Flu and Salmonella at high levels already! Clostridium, mumps and even measles are roaming and active. They and everyone around them believe the patients are dying from cancer. I see no attempt being made to identify and treat these infections. They are, after all, only infections! and should be treatable. In this program we will treat all such infections very vigorously until they are gone.

It is obvious that the clinical care the patients received is helping…helping enough to empower the body to begin killing its own parasites again. But it is not enough for survival without stopping the chlorox-water and removing the cancer-complex.

Surely, it should never be said that you died of Flu and Salmonellas! It is like giving in to a mouse when it runs into your kitchen, by running away and screaming instead of acting. Mice are certainly not to be tolerated, and yet to be expected, repeatedly. All your symptoms of illness are due to "everyday pathogens" like E. coli, Salmonella, and Flu. The more fierce ones are Streptococcus G, bread yeast, Shigella and malaria (a subclinical type). The stealthy ones are Clostridium, and Staphylococcus aureus. Streptococcus pneumoniae announces itself with pain…the only one. The viruses seem stealthy too, not knowing just what symptom they cause. Chronic mumps and measles must certainly be attacking you somewhere if they are active. Half a dozen oncoviruses, including EBV, CMV and Adenovirus must be doing some harm when they get systemically activated, even though they are acting differently in the chronic state than the acute state. But they can all be conquered in days.

It is understandable that you can feel very very ill, with nausea instead of appetite, weight loss when you are eating to fullness, bloating, headache, insomnia, a feeling of weakness besides fatigue, and sometimes diarrhea or vomiting and even fever from everyday bacteria. You could certainly die from so many untreated infections.

Dr. William Koch, an early cancer therapist, developed benzoquinone, rhodizonic acid, and several more "oxidizers" that he gave in a mixture by shot. A single shot cured his patients. His books are full of notarized accounts and photos used at his court trial, showing patients years later, after their "single shot". His theory was that he had oxidized bacterial toxins. We should review his treatment. His patients also became immune to cancer, later.

How could you have so many infections without your doctor noticing it? Certainly the clinical method was never meant to "notice" many things. It was meant to astutely suspect just a few possibilities. In fact the deepest lesson a bacteriology student learned was that there may be many pathogens (bacteria or viruses) present, but the clinical task is to find which one is responsible for your illness. And you do this by discreet culturing. Finding the major one this way would surely not benefit you much now, though. You need to kill them all as fast and decisively as you can. That is why we will use herbs. This will not give you more detox symptoms. It will give you less.

There is another possible explanation why doctors at the most prestigious hospitals have not found your half-dozen infections. Maybe pathogens that could be easily cultured in a non-cancer patient cannot be identified in a cancer patient when so many others are sharing the culture broth. The Syncrometer® does see that each of these pathogens is radioactive, having polonium, radon and its daughters, besides lanthanides attached to themselves. Until there is enough vitamin C, germanium and selenium to remove the radioactivity from these common pathogens, they might not be recognizable.

The Gold Intruder

The recent discovery of a new kind of very virulent Flu is another example. The Syncrometer® finds gold is attached to each virus. This could make it unrecognizable to your immune system. It can multiply unchallenged. The Syncrometer® has found gold attached to Staph aureus in breast cancer and to Strep pneumonia in excruciating pain. The search is on for more gold mutants.

Certainly research is needed to answer the profound question: "Why are cancer-bacteria not identified clinically?"

If all your common pathogens could actually be found clinically, your clinical treatment would be one antibiotic or similar drug for <u>each</u> pathogen. There would be quite a few side-effects. It is very fortunate that we still have some, although very little, herbs to try instead.

Herbal Secrets

Herbalists of ancient times did not know which "bug" they were fighting. "Bugs" were not even discovered then. But they knew which symptoms they were fighting. They had to deal with mixtures just as we have them now. They knew their mixtures (syndromes) quite well, although names and terms interfered with accurate interpretation, at that time, just as now. As few as possible concepts were used to classify many problems, such as "too acidic, too alkaline, too scant, too plentiful, too active, too inactive, too wet, too dry. Helpful it was but mostly for the therapist, so all treatments could be turned into simple protocols.

To cure all your symptoms together, without a need to culture or identify them we will take advantage of the ancient herbalists' knowledge. For this, we should not be too attached to our clinical concepts or even to names of pathogens or symptoms.

We will be able to kill most of your pathogens and a dozen symptoms with our powerful collection of herbs called *Protective Herbs and Teas*. Only using them together will they have so many overlapping actions as to be able to kill so many bacteria and viruses, and even unknown ones.

The protective tea recipe is to be taken both preventively and curatively. The concept is not clinical. But it is biologically correct. If a little bit, such as a cup of tea, can kill a few bacteria or viruses, we should do it promptly because it will prevent a buildup with worsening of symptoms. Clinically we do the opposite. We wait till the symptoms are bad enough to outweigh the harm done from a drug that treats it. By then it will be needed a longer time and in larger (maximum) doses to be effective. If it is no longer effective, due to delay, you have lost valuable time while the condition gets worse. Drugs nevertheless have their place and are very important to us.

And not everyone can turn to herbal remedies; in fact the earth would soon be denuded of them. We would consume them the way we have consumed the forests and the woolly mammoth.

I would suggest growing these in our gardens, domesticating them to preserve them, and not fertilizing or hybridizing or extracting them.

They must, of course, be sanitized before use. I find the best method is freezing the dried or encapsulated herb at -20° F or colder for 24 hours or longer. This must be exact. Other details are with the program.

> Herbs should be tested for chlorox bleach, disinfected by freezing correctly, and tested again for Salmonella and E. coli.

There is no need to wait any longer to start the curing program. If you have the proper freezer, tested with a thermometer, a stainless steel saucepan, the protective herbs or teas, and the WBC supplements and *Kidney Cleanse* or drop set, you can start.

Do <u>not</u> start if your water is not yet changed. If you do start prematurely you will be putting a lot more polonium and ferrocyanide-containing water into your body than before, from drinking much more. This is harmful. Also, do not start unless the herbs have been tested for chlorox.

If your hot water heater is not contaminated, remove all filters and softeners and run 3 tankfuls of very hot water (30 gallons each time) through your pipes, both hot and cold. It will be a huge improvement and you could send your new cold kitchen water to be tested by a Syncrometer® tester.

Remember to find dishwashing liquid and laundry detergent of a safe kind besides NSF bleach before cleaning up the house. It would be good to get help for this. If your family is casual about supporting your new needs, find a friend who would take you seriously. It is a very demanding discipline. But be kind. These are new concepts and can even be difficult for a scientist to give attention to or a professional person who has never encountered them.

It is also a good idea to fill 1 or 2 pages with symptoms for yourself before starting. It will help you keep perspective as well as tracking progress.

When you do start and you feel disoriented or slightly woozy, you will be experiencing your first detox symptom. It means the program is already working for you! It is an occasion for joy. You will certainly succeed if you do it <u>all</u>. Doing it all means these 4 things:

- getting the ferrocyanide out of your body
- getting the ONION-GARLIC-MUSTARD oils out of your body
- killing Fasciolopsis buski because it makes ONION-GARLIC-MUSTARD compounds and links its own metabolism (reducing power) to your DNA
- getting the polonium and uranium out of your teeth

After killing some invaders, starving some, creating metal deficiencies for some and blocking the reproductive cycle for others you have made a powerful start.

In 2 weeks all your invaders can be reduced so much, you feel decidedly better, your cancer crisis could be over, and your tumors visibly shrinking.

We will use some of the best herbs known to kill flu viruses and cold "bugs", besides Clostridium and E. coli.

We will take the best homeopathic medicine for Flu, besides, although it does not combat Avian flu. Some of the herbs can kill Avian flu, though.

Our best help for Salmonella comes from Lugol's iodine…just 6 drops…for action within one hour.

When you take all these <u>ahead of time</u> it is powerful <u>protection</u>. But if you think the discipline will be too much for you, ask a friend to be your police-person while you promise to take everything handed to you without a word or stall. You will need this powerful protection most when you are most successful at killing parasites! It will be gratifying to see that the Syncrometer® finds you full of Flu and Salmonella, evidence for "buski" killing, but not feeling one bit sick.

Clostridium Illness

As soon as you have killed a Fasciolopsis parasite, one nearby family of bacteria takes notice; they are the dead flesh eaters, Clostridium varieties. Their poisonous products can even be seen on your blood test; they give you a low uric acid level. If you see that, act quickly. Oregano oil and pomegranate seeds (freshly ground) are swift and sure (see *Sources*).

There is a silver lining to sudden Clostridium invasion. You must have killed a buski. You have at least one wherever there is a malignancy.* Each one killed removes a cancer-complex and its malignancy. Washing away the pieces of the complex is all that is needed to let the whole tumor get carried away by the WBCs. Clostridium does not make you feel sick so it does not warn you that their deadly toxins are forming. Because you can't feel the Clostridium attack, it is not considered part of detox-illness, but it is even more important. Be sure to protect yourself from Clostridium attacks even though they bring "good news".

Starved WBCs

Cancer patients' WBCs have been so busy fighting off the long list of chlorox bleach toxins that they have

* Testers, when you search for the OPT locations, list them carefully. Next day, if you find OPT missing you should find Clostridium *Positive*. This can be used to verify that a buski-parasite got killed. Clostridium will only be there a day or so, if the protective herbs are being taken.

depleted all their own "vitamins and minerals". They need 3 essential supplements:

- organic germanium
- organic selenium
- organic vitamin C

All cancer patients have starved WBCs.

These are the most important supplements of the whole program.

A teaspoon of hydrangea root or raw nuts or safe peanut butter supplies the organic germanium; an equivalent supplement would need to be huge and expensive.

A large Brazil nut, freshly cracked, has 50 mcg of organic selenium, but seems to replace a much larger dose of pure sodium selenite.

A teaspoon of coarsely ground rose hips, seeds included, supplies the vitamin C power of about 2000 mg. But often this is not enough and we will be tempted to add synthetic vitamin C. It is a dilemma because nearly all synthetic vitamin C has radioactivity from its chlorine disinfectant that gives it "food grade" status. Search for unchlorinated vitamin C.

Add currants to your diet, 1 tsp. 3 times daily. Now you can take up to 10 grams of synthetic vitamin C and hope to use it all for uranium and polonium removal. But the organic components are extremely fragile. They must not stand in water or be heated. Eat them out of hand, after freezing.

If you prepare and grind supplements yourself you must promptly eat them, or promptly encapsulate and freeze them. They must only be coarsely ground to avoid putting chromium and nickel into them from the grinder as the blades get hotter.

Nuts must be tested for laundry bleach even if they are in the shell. Pecans, in particular, let the chlorox penetrate.

And before you allow yourself fresh nuts, which could supply both germanium and selenium, you must ask yourself: Do I have a chronic cough or a cold I cannot get rid of?

If you do, nuts are not for you, yet.

A quick check of the table on page 233 (*Parasites Bring Oncoviruses*) shows you that most viruses require the exquisite unsaturated oils from plants, such as nuts, to reproduce themselves. It is best to wait till no evidence of viruses is in you, and even then, be watchful.

As soon as your WBCs are fed, within 10 seconds, they are at work eating your Flu and Salmonella. They will have used up their supplements soon and need more.

Just feeding your white blood cells starts the body killing its parasites automatically. This is especially true in children. Often their colds are really a detox-symptom from killing Ascaris.

In the first week of the program we have changed the water and the diet. We have fed the WBCs and taken half a dozen teas to protect you from detox-symptoms and to cure you from half a dozen simple infections. We still need to "open", that is, unblock the kidneys, so they can bring everything the WBCs will pick up for you to the bladder.

After this we can kill parasites in earnest, in 4 ways: with herbs, by zapping, with homeography, and by starving them. Dogs, elephants, birds, and whales use multiple approaches, too. They bite them, lick, scratch, attract helpers like birds and fish, throw dust, go swimming, and eat specific plants. Every bit helps them, like us.

The Herbal Way

How to make your own green Black Walnut Hull tincture was described in earlier books. It is best to make it yourself because you understand the water pollution problem better than others. Use the recipe on page 581. Be sure you are not using chlorox-contaminated water. Rainwater would give you certainty.

The Black Walnut Hull way of killing parasites includes 3 herbs:

1. The green hull of the Black Walnut extracted in ethyl alcohol

2. Freshly ground cloves (each capsule with 400-500 mg. cloves) in capsules or ¼ cup in bulk. Store bought sources do not work. Immediate encapsulation after grinding does keep it potent. Beware of nickel, chromium, and vanadium from grinding; test them.

3. Wormwood, encapsulated (each capsule with 200-300 mg. of wormwood), or ½ cup of Artemisia leaves gathered from the shrub.

These herbs must be taken together as a single treatment within ½ hour (preferably within 5 minutes). But they should not be extracted and premixed because they interact with each other to destroy their potency. Even extraction is damaging.

The 3 herbs kill different stages; cloves kill eggs, wormwood kills cercaria and the tincture kills adults. But they don't all reach every place in the body. That is why repetition is necessary.

It is only the green hull that has this amazing parasite-killing power. A few days after opening a bottle it may already be much darker and less potent. Use the one-serving (1 or 2 oz.) bottle to maximize potency and results. Store in freezer before and after opening.

Beginner's methods, using only drops of green Black Walnut Hull tincture, are described in earlier books. You may use those if you are just preventing cancer or have very early cancer. In an extremely advanced case, almost terminal, where every hour of every day is precious, we will use one whole bottle in a single dose or as much as you can take comfortably. Always check beforehand or some days earlier what 1 tsp. of green Black Walnut Hull tincture would do, if anything, to give you some discomfort. If only the taste is objectionable, search for solutions. Add an equal amount, approximately, of heavy whipping cream, syrup, or a juice. Then sit down to wear off the alcohol. Do not drive a vehicle or do anything complicated for a while. Take niacinamide (1 capsule, 500 mg), too, if available, to help the liver detoxify the alcohol.

In spite of this large dose, you can easily miss one or two adults attached to the esophagus or stomach or bladder. You will routinely miss those that are being protected by the polonium coming from your tooth fillings. These must wait for dental work that removes polonium.

The Six Fresh Seeds Way

…was mentioned in earlier books, but not till now was its full potential known.

Only 3 seeds, pounded to shreds and given as a suppository for 3 nights kill one tumor, namely, the F. buski parasites responsible for one. This will remove the source of alkylating oils and the living connection to your DNA provided by the live buski. This takes less than a day. Another 3 seeds, taken by mouth, treats the upper half of the body, especially in brain and mouth cancer. But the upper and lower treatments should be done together so there are few escapees.

In fact, the two herbal methods, Black Walnut Hull and apricot could be done together to reduce the time still further, only being aware of the need for more protection from detox-illness first.

When you can clear 2 liver cancers in less than a week and then move on to other cancers at the same speed, I believe you have the best method so far developed (except Dr. Koch's on page 580.), including all the clinical methods known. In fact, you could have yourself cured by the time the 2 week wait for the clinical appointment is up.

But it is neither a gift nor a miracle. You must tend to every detail required without making loopholes. You will not have removed polonium-containing teeth. You will not know how many more tumors you have, oncologist's numbers are far short. Taking shortcuts will plunge you into risk, the very opposite of the certainty you want for your life. Over compliance is much better advice.

There are, no doubt, other herbs besides these that can cure a cancer quickly. Many have been known in the past. But they became overexploited, or were given the wrong commercial treatments, so they are no longer used. I see our herbal treasures eroding with passing time. There are those who would prefer to make extracts and concentrates from them adding manufacturers' pollution to every tablet or capsule. There are those who would like to frighten us that they have great toxicity. Always use a recipe till you have found your confidence. And use your plain intelligence before accepting advice from authorities all around you who have something to gain by it.

There are those who believe herbs have insignificant effectiveness. That is correct if they are not well matched to the problem or have aged.

Using 4 or 5 herbs together is more likely to produce a perfect match for your problem. I would rather use a set of

6 herbs, taking 1 dose of each 3 times a day for 2 days than take a drug at the prescribed level for the usual long period of time.

But I am concerned about overusing our herbal treasure as more people see the wisdom of turning to it for our most common ailments. I am concerned about radioactive fertilizer to be used on domestic fields of herbs. We must learn to cultivate our own as our great-grandparents did. The two most important ones, Black Walnut Hull and apricot trees can be grown by anyone. We must grow our own sheep sorrel, eucalyptus trees, wormwood, Ginkgo tree, rhubarb, currants, and red raspberries. We should learn to use the "weeds" of our own neighborhood, grown safely, instead of imported herbs when possible. Again, we should grow our own to avoid pesticide and test for radioactivity yourself before using.

Exact amounts of the Black Walnut Hull tincture, wormwood, and other herbs that we will use are given in the *2-Week Program*. Try to make them pleasant. You have nothing to lose but illness and this should be enjoyable.

Killing Roundworms

We have been focused on killing the intestinal fluke and this will include most other flukes. For roundworms like Ascaris, Strongyloides and filaria we use a common medicine, levamisole. This has the advantage of also clearing the ferritin off WBCs caused by asbestos. Ferritin coats the outer membranes of the WBCs of cancer patients. Levamisole cannot kill our roundworms completely, so we will also starve them.

Tapeworms

We all have tapeworms if we owned a dog or cat. In fact, the house dust at any spot has dog and cat tapeworm eggs. These tapes may only be 2 or 3 inches long but can do incredible harm to babies in the crawling stage. **As this book went to print**, a breakthrough on killing tapeworm safely arrived. It will be possible to kill all our tapeworms with culinary herbs. They do not seem to return, suggesting the scolex (head) was removed. But more research is needed to make failsafe recipes even for babies. It will astound us all to see "the grey tape pudding" in a diaper or toilet bowl.

Summary — Chapter 5

1. There is a limited list of parasites, bacteria, and viruses to get rid of, besides prions and yeast spores.

2. Parasites have a requirement of their own for food factors they get from the food we eat. It is surprisingly simple and quick to starve them and drive them away, instead of killing them. This produces no detox-symptoms.

3. Cancer patients have blocked kidneys in at least 7 ways. Unblocking these specifically lets the whole body detoxify itself.

4. The most important part of this program is feeding the WBCs organic germanium, selenium and vitamin C.

5. Detoxification illness should be prevented before starting actual parasite-killing.

6. The major goals of the program are to remove ferrocyanide, ONION, GARLIC, and MUSTARD oils, polonium, cerium and uranium from your body, as well as killing Fasciolopsis.

CHAPTER 6

ZAPPING PARASITES

Many variations in zapping technique have been discovered since the first one found around 1990.

The original technique showed that very small animals, like our parasites, could be killed with a very small voltage. But only IF the voltage is 100% *Positive offset* and only IF the voltage is varied up and down repeatedly.

If the varying voltage becomes *NEGATIVE*, even momentarily, it supports and maintains their lives! This must be avoided. You cannot take this for granted when you purchase a zapper. The maker must assure you that it has been checked on an oscilloscope and not even the briefest spike of *Negative* voltage found. Preferably a picture of the zapper output on an oscilloscope should accompany the device together with an arrow pointing to the zero line. If the circuit parts used are exactly as given on page 520, there will be no mistake.

If the voltage is applied in pulses, to produce a "square" wave, it will affect many parasites at once so that the rate of pulsing, called frequency, is not critical. Even though these tiny animals undoubtedly have a "mortal frequency" (a frequency that kills), this rate does not need to be known or used when a square wave of electricity, **totally *Positive***, is used.

A *Positive* electrical force that pulses up and down not only appears to kill tiny invaders; it also seems to energize your white blood cells to go on an all-out attack on your enemies: your parasites, your toxins, your bacteria, everything, in spite of their immunity blockers. In spite of benzene, PCBs, metals, dyes, and asbestos! For a time, your WBCs turn into Super-WBCs. That is why I recommend eight hours of zapping daily until you are well. Using your feet makes this possible.

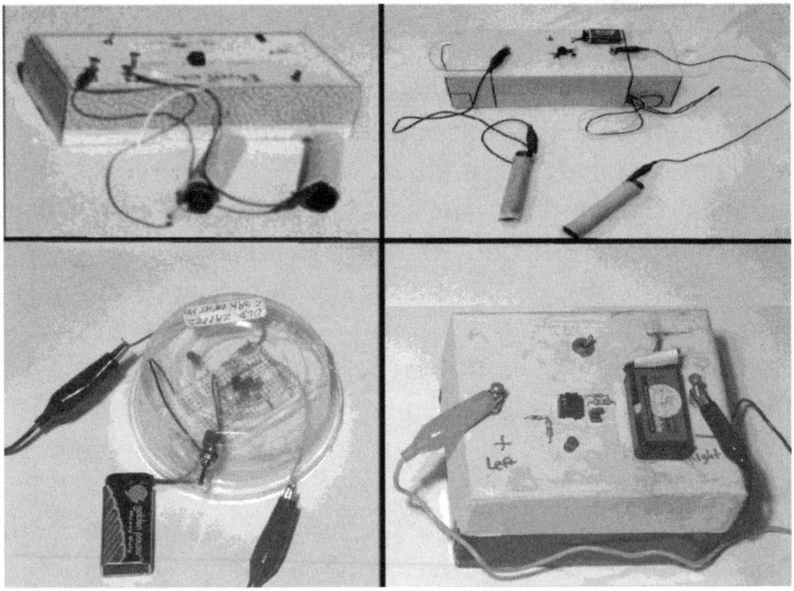

Fig. 43 Homemade zappers

Remember that killing parasites, as we can do with herbs, removes the source of OPT, and oncoviruses, but this does not return immune power. Only removing the immune destroyers does that. A zapper, on the other hand, not only destroys parasites; it does so by turning on immune power, at least temporarily. Each method has its advantages.

With this knowledge you may build or purchase a zapper. It is energized by a 9-volt battery. This is too small a voltage to harm you, or even to feel, although some people can feel a weak tingling sensation. Most of the current is flowing through the blood in your arteries and veins, but a fraction of it reaches every organ in your body. Except when this organ is saturated with a liquid *insulator*! Insulators do not let current pass.

Cancer victims are particularly full of insulators because they have been drinking and cooking with water that is polluted with PCBs, benzene, motor oil, and wheel bearing grease. These are insulators. They accumulate in the thin layer of fat just under the skin and surrounding internal organs. They do not let the current pass through the skin or into an organ easily.

PLATE-ZAPPING

Automotive Oils And Grease

Cancer patients are full of automotive oils and greases. They are in the bleach that is added to the water. Filtering the water does not remove them anymore after 1 week of use. I believe (this is only a theory) the oils coat the activated carbon particles to make them slick and not adsorptive. I believe that a new kind of zapping, called plate-zapping can overcome the obstacle of grease insulation. Any sample organ placed on the plate will be in resonance with the same organ in your body, giving you a higher voltage and current at that organ. For instance, by placing a sample of liver on a 3½ inch square aluminum plate in the

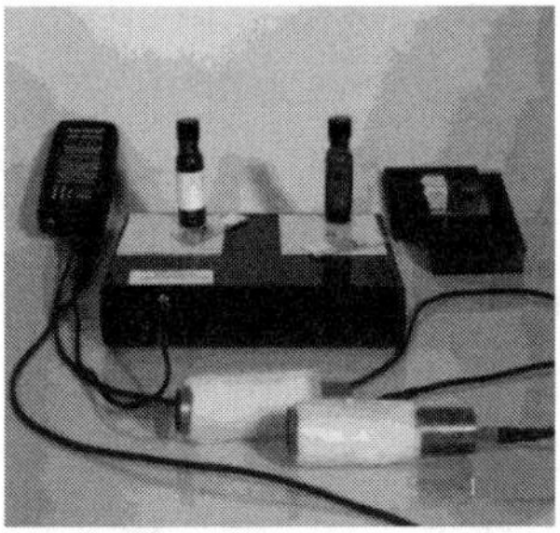

The location to be zapped is on the plate. Bottles or microscope slides can represent them. Escaping tiny pathogens can be placed here, too.

Fig. 44 Plate-zapper

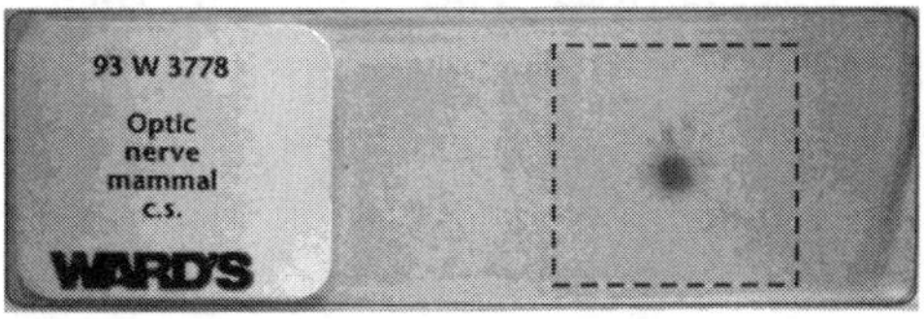

Fig. 45 Microscope slide with real tissue under glass square

path of the zapper current, the two similar organs (your liver and the liver sample on the plate) will be in resonance. I think this maximizes the current through your liver. The liver sample you put on the plate can be in the form of a microscope slide, meant for study by biology students. Microscope slides can be purchased from biological supply companies (see *Sources*) and are safe to handle.

Bottled Alternative

Instead of an actual sample of an organ, like on a microscope slide, it is possible to use a virtual copy. A virtual copy is a sample of water that has the frequency pattern of an organ in it. This bottle of "patterned" water can act like the slide or real sample and has the advantage of convenience and availability. The zapper circuit uses the frequency pattern in the bottle-copy to find an identical one in your body. Whether you use a slide, bottle-copy or a piece of real tissue does not matter; it provides the location where you want to maximize the zapper effect.

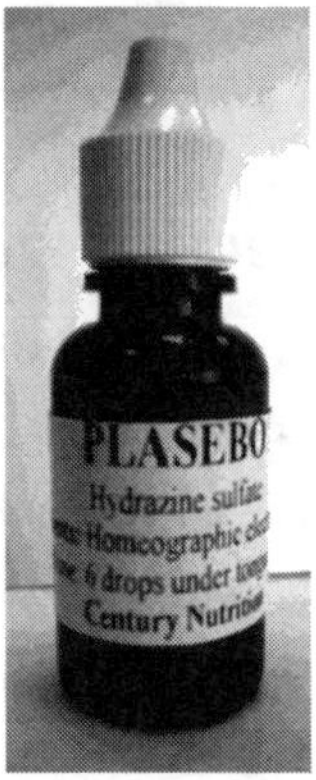

The frequency pattern of any item can be copied into water.

Fig. 46 Bottle-copy replaces the real item

Bottle-copies are easily made from slides or real organs, even by a totally inexperienced person, using a regular zapper (30 kHz or more) see page 189. Extra details are given in Experiment #96 in the *Syncrometer® Science Laboratory Manual* (see Parts Kit #96 in *Sources*) by this author.

White Blood Cells Respond…

With the sample of liver placed in the pathway between you and your zapper, the current has an instant effect on the white blood cells of your liver. Immediately they are energized and begin to eat the PCBs, the benzene, the heavy metals, the dyes, and the malonic acid in your liver. They even eat wheel bearing grease!

Like a fairy godmother that has waved her wand, all toxins are quickly taken out of the liver tissue and imprisoned in the liver white blood cells. They have eaten, although they could not earlier. If they have been fed themselves, they can unload all this into the urine. Then they continue to eat toxins without zapper help until they run out of food: germanium, selenium, and vitamin C. Hundreds of toxins, heavy metals, fungus spores, mycotoxins, all are eaten in one big frenzy.

However, it can all come to a screeching halt if the voltage of the battery has dropped below 9.0 volts. To do this superb job the battery must not run below 9.0 before the job is done. And it takes 20 minutes, not just seven as it does for regular zapping. Only the locations placed on the plates are zapped by this method, not the whole body as for regular zapping.

…But Only If Fed

What will happen to the gorged white blood cells after they have "eaten" all this toxic waste? Will they unload their super toxic cargo in the proper place (bladder)? It all depends again on being fed! Only <u>selenite</u>, <u>organic germanium</u> and <u>vitamin C</u> are useful. These three enable the white blood cells to transfer their toxic load to the kidneys' WBCs, and then to the bladder and from there to appear in the urine. A Syncrometer® urine test will now be *Positive* for PCBs, asbestos, lanthanide metals, nickel, mercury and all the others identified before, even Fast Garnet, and Fast Green dyes.

If there is not enough of any one of these three supplements, the white blood cells simply stop; they wait as at a dock, for a day or so, then some of the toxic cargo escapes to the kidney itself, clogging it, changing its polarization to south, and stopping its ability to put toxins into the urine. You are back at the beginning now. The toxins escaped and will have to be "eaten" again. Much time is lost this way. These supplements are top priority.

Throughout the day, the organ with a tumor should be plate-zapped in various ways: combined with arteries, combined with veins, combined with white blood cells, each for 20 minutes. These zaps are followed with zaps to clear blood, lymph and the white blood cells themselves. Or these zaps are done at the same time if you are using a double plate-zapper. And, of course, the kidneys are zapped or given special homeographic drops to keep them from clogging repeatedly with heavy metals and industrial greases. Twenty-minute zaps can be kept up for eight hours or more this way.

A miracle has been done for you in one day. The battle for your sick organ has been won. Continue protecting and helping the kidney white blood cells. Be patient with the after-effects due to dead parasites. Be sure to take your protective herbs.

What happens to the dead carcasses of large flukes lying about like dead rats? They will soon be enveloped in mold. Watch what happens to a tiny dead fish at the bottom of an aquarium at a pet store. Within a day fine fuzz appears all over the surface, like velvet. In a few days, if it is not scooped out, a halo appears around the dead fish. Fungus has taken over the entire fish and is now going through its own stages of development, glistening under the aquarium light. The owner will scoop it out.

Who will scoop up the dead flukes in your organs? If you had zapped flukes in the intestinal tract or liver or pancreas, they could have been pushed out through their ducts into the intestine and finally into the toilet. But most organs have no such ducts; dead parasites will have to rot on the spot. They will be fought over by scavenger Clostridium bacteria and its competitors, **Aspergillus** fungus and yeast. Clostridium will produce isopropyl alcohol, DNA, and DNA polymerase. Aspergillus will produce **aflatoxin**. Even if it has to share the carcass with **Penicillium** mold, it does not help; they both produce aflatoxin. The aflatoxins are very sinister **mycotoxins** (fungal toxins). They precede all **jaundice**. A much better solution is to digest the dead flukes before these scavengers get them.

Fifteen capsules (about five or six grams) of mixed enzyme powders can digest the dead matter coming from four hours of zapping. Eight hours require two such doses. More is better.

In advanced cancer nothing less than eight hours of zapping daily can catch up and exceed the rate of spread of disease. Zap eight hours daily until you are well. There are reports from victims who zapped without stopping for a whole month; symptoms came and went while they cleaned up their environment and suddenly the disease was gone.

The Flu Again

You will keep getting Flu and Salmonella attacks throughout your parasite-killing efforts, if you are successful! Remind yourself immediately to catch up with detox-protection even though it is too late. It is a time for your helper to insist that you treat yourself instead of doing nothing about them. As the Flu and Salmonella sweep through you they will enter your tumors, lesions, lymph nodes, making them all look and feel worse, and any scan will look denser. If you awaken to see the ceiling rotate and find it necessary to hug the walls as you search for the bathroom but your mood is just fine, it is the **prion** part of detox-illness. If your caregiver would quickly make a cup of birch bark tea and give you Reishi mushroom, you would soon be "set right" again.

Prions are associated with gold. Remove all gold metal if you had forgotten, that very day. Remove crowns and inlays, rings and necklaces. Stop eating out of glass or Teflon dishes. Stop eating store bought bread, beef, and honey. They all have gold. Then wait till the gold is out of your teeth before continuing to kill parasites.

If, instead, you begin to shiver, ache all over, cough and feel a sore throat, it is the Flu, with or without Adenovirus, the common cold. You immediately know you killed a "buski" and an Ascaris. F. buski presented you with the Flu, and Ascaris gave you the cold. You must stay warm in bed and drink Boneset tea, Eucalyptus tea and small sips of the other teas throughout the day. These can have you feeling fine again in hours. Also take a dose of Oscillococcinum at bedtime, homeopathic medicine for Flu, to feel normal next day.

But if you get a fever, nausea and diarrhea, you have mainly Salmonellas. These can be terminated with 6 doses of Lugol's, 6 drops each in ½ cup water (or 10 drops if you are using diluted Lugol's, (as in Veggie Wash), and Burdock tea. Salmonellas use gold, as did the prions. Killing Salmonellas releases the gold they have been using. Then prions can snatch it. Without gold in your body, you could not get Salmonella illness, nor prions!

We will use homeographic drops to remove gold from your organs after it has been removed from your dentalware.

Prions

It is not known yet where prions really come from. My preliminary evidence is that the cells set free by the hypothalamus turn into prions. Prions appear to be the companion-pathogen of Macracanthorhynchus. This parasite uses gold too. Prions are always ready to snatch gold away from "Macra". Prions are forced to share this gold with some Salmonella types, the new Avian flu, SV40, HIV and most recently, Staph aureus and Strep pneumonia! Prions should always be taken seriously. They stop nerve function by simply blocking them. Then no neurotransmitters can travel along them. They can lead to dementia. Early symptoms are breathing and swallowing problems.

If you can't test to identify these detox "bugs" yourself, you must treat yourself for all of them…or miss several days of cancer-curing till you are back to normal again. This time resolve to take all your teas (or capsules) and if you forget to take your protective supplements again, this time you might be able to smile as you feel ill, while gloating over your "real" evidence of progress: detox-illness…you did reach and kill some F. buski's!

But if you get quite ill and lose weight over it, ask your caregiver to take over the responsibility of preventing detox symptoms while you agree to dutifully sip, swallow or take whatever is put before you.

Your cancer does not get worse from a bout of detox-illness. But it appears that way and it is rather demoralizing to add new symptoms. Losing weight, though, is serious. Make a special effort to eat all your food and gain it back. If you cannot gain it back, switch to blended food that you can drink so all food is consumed at each meal.

It is important to know that if you develop <u>any</u> after effect from zapping, however small or large, we have always found it to be due to Flu, Salmonella and occasionally Prions, not a worsening of the cancer, or anything harmful. For some persons, weeping plays a role in detox-illness, too. This is caused by a special Clostridium variety, C. botulinum. It appears after killing human liver flukes. If you kill very many, the C. botulinum "undertaker" bacteria can reach the hypothalamus, so weeping starts. If you are a "weeper", be sure to take drops of oregano oil (in capsules) and to drink Eucalyptus and Birch bark tea, kill all Clostridium daily to stay cheerful while you zap and starve the flukes.

The most agonizing part of detox-illness is not knowing that it is detox-illness, not the cancer worsening. Cancer does not worsen all over the body at one time. It could worsen in one or two locations at a time, increasing pain or pressure or swelling. But when many places develop symptoms together, it will be due to bacteria or viruses.

After plate-zapping the organ that made the tumor, zap the tumor itself. Follow these detailed instructions.

The Plate-Zapping Method

First of all:

1. Identify the "hot" (+) lead from your zapper. If you accidentally choose the (-) lead you will get no benefit, although it does no harm. If your zapper is not clearly marked with a (+) sign take it to any electronics shop. The technician will gladly check it for you. Ask to be shown how to use a voltmeter for this detail.

2. Do not use a wall outlet as power source. Do not use a frequency generator without supervision by an electronics expert.

3. Purchase a voltmeter and test your batteries before beginning and after every two zaps afterward. Make sure

the voltage is not below 8.9 volts at the end of each zap or it will have to be repeated. Start at 9.4 volts to be sure of this. Be careful not to stress the battery holder as you take the battery out repeatedly for testing.

4. Purchase a battery charger for metal hydride batteries that will charge to 10 volts and two to four metal hydride rechargeable batteries.

You will need:

1. Zapper with continuous running capability instead of seven-minute sessions; this is for convenience only.
2. Plate box that can be attached to the "(+)" lead of the zapper with proper leads. Do not buy imaginative "improvements" in design that combine the zappers with the plates. Do not buy zappers with special features or new shapes.
3. Two copper pipe electrodes and two banana-to-alligator clip leads (wires). Do not buy flat electrodes for the feet.
4. A kitchen timer.
5. Four packages of 1 pF capacitors and 1 μH inductors.
6. Microscope slides of body organs (anatomy set), and digestive tract organs (see *Sources*).
7. Bottle-copies of any tissues that cannot be purchased as slides (see *Sources*). These are white blood cells (WBC), lymph (the fluid), and others.

Digestive System Slide Kit

Appendix	Liver
Bile duct	Pancreas
Colon	Parotid gland
Duodenum	Rectum
Esophagus lower	Stomach, cardiac region
Esophagus upper	Stomach, fundic region
Esophagus-stomach junction	Stomach, pyloric region

Gall bladder
Ileum
Jejunum
Sublingual gland
Submandibular gland
Submaxillary gland

Anatomy Kit

Brain, composite (cerebrum, cerebellum, medulla)
Bone marrow, red
Bladder
Blood, smear, human
Hypothalamus
Kidney
Thymus
Lung
Lymph node, human
Mammary gland (breast)
Pineal
Pituitary gland

Anatomy Male Slide Kit

Ductus deferens
Epididymus
Penis
Seminal vesicle
Sperm
Testis

Anatomy Female Slide Kit

Cervix
Fallopian tube/Oviduct
Fimbria
Ovary
Uterus
Vagina

Miscellaneous Specimen Kit ("B.C." means bottle-copy)

Lymph (fluid), B.C.
Saliva, B.C.
Artery combination, "A", arteries, veins, nerves, B.C.
Lymph vessel combination, "L", lymph vessels, veins, B.C.
Cerebrospinal fluid, B.C.
Heavy metals, about 40, from amalgam plus cobalt, strontium, gold, antimony, uranium, chromium, radon, ruthenium and rubidium
Prion, B.C.
Copper (atomic absorption standard)
Mercury (atomic absorption standard)
Thallium (atomic absorption standard)

White blood cells, B.C.
Dye set, assortment, B.C.
Motor oil, B.C.
Wheel bearing grease, B.C.
Tricalcium phosphate
Malonic acid, maleic acid, maleic anhydride, methyl malonate, D-malic acid
alpha radiation (α), B.C.
beta radiation (β), B.C.
gamma radiation (γ), B.C.
polonium, B.C.
cerium, atomic absorption standard
potassium ferrocyanide, B.C.
potassium ferricyanide, B.C.
methylene blue (dye), B.C.
radon, B.C.
promethium, B.C.
plastic, white & black, B.C.
rubber, white, black, green, B.C.

Basic Vascular Set

Blood	WBC
Lymph	cerebrospinal fluid
"A"	"L"
Four 1 pF capacitors	Four 1 μH inductors

You do not need to purchase all the items listed. Use the schedule to guide you. You are now ready to start zapping every organ for which you have a specimen, slide or bottle.

Setting Up:

Wrap a single layer of paper towel around one of the copper pipes. The paper towel should not have chlorox bleach disinfectant. It should not cover the pipe all the way to the ends. It should stay ¼" away. The water should have been tested for chlorox bleach beforehand. Wet it under the cold faucet and place it under your foot, near your heel. Protect the carpet with a paper plate pushed into a plastic bag.

Connect the ***Positive*** side of your zapper to each plate (in "parallel") on your plate box. (Notice how easy it would be to make your own box.) Then connect each plate, in parallel, to your left foot, meaning the copper pipe under your left foot. (Although the *Positive* current is coming to your left foot through the plate box, it doesn't really matter which foot gets the *Positive* current. You may alternate feet every day if you wish.)

Connect the ***Negative*** side of your zapper directly to your other (right) foot.

Now the current will be guided to whatever organ (location) you put on the plate. You could use a body wipe, too.

On each plate you must choose only one location. If you choose more than one the current must divide itself between them and neither one gets enough to do a good job. However, if you put on two locations that touch each other, such as liver and arteries, the current goes to your liver-arteries, not foot arteries or any other arteries.

The Left Plate

Your blood and lymph system is the most important place (location) to zap, because this is the river-system that all pathogens use to spread themselves. Whenever adult parasites are killed, in any way, they release their eggs, which immediately enter the blood and lymph system. Fortunately this body fluid conducts electricity best, even when PCBs and benzene are everywhere. It is called the *vascular system*. By zapping one of the body fluids at all times, all released eggs are promptly zapped. We will use the left plate to zap the vascular system, but this is only a convention.

With regular zapping instead of plate-zapping, the current already goes mostly along the vascular system and is therefore very useful, especially after taking parasite-killing herbs. With plate-zapping you must specifically choose the vascular system to accomplish this. Simply leaving one plate empty also accomplishes this since the whole body is reached through it.

Plate-Zapping Schedule

Each zap will be 20 minutes long. In earlier methods you were instructed to attach kidney magnets before starting. I no longer do that because occasional errors were made. Our present kidney "drops" replace the magnets. Set your supplements, voltmeter and charger on the table nearby. Find a comfortable chair, warm blanket, and begin.

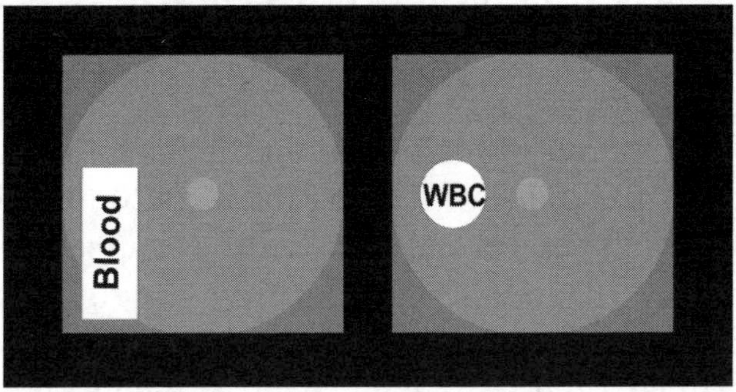

Fig. 47 Plate-zapping arrangement for #1

#1. Put the blood slide on the left plate.
Put the WBC (white blood cell) sample (bottle) on the other plate. Turn on the zapper and put your feet on the copper pipes for 20 minutes. Three 7 minute sessions are fine, too.

#2. Exchange the blood for the lymph sample (bottle). Exchange the WBC for the "A" sample (arteries, veins, nerves). Also place a 1 pF **capacitor** on the plate, but not touching A nor hanging over the edge of the plate. This capacitor somehow creates a preference for the **right side** of your body. In this case, it is the arteries, veins, and nerves on the right side of your body. Zap for 20 minutes. Keep notes on locations you have zapped (blood, WBC) and check the battery.

#3. Keep "A" on the plate, remove the capacitor, and replace it with a 1 µH **inductor**. The inductor creates a preference for the **left side** of things. In this case, it is the arteries, veins, and nerves on the left side of your body. Remove lymph from the left plate and place the bottle called "L" on it, and a 1 pF capacitor beside it (without touching each other). Now you are focusing on zapping the lymph vessels and more veins on right side of your body. (The lymph vessels are different from the lymph fluid sample used earlier.) Zap for 20 minutes. After 20 minutes you will have completed your first hour of plate-zapping. It is unlikely that you will feel anything yet. Remember you can take a break between 20-minute zapping sessions.

#4. Keep "L" on the left plate and replace the capacitor with your 1 µH inductor. During the next 20 minutes your left side lymph vessels and veins will get zapped.

Remove "A" and the inductor from the right plate and place the bottle called "CSF" on instead. This stands for cerebrospinal fluid. It is equivalent to lymph, but bathes the brain instead of your other organs. In fact, it is the same as lymph plus 3 pF. Zap for 20 minutes.

On the next day go back and do the basic set, first. You will do the basic set, first, every day. We will continue zapping a part of the basic set at the same time as other organs throughout the day with a double-zapper.

# Zap	Left Plate	Right Plate
1.	blood	WBC
2.	lymph	A + 1 pF
3.	L + 1 pF	A + μH
4.	L + 1 μH	CSF

The order of these locations does not matter.

These four zapping sessions form the **basic set**. Do these every day. They consume a little more than 1¼ hours, leaving seven hours for you to advance into your other organs and tissues. Even if all you do on the first day is the basic set, you are off to a good start. You do not need to wait for a complete set of slides or supplies. Use whatever you have as soon as you have it. You may make your own organ samples, too, using animal parts from the meat market. Even a drop of blood squeezed from a slice of beef liver into a plastic zippered bag works well for a blood sample.

#5. For the next zap, place the blood slide on the left plate again. On the right plate place the organ with your problem. For instance, the liver if you have liver cancer, or the prostate if you have prostate cancer. It is the organ that has the cancer, not the cancerous part itself. We will zap that later.

#6. Replace the blood slide with WBC on the left. On the right plate add the arteries to the liver sample by touching bottle "A" to the liver sample. They must touch to make a single location, namely the liver arteries.

#7. Replace the WBC with lymph on the left. On the right, replace the arteries with the lymph vessels, bottle "L". It should touch the liver sample.

#8. Replace lymph with the arteries (A) on the left. Then ask yourself, "How can I reach more parts of the liver"? You could move to the right, 1 pF at a time, and then move down by 1 μH. Follow the scheme used on page 176. Zap each location 20 minutes.

For each new location on the right plate, choose another part of the vascular system on the left. It does not matter in what order you zap the vascular set; you could rotate them all or just a few; you could even stick to one if that is all you have.

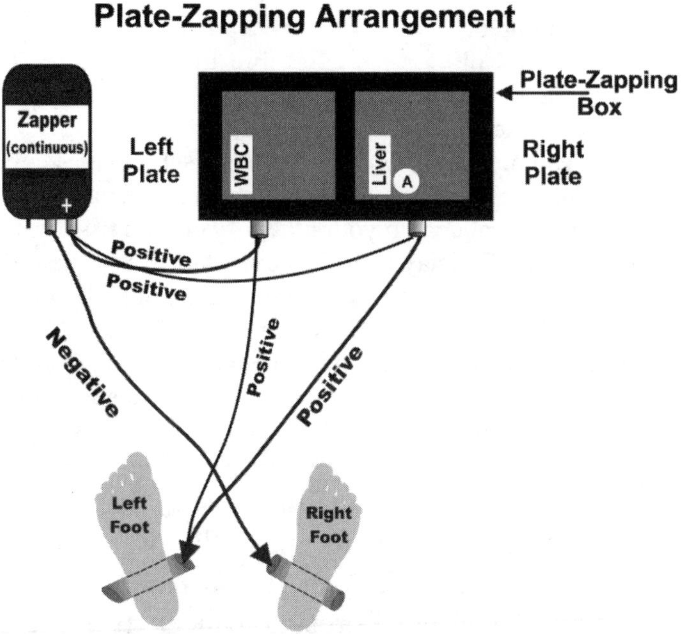

Fig. 48 Plate-zapping arrangement for #6

You are sure to have an attack of detox symptoms by now if you have not taken preventive measures. The liver is heavily parasitized. Keep your WBC-food handy on your zapping table. Keep your detox-teas and Lugol's handy, too.

Zap your organ with the tumor every day after the vascular set. Then zap the tumor itself.

The tumor does not have the same frequency pattern as the organ with the tumor. To identify the tumor we must add tricalcium phosphate to the organ. Virtually all cancer cells have tricalcium phosphate deposited in and around them. By touching the organ with the tricalcium phosphate bottle we are selecting tumor cells for zapping.

For example, to zap a left breast tumor, first place a part of the vascular set on the left plate as usual. Place a slide or bottle of breast on the right plate. Beside it, touching it, place your tricalcium phosphate sample. Place a 1 μH inductor on the right plate, too, to indicate the left breast tumor. It should touch nothing and not hang over the edge.

To zap the prostate gland thoroughly, zap both sides separately.

For the right side, place a 1 pF capacitor beside the slide. For a right side tumor, place the tricalcium phosphate bottle touching the prostate slide with the 1 pF capacitor nearby.

Get all the rest of your program done while you are zapping. You can even get IV's while you are zapping.

If you cannot sit, put the pipe-electrodes under you, each on a large zippered plastic bag. Move them from place to place to stay comfortable. By lying on them you will have the necessary pressure to internalize the current. Otherwise it travels along your skin. Do not switch to flat electrodes, unless you need to contact an area with a tumor just below. Flat surfaces do not make enough pressure and this makes the skin resistance higher, to cause small electrical burns. Watch flat electrodes for tiny stinging sensations so you can move the electrode before getting an electrode burn. If you do accidentally get one, do not bandage it or treat it. Merely keep the skin sterile with 1 or 2 drops straight Lugol's each day.

If you zapped the vascular set on your first day and the organ with the tumor on the second day, followed by the tumor itself on the third day, you are off to an excellent start.

If you lost no time to detox-illness you are very fortunate. But do not leave this to chance.

Next clean up all the locations of your digestive tract. Do one a day. You should have a set of about 20 digestive slides. Most of these organs do not need to have left and right sides zapped. For those, you can do two organs in one day.

If you cannot purchase slides, use raw meat samples from the market place. A whole chicken gives excellent substitutes for human organs. The bones can be salvaged from a cooked chicken; they do not lose their identity. Do not clean them up too carefully; you want the cartilage and tendons to stay with the joints. Small bones can be left together. Set them in a warm place to dry for several weeks, after labeling each large bone.

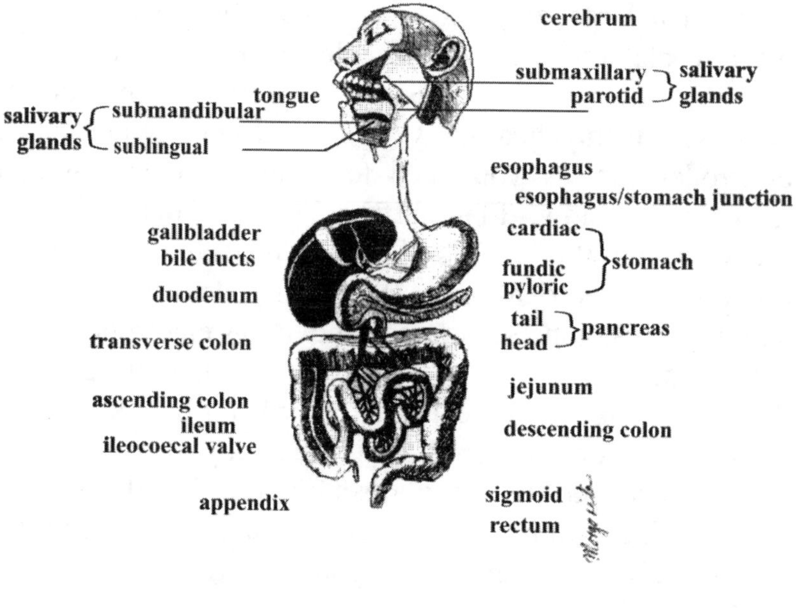

Fig. 49 The location of your digestive organs

Bones you can't identify can be used anyway. Use them to test for OPT, then use them to zap the correct location. They can be stored together in a zippered plastic bag in the refrigerator.

After zapping the colon, repeat it. This time add <u>two</u> 1 pF capacitors. This targets a spot halfway down the descending colon, which I have found to be especially favored by flukes.

If you are suddenly attacked by detox-illness, write down immediately which new organs you zapped that day. They obviously had a significant number of large flukes. As soon as you are ready to continue, repeat these several times to be sure there are no parasites left there. This time be more prepared.

Eliminate Fasciola

- Link #9 -

Expect to see parasites in the toilet bowl while zapping the digestive organs. This doesn't happen when you zap other organs, but when parasites in the digestive system die; they can leave with your bowel movement. Try to identify yours.

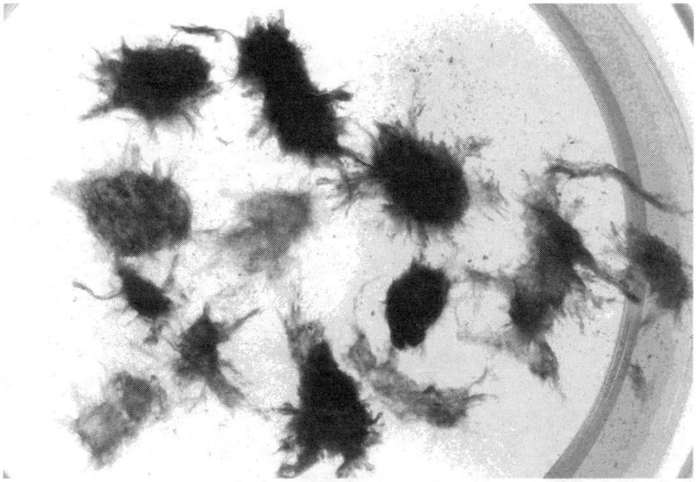

Fasciola is pink, which tests *Positive* for vitamin B12 by Syncrometer®. It has consumed your vitamin B12. See *Practical Parasitology*, page 181 to preserve it as a specimen.

Fig. 50 Photo of Fasciola

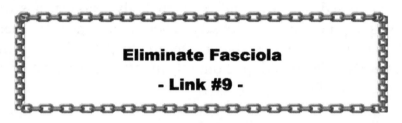

Fasciolas and Fasciolopsises are often an inch long but can also be much smaller. They can be distinguished by color. Their edges are ragged, like torn pieces of bread. This is due to having burst in the toilet water after falling into it. The difference in osmotic strength between their body fluids and the water outside is probably responsible for bursting. A few do not burst and resemble wrinkled canned grapes or rectangular blocks if they were compressed by crowding. As their body tears, strings of eggs slip out, hanging loosely. Their appearance is rather translucent under a binocular microscope but when Lugol's iodine is dripped onto them, many tissues take on clearer outlines.

Eurytrema is much smaller and rounder, about $^{1}/_{8}$ inch in diameter. There are actually 3 red dots, but one is much less visible, on the side. Two of them appear to be round at one end, close together, possibly the mouth and a sucker attachment. It too is in burst condition, letting egg strings hang out.

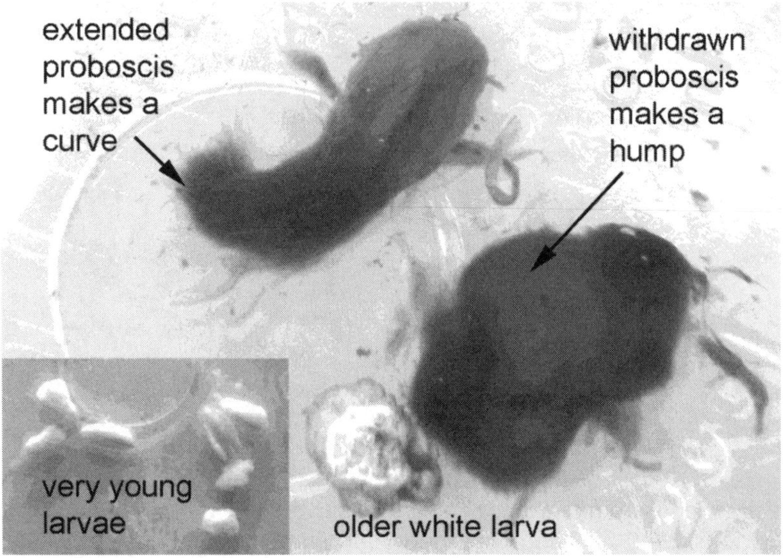

Fig. 51 Different Macracanthorhynchus appearances

Macracanthorhynchus is easily identified by its white color. It does not burst. The very tiny ones look like styrofoam "dust", afloat. The larger ones have a "trunk" which can be pushed out or drawn in. When it is pushed out it forms a curve so it looks like a tiny shrimp. The main body has a white area, easy to spot. When it dies or is prepared in formaldehyde, it turns brown.

To keep toilet bowl specimens from disintegrating you should prepare them with Lugol's solution or formaldehyde. This may keep one or two intact specimens from bursting. To preserve them for a few days let several drops of Lugol's solution fall right on top of them. For permanent specimens purchase formaldehyde. You will need 10 to 15% formaldehyde. Large parasites need the 15% formaldehyde to stay preserved for a long time.

Formaldehyde is a very toxic and dangerous chemical. Use great care, avoid breathing, and keep away from children.

Practical Parasitology

This is a method for finding your own parasites and preserving them. Do not start this project unless you have formaldehyde, Lugol's iodine solution and screw-type small jars such as baby food jars. You will also need a strong flashlight and white plastic cutlery with the longest handles you can find. You may tape a straw to the handle, very securely, to make it longer. Throw it away after each use.

Prepare Lugol's solution for hands, 20 drops in 1 cup water. Do not use gloves because they trap drops of toilet bowl water.

Get formaldehyde from pharmacy or your doctor. It will say 37% formaldehyde. You must dilute this.

Find a very sturdy plastic bottle with screw on lid to hold about 1 quart diluted formaldehyde. Work in the bathroom with door and windows open. You do not need to be extremely accurate with this recipe. A measuring cup will be fine.

Pour ½ cup cold tap water into the bottle. Add again as much 37% formaldehyde. You do not need to measure it. Just make a mark on the bottle where you will stop pouring. Close the bottles. You have diluted it in half; ½ of 37 is not too far from ½ of 40, making about 20% formaldehyde. To make a 10% formaldehyde solution, repeat the recipe. You already have 1 cup in the bottle. Now add another cup of water to make 2 cups total. This is your 10% formaldehyde. Label it and store it safely. Store in a locked cupboard.

Eliminate Ascaris

- Link #10 -

Make 15% formaldehyde in another bottle. Pour ½ cup cold water into it. Add again as much 37% formaldehyde. You now have 1 cup total of 20% formaldehyde. Add 1/3 cup more cold water to make 15% formaldehyde. Close securely and label. Metal lids will rust. Cover the jar with a sandwich bag first.

Keep formaldehyde safely on sink while you are using it. Do not keep it on back of toilet.

Pour about ½ inch of 15% formaldehyde in a small jar with a screw-on lid and also that much 10% formaldehyde in a 2nd jar. Label them beforehand. Keep these jars in a tray on the toilet tank to be handy. If there are children in the house keep them all in a locked tool box or tackle box. Wait for a soft stool because the parasites will be tightly stuck in a hard stool. Take advantage of any diarrhea or a liver cleanse.

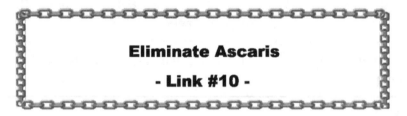

Stir toilet bowl contents round and round with plastic fork. Let settle from time to time. Put anything suspicious in a jar with formaldehyde already in it. The 15% formaldehyde is for larger parasites. The 10% is for smaller ones (less than ¼" long). Cover the jar with paper till done searching.

When done throw away the cutlery and wash hands in Lugol's water. Do not brush hands; it scratches them. Just wash continuously for 1 minute. Help Lugol's get under each fingernail.

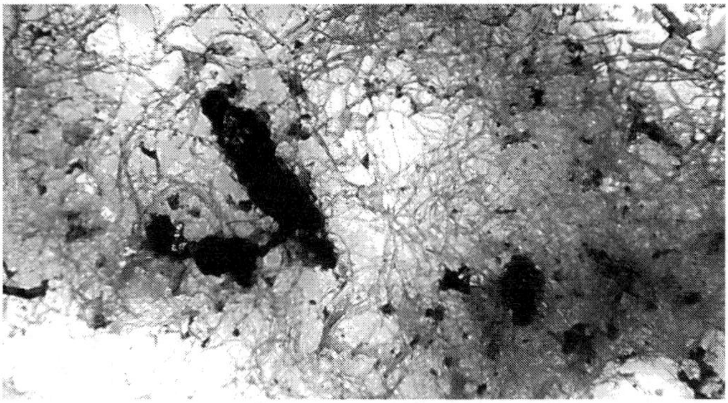

All the fine lines could be one worm(!) in the background. The black shadows are trapped debris.

Fig. 52 Onchocerca is a filaria roundworm

Onchocerca makes a hair-like thread around the plastic fork, like spaghetti when you swirl the fork round and round. If they are dead they will be brittle and break very easily into short pieces or small "snarls". Notice that the one in the photo has "captured" assorted debris just as it does in the body with a lymph node. The result is Hodgkin's or non-Hodgkin's lymphoma. You must kill the extra parasite in each cancer type. Onchocerca, wound up on a fork, looks like a scouring pad when it slides off your fork into formaldehyde.

Fasciolopsis buski looks like Fasciola but is grey and slightly larger, with short black threads spread around it (see also page 32). But you can also get more perfect ones that didn't burst (see page 119) if you use the *Gary Technique*.

The Gary Technique

Find small clear plastic bowls, like food containers, to show off your perfect specimens. Press on lids will be fine since these bowls are only temporary containers, allowing you 2 or 3 days to find a suitable camera and to identify them. Try to study the first diarrhea of a liver cleanse. Make a urine sample into the plastic bowl during your diarrhea session (only ½" deep). Later, fish up parasites directly into the urine sample, not the formaldehyde. They may keep for days without changing shape with just 10 drops of Lugol's. Later, you can fish out the identified parasites into a formaldehyde jar for labeled specimens.

The *Gary Technique* avoids the bursting action of the osmotic pressure difference. When convenient drain the bowl and pour on a formaldehyde solution. Let drops of regular Lugol's fall on them if you want to stain them darker.

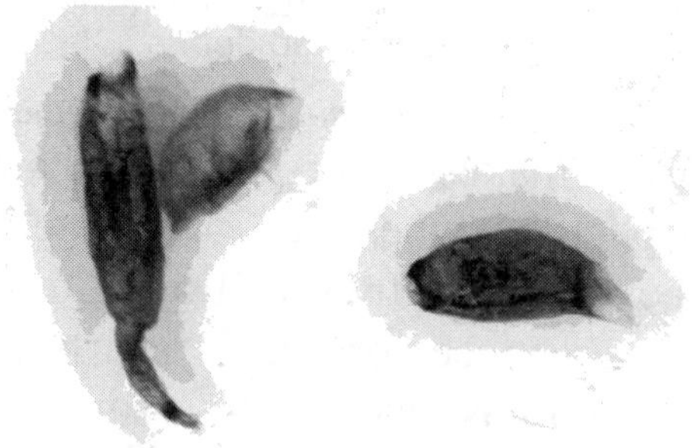

In the toilet bowl E. revolutum is usually missing the organs at the body ends giving it a pot-bellied look. A microscope slide of it shows a curved "tail" and a tuft at the opposite end. They have different appearances at different times.

Fig. 53 E. revolutum

Acanthocephala (see page 120) looks like amoebas, floating or sinking, connected by many "isthmus-like" branches. Soft, tiny "fingers" stick out of a soft body that glistens in the light. It is very slightly pink and glossy, about ¼ to ½" across each "body". It seems to have several different appearances, possibly stages.

To keep your specimens from drying out over the years, keep each jar in a plastic bag tightly zipped. Line the lid with a sheet of thin plastic.

E. revolutum may be missing the angled tip at one end and the tuft at the other end.

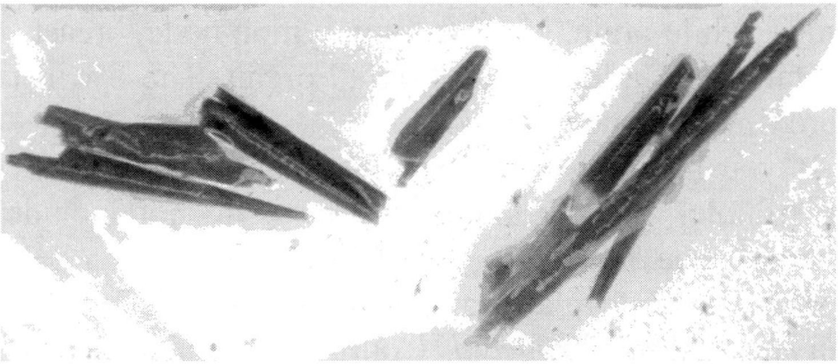

Parasites do not always look similar even though they are the same.

Fig. 54 E. recurvatum

E. recurvatum may have 3 or 4 quite different appearances. The most common is not the straight match stick as seen on a microscope slide. It is the long brown triangle, furled like a curled up leaf. Two such triangles are often joined at the wide end. Sometimes 3 are joined, making it up to 3 cm long! Another appearance is redder, like a curled up tomato skin. A fresh one, put quickly into the urine, may tighten its furled "sail" as you watch it. Very small ones have sharply pointed tips and a bulging belly in the middle.

Keep your parasite "treasures" locked up away from children because formaldehyde is very toxic; read the label. But the parasites themselves are dead and safe to handle or "show off" as you continue to plate zap your digestive organs.

Week Four Plate-Zapping

Depending on how many slides you have, and how long you spent on problem areas, you have been plate-zapping about three weeks. Now we are going to finish with various other locations of your body. An anatomy set is available as a slide kit (see *Sources*). Zap all locations you can acquire.

Bladder, hypothalamus, and pineal are all "single" organs, while brain, kidney, lung, lymph node, breast, and pituitary have a "left" and "right" organ. These will take approximately one more week.

If you have an organ or body location that is giving you trouble, and the slides you have do not include it, **order it!** (See *Sources*.)

The complete plate-zapping program will last longer than the *2-Week Program*. Continue steadily. Going too fast invites detox-illness. Hopefully you have seen at least a few parasites of your own, and have positive evidence of getting better.

So far we have discussed three ways to kill parasites on a grand scale: the starving way, the herbal way and the plate-zapping way. But there is another, simpler way that uses homeography.

I believe it is the body's <u>own</u> way, although we knew nothing about it. The body normally uses benzoquinone (BQ) and rhodizonic acid (RZ), besides its own methyl sulfonyl methane (MSM) and a host of other very powerful chemicals I call WEAPONS. It makes these itself, but in extremely tiny amounts, similar to vitamin B_{12} or a hormone. And it can use the body's own electricity to make these, as we will see.

In cancer, as well as HIV and other diseases, large parts of the body are no longer making BQ or RZ nor the other powerful chemical "weapons". We will find a way to help the body make them again through **homeography**.

Summary — Chapter 6

1. The body can benefit from a very low voltage applied at radio frequencies if the wave form is a square pulse and it is always *Positively* charged.

2. The tiniest *Negative* voltage aids a pathogen out of proportion to its size.

3. The mechanism is not understood but obviously the body can respond to such electrical signals. One response seen by Syncrometer® is the WBCs beginning to eat the pathogens around them.

4. Plate-zapping concentrates the current and the action at a particular organ.

5. Follow the *Practical Parasitology* instructions to find, identify, and preserve your own specimens.

WANTED DEAD—OR DEADER

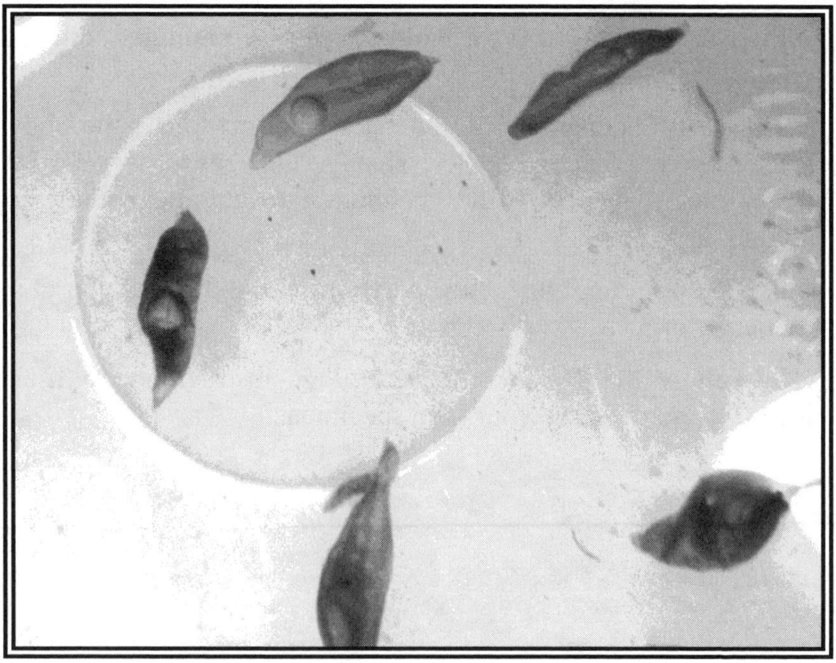

Five Hymenolepis cysticercus look like grey squash seeds. Squarish ends are replaced by "purse-string" ends. This cat-tape is smaller than other varieties. We probably <u>all</u> have these.

***WARNING: DO NOT EXPERIMENT ON YOURSELF** to remove tapeworm. The recipes were not complete at time of publishing.*

CHAPTER 7

HOMEOGRAPHY

Homeography is a new science. It uses electronically prepared drops of water taken by mouth. It depends on the ability of water to incorporate a frequency pattern of some object or chemical or living thing and to hold it in a stable way for a very long time (years). More than one frequency or frequency pattern can be stored together.

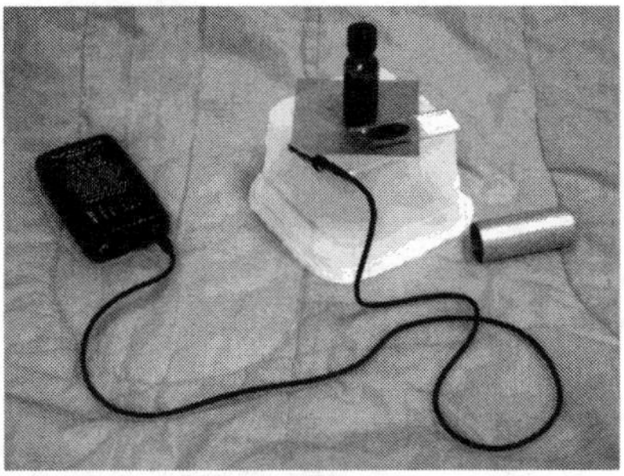

Place the bottle touching the slide or object.

Fig. 55 Making a bottle-copy

In fact, water seems to have a large capacity to hold frequencies without getting them mixed up or weakening. These discoveries are too new to be able to answer even simple questions. What kind of energy is being held in the frequency pattern? We have seen that a purely electrical force and a static magnetic force can be held. Could a pulsing magnetic field be held and detected somehow, too? Only further research can shed light on these questions. But the electrical frequency pattern that we will use here is surprisingly simple to see and produce by anyone.

How To Make Homeographic Drops

You will need a source of *Positive* offset square waves, at least 30 kHz, close to 50% duty cycle and at least 9 volts from a fresh battery. This is what a zapper produces, so you may already have the most important item. You will also need a 3½ inch square of aluminum sheet, about $^1/_{32}$" to $^1/_{16}$" thick, called the **plate**. You may find the aluminum at a hardware store; just cut to size and drill a hole for a small screw in the middle. The plate is fastened to a plastic stand such as a disposable food container. A wire comes from the *Positive* output of the zapper and connects to the plate. The *Negative* output is not used. If it is accidentally used, the signal arriving at the antenna-like plate would be grounded to the *Negative* side and disappear. There would be no results.

To use the copy maker, place a bottle of plain pure water on the plate. The bottle may be brown glass or brown polyethylene plastic. The brown color keeps out intense light, which could switch the polarization of the contents at any time. It should contain about 10 to 15 ml (2 to 3 tsp.) water. Place the item you want to copy right beside it. Surround each bottle being used with a metal tube as a shield* (aluminum or aluminum-steel pipe, see *Sources*) to make the effect stronger, although it is not strictly necessary. The two items or tubes must touch. Now zap for 20 seconds (this is not precise but should not be longer than 30 seconds). The plain water now becomes a **bottle-copy**.

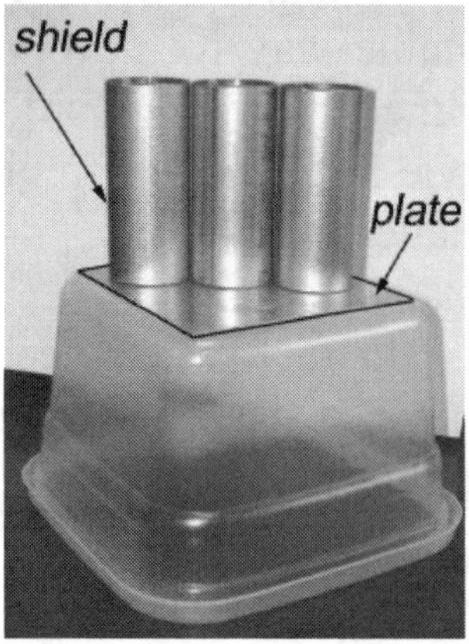

Place metal (aluminum-steel) tubes over bottles to shield them (see *Sources*).

Fig. 56 Shielded bottles make stronger copies.

After incorporating a bone or other substance into a water sample, its presence should be, ideally, verified

* Testers, use these pipes as amplifiers too. It approximately doubles a signal from a Syncrometer®. A bottle that was *Negative* in a test can be *Positive* with a metal tube around it! Repeatability is much greater, consistency much better.

using a Syncrometer® or more rigorously, using a digital frequency synthesizer in conjunction with a Syncrometer®. These optional details of copy-making are in the *Syncrometer® Science Laboratory Manual.* Realistically, you must be able to trust the copier. How could this be useful?

Many purposes can be achieved with electronically made bottle-copies. You can use them when testing with the Syncrometer® or when plate-zapping, as we saw in the previous chapter. Further, the water copy itself can be taken by mouth in the form of **drops** under the tongue. But for this purpose you should <u>make your own</u> so you could be sure of the water quality. Even a minute toxin would build up to hurt you even if it is only water. Other goals can be achieved, too.

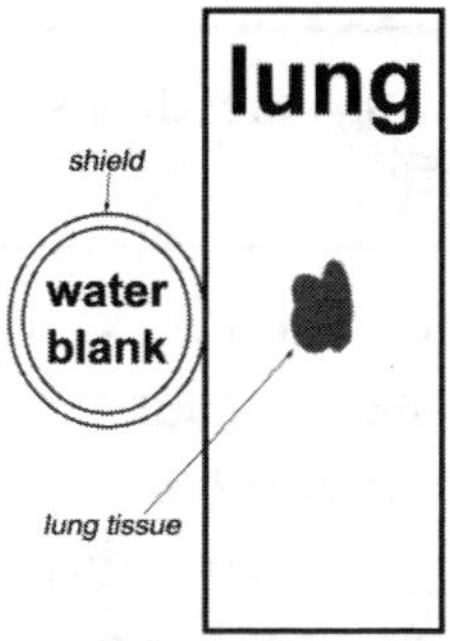

Strengthen your lungs with their own frequencies copied from a lung slide and taken as drops of water.

Fig. 57 Making organ drops

Homeographic Drops Can Strengthen

The most important goal is to clean your organs of all the toxins, pathogens and parasites accumulated there. Simply making a copy of each organ and taking this as drops many times a day accomplishes this. For a few hours the Syncrometer® sees the new frequency pattern superimposed on your own organ's pattern. For a short time you are not missing any frequencies from your own "sick" organ. Sick or merely old organs regularly miss many of their frequencies. You can find the missing ones precisely with a high quality frequency synthesizer. (This is described in the *Syncrometer® Science Laboratory Manual*). Does taking these as drops strengthen metabolism?...impart energy to that organ? The WBCs in this organ get activated, as if you had zapped this organ. The Syncrometer® sees the WBCs are soon full of their surrounding toxins. Sometimes you can feel the effect immediately.

Taking drops of harmful invaders would surely reach them and strengthen them! Use only the goals and formats given here. This is not the same as homeopathy.

> Never take drops of a parasite or a virus or anything harmful.

The dose is six drops taken 6 times daily for two days. Drop them under your tongue just behind the lower teeth. Leave them there to slowly absorb before swallowing them. After two days reduce the dosage to 3 times daily. No food should have been in your mouth for five minutes, nor eaten afterward for five minutes. Two bottles should be kept at least 1 minute (60 seconds) apart. Swallow any remaining drops before giving yourself new ones.

Do not touch your mouth with the bottle. It is instantly contaminated with E. coli or Salmonella. Do not touch the nozzle with your fingers. Hold the bottle about 10 inches above your mouth to be able to count drops as they fall.

You can combine slides or bottles (not drops) creatively to match precise locations. In the example shown we make drops of the CD14 cells in the liver. The CD14s are the macrophages, our huge white blood cells, always immobilized and coated with automotive greases in cancer victims. Taking these drops would strengthen them specifically.

Placing 2 tissues on the copy plate so they touch each other represents a "series" type circuit. This implies that they touch each other in real life. If they don't really touch in real life, but are close to each other, you would leave a space between them on the plate. For example, to create the location of a mediastinal tumor, which is between the upper lung and the esophagus, you would place these 2 slides on the plate, separated by a space of about ¼". It is a location. The blank (for copying) touches one of these. This location can be searched and if found could be zapped. Slides that are placed more than 1" apart are for organs that are definitely not in contact in real life. Two tissues placed at different corners act as if in "parallel" electrically. As you place them closer together, you are assuming they are partly in "series".

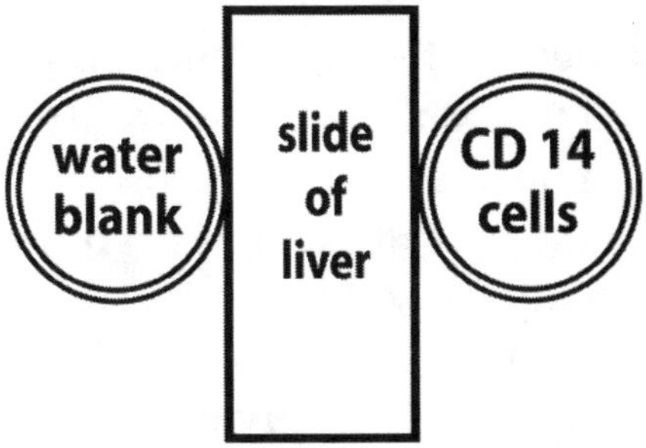

This combination puts the liver-CD14 cell pattern into the water blank. Reversing them contaminates your CD14 bottle by passing the liver through and into, the CD14 bottle on its way to the blank.

Fig. 58 Combinations should mimic reality

Many of your organs have a left and right partner. For example, you have two lungs and two kidneys. Your brain has a left and right side. In the case of the liver there are many lobes (see page 462). Your pancreas has left and right portions that are not symmetrical. The more precisely you can imitate the real life situation, the more effective the copy will be.

Capacitors and inductors are electronic components with a precise amount of capacitance or inductance. By putting them on your plate, along with an organ sample, you change its electrical properties slightly. I have found by adding a 1 pF (picofarad) capacitor you can adjust a location more to the right or further up. If instead you add a 1 μH (microhenry) inductor you can structure a location more to the left or further down.

For example, suppose you know your right lung is worse than your left, and you want to zap the right lung first. You would make a bottle-copy of a lung slide with a 1 pF capacitor laid near it. The resulting drops would strengthen the right lung only. The bottle made could be used to zap the right lung only.

You may make drops of all the organ samples you can buy or somehow locate. You may have 30 or 50 bottles to take, **giving one minute to each**. You can do this while you are zapping. There are no side-effects although you may feel new body currents in locations of disease. If you take these drops more than 6 times daily, the effect may be much stronger. And, if you give yourself detox-illness you have evidence (though uncomfortable) that you even killed large parasites. How did your body do that with only 6 drops of water?

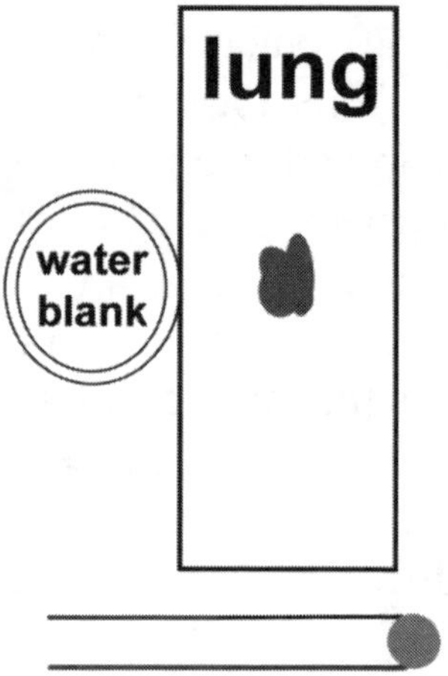

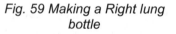

To make a right lung, place a 1 pF capacitor on plate.

Fig. 59 Making a Right lung bottle

Homeographic Drops Can Supply (Add)

Homeographic drops can <u>add missing things to a particular organ</u>. The things we want most are the immune weapons benzoquinone (BQ), rhodizonic acid (RZ), glyoxal (G), and glyoxylic acid (GA). These mega parasite-killers are by far the most dramatic and versatile chemicals in our bodies, as impressive as the power of our neurotransmitters. They have the most responsible job—to kill large parasites. The cancer patient's body is full of parasite eggs and stages because there are no mega killers at most locations. Children do have them.

Never try to obtain real BQ or glyoxal or glyoxylic acid. You would surely overdose yourself because the body only makes picogram quantities of them.

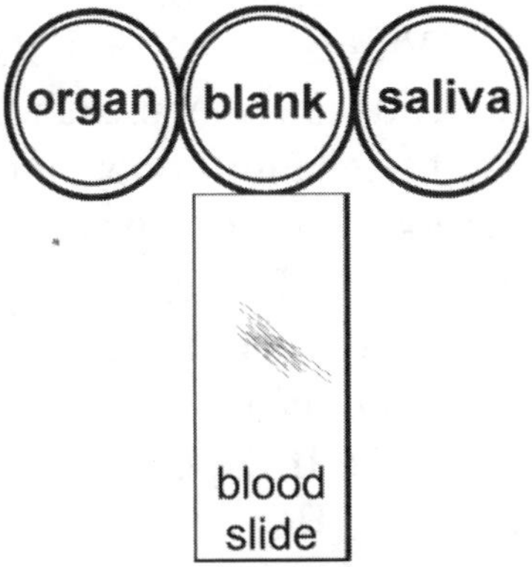

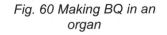

Each item touches the blank, but not each other.

Fig. 60 Making BQ in an organ

You can instruct your body to make BQ by using a homeographic combination. A different combination makes RZ.

To make BQ, which kills one of our Ascaris varieties (Ascaris lumbricoides), we must combine the organ where you wish to install it (such as the organ with a tumor or other problem), with saliva and blood all together in one blank bottle of water. The saliva and blood samples should come from a different person or an animal. Bottles have shields placed around them; slides do not. After taking these drops several times you will find BQ present in this organ. It will be ready to go to work for you.

One could, of course, copy some real benzoquinone into a bottle of water and take those drops. We call this "cloned BQ." These drops are quite powerful, too, but only for a short time. Inducing your body to make BQ using the combination of saliva and blood and organ is superior! BQ may be our most powerful and multipurpose weapon, killing many other kinds of larvae, as well.

To make RZ, the organ to be replenished (your organ with a problem) is combined with saliva and lymph. The saliva can be in bottle-copy form, originally from a fairly healthy person. Bottle-copies of all these supplies can be purchased (see *Sources*), but are easily made, too (see page 619). Notice that the three ingredients must not touch each other, but all must touch the blank bottle.

Why are BQ and RZ missing in the first place? It depends on the presence of Ascaris-chemicals, such as 1,10-phenanthroline, guanidine, methyl guanidine and others. Ascaris produces a host of such abnormal chemicals. Evidently they use up BQ and RZ.

If BQ can be made abundantly, until no Ascaris or their chemicals are left, the body can continue to make its own BQ. If not enough is made and Ascaris chemicals are leftover, BQ continues to be missing and now parasites can grow large, mature, and shed eggs. Parasitism continues.

As soon as you take six drops of the saliva-blood-organ bottle-copy your body starts making BQ at that organ. This destroys the Ascaris-chemicals as well as Ascaris itself at that one location. Within the day, this tissue is freed from Ascaris parasitism. You may suddenly feel like a brand new person. Ascaris was bringing you night sweats from its bacteria.

As soon as you feel better you may reduce the dosage to 3 times a day. Because of the possibility of reinfection from the environment and also from other parts of the body, it would be wise to continue taking these drops 2 or 3 times per day for weeks. Afterwards, test your ability to keep making BQ and RZ yourself.

Making G and GA requires combining other body fluids, including bile and urine. Many combinations are possible. Each combination kills a specific large parasite. Two more are MALDE and MALDM (tetra ethoxy and tetra methoxypropane). These can kill Fasciola, which I believe to be our most prevalent fluke. Until research on these is complete take the cloned weapons themselves, which you can easily make from a master sample.

You now have a very easy way to improve your most important organs by adding something to your body. It is not unusual for a cancer patient to be taking 30 or more homeographic bottles continuously while zapping for eight hours a day.

> Zapping an organ while taking drops for that same organ seems to be especially beneficial. Try to arrange for that coincidence.

But could you add something, precisely, to one location in your body, as tiny as the retina or your left little toenail, instead of adding it to the whole body?

Homeographic Drops Can Add Selectively

To send a hormone precisely to one place, like a gland, you need to copy them "in series" into a water bottle, both the hormone and the gland. This means they must touch each other before they touch the blank bottle. Remember that any bottles touching each other share their frequencies, so the hormone bottle enters the gland bottle and vice versa. They have contaminated each other in the process of fusing in the blank. You no longer have pure hormone or pure gland bottles! To avoid losing your "master" bottles this way, copy each one first. Mark the copies "for throw away" before you use them. Then line them up, with the blank at either end to be used for drops.

Homeographic Drops Can Remove (Subtract)

We saw how we can put things into the body, by supplying it as a single item or by sending it to an exact location. Can we also remove things?

We can take something out of a body location by copying each "in parallel" into a blank water bottle. The item to be removed and the location must each touch the blank, but not each other. Setting them exactly across from each other on either side of the blank works well.

The most important things to take out are wheel bearing grease, azo dyes, nickel and other heavy metals. When the body's immune system can not recover fast enough to remove these major toxins in time to save the liver or kidneys, making *take-out* bottles for them brings emergency relief in 1 to 2 days. Because of their power, you must not make a mistake with them. In the examples given, *take-out* bottles are left to the last so you can gain experience making other bottles first. Do not leave such big responsibilities to others. You can reverse your jaundice, kidney failure, seizures, anemia, and other emergencies in this way, but only if done correctly.

Homeography in Perspective

Homeography, like zapping, can be systemic in scope or focused on specific organs. Taking six drops of electronically "patterned" water mobilizes the white blood cells; that can be easily seen. It adds things or subtracts them. That is easy to test for, too. Fortunately the body makes its own decision on amounts and does not use our "units" like grams or teaspoons. That gives us some protection from our own ignorance. It may be able to do much more, but that must wait on research.

For you to be able to interact with the body using electrical and homeographic methods suggests that the body understands and acts with these same methods or "languages". Does a mother cat not lick her kitten from top to toe—combining saliva with nasal secretions, eye secretions, mucous, sweat, even anal and urinary secretions? Certainly a wound is immediately treated by combining it with saliva, right at the needy and bleeding organ, so blood and lymph are immediately added.

Negative voltage frequencies do not have this beneficial effect, although they can be copied, too. If you are purchasing ready-made bottle-copies, be sure to specify and ask for assurance that a *Positive* offset voltage was used and how much offset there was. If they don't understand the question, purchase elsewhere.

You cannot take out what you are putting in.

I do not understand the physics or chemistry of water enough to explain these phenomena. Questions must wait. But you can harness the forces involved to "boot-up" your own immune power even when all the blockers are present. The organ chosen can begin to clean itself up provided you stop taking the toxin in. You cannot take out what you are taking in!

For instance, taking kidney drops can send you directly to the bathroom. You can even get a mild detox-illness. Perhaps the electronic language of adding and subtracting frequencies (called heterodyning) or riding along on other frequencies (called modulation) is native to life. Perhaps water supplies the "mixing" where these electrical forces can meet and interact. Water, being the unifying chemical for life has its electrical charges, called ions, which then make it susceptible to voltage influences. Only more research can help us understand.

You must be very careful not to set your drops near a magnet. The magnetic field destroys the pattern in them. Always keep magnets in their own container, to separate them. You must be careful, not to freeze any bottles. It causes them to become jumbled, and resonating with all others. Don't even refrigerate them.

Shipping And Traveling With Bottles

Ways to salvage damaged bottles will be found as the science progresses. Meanwhile, ship your bottles packaged in air bubble wrap first and then aluminum foil for airplane shipment or in the middle of your suitcases wrapped in clothing. Label them all homeographic pure water. Test them on a Syncrometer® when they arrive.

Do 2 tests on each bottle that has traveled or been shipped by air.

1. Test each bottle for resonance with its own kind. It should be *Positive.*
2. Test each bottle for resonance with a different kind. It should be *Negative.*

If both tests fail: Set each bottle, one at a time, on the copy plate without a shield. Give it 20 seconds of the usual frequency from a zapper. Turn zapper off before taking the bottle off. Repeat the 2 tests. Label carefully.

Please inform author of your results.

Making Drops

The first drops to make should be the "protective set" for the lymph and kidneys. These are both organs. The lymph needs cleaning more than other fluids and often rewards you with pain relief instantly or extra energy. The kidneys will be the first to get help for their white blood cells. Take these drops continually, for weeks, at least until you are done plate-zapping.

> Mobilizing the WBCs is not all that is involved. You can often "taste" the action. Sometimes you can feel the organ respond.

The Water

In earlier books I recommended distilled, filtered or bottled water. I no longer do that. Since then I discovered that all bottled water has radon even though it may test *Negative* for it. I had neglected to test for radon's daughters, (Pb, Bi, Th, U, Po, Ra) and one or more of these very harmful radioactive elements is always present.

Now I recommend rainwater that has been stored in 1 gallon HDPE water bottles (used is fine) in a cool place. It should not be used for copying until it is at room temperature, though. It can be filtered through boiled cheesecloth that was tested first for chlorox bleach. The water only stays clean if you store it in a non-seeping container! Well water nearly always has a bleach or other disinfectant added, sometimes at a low level. Do not trust it. Bleach, whether the laundry type or NSF "good" type, still gives you sodium hypochlorite and ferricyanide, which will get highly activated by the homeographic procedure. Don't use any chlorinated water. You cannot filter water or "let it stand" and expect to get rid of chlorine. Boiling it "out" does not work. The drops you make and the drops you buy should be tested for bleach before you take them, also for E. coli and Salmonella.

To clean and store rainwater for drop-making, collect it in an opaque polyethylene bottle, preferably a used one that had held water marked with a kosher symbol on it at the supermarket (this would identify it as chlorine-free). Make a funnel out of another such bottle or purchase a stainless steel one. All plastic funnels will seep very toxic metals into your rainwater. Test its conductivity with an indicator (see *Sources*). It should be zero. Also test for strontium, beryllium, vanadium, and chromium, the common air pollutants. If these are absent, you are very fortunate. It is healthful; you can drink it and make drops with it. **It will not test accurately at refrigerator temperature, though.**

Place each rainwater collector in a bucket that is suspended in the air, or weighted down by a rock in the middle of your lawn. You may also use plastic bags of the zippered kind that can be suspended with clothespins or used to line a wastebasket. Guard against clothespin drippings or roof runoff.

Most efficient and failsafe is a set of buckets lined with zippered bags held in place with bungee cords on 2 chairs. Set them away from trees and buildings (see page 360). Do not leave your collections open and unattended. Air pollutants could fall in. Also protect it from bright sunshine; this changes it to southerly, but is reversible.

The Rain Filter

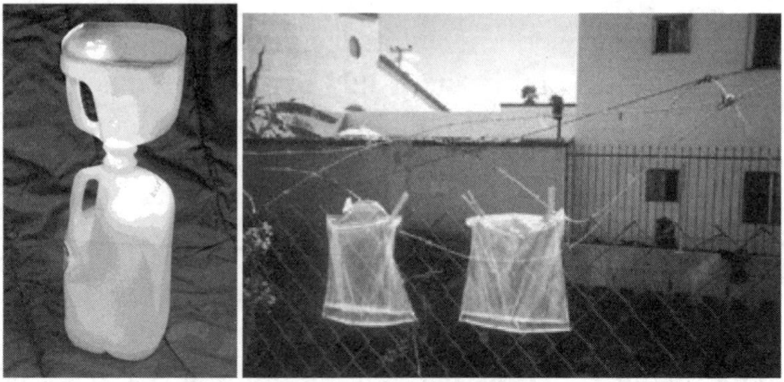

Fig. 61 Collecting rainwater

Wait for 1 hour of raining before starting to collect so that smog particles, bits of foliage and dust will have rained down. Test it first for pollutants. If there are none, and you can see no particles in the water, use no filter. Any regular filter would remove beneficial elements while adding its own toxic ones. These will be potentized by the homeographic treatment. Cheesecloth and "cotton wool" from vitamin bottles can be tested for both bleaches first. Choose a bleach-free kind. Wash it in rainwater several times and squeeze dry, then boil in rainwater for 5 minutes at a rolling boil. Rinse with rainwater. Use it as a loose fitting cork in your homemade funnel to filter the rain as it comes down. You could also use the white cellulose fiber from a filter pitcher, squeezed dry several times under hot tap water and then boiled 5 minutes and rinsed in rain.

The Taste Of Rain

Rain tastes best in the first 5 to 10 minutes. The zest of its ozone reminds us of snow. It is medicinal in an unknown way since you can get detox-symptoms from it. If it is kept open to air it absorbs carbon dioxide and soon tastes "sharp", namely acidic from CO_2. This is not harmful. For original freshness keep it zipped shut or capped in a refrigerator. After 1 year of storage in a HDPE gallon jug it had no oxidized minerals and tasted fresh.

The Bottles

Buy ½ oz. amber glass bottles with caps that have a polyethylene protected surface inside (see *Sources*). Do not buy droppers for them. The rubber end of the dropper seeps heavy metals, cerium and malonic acid. You may buy a separate polyethylene drop dispenser (pipette) used by chemistry students (see *Sources*) if it is free of chlorination. Keep each pipette with its own bottle. One wrong dip would destroy the bottle! It is always wise to transfer any bottle of liquid to a bottle with built in dropper to prevent all mistakes. Buy ½ oz. amber polyethylene bottles with 2 kinds of caps: a flat one and a dropper variety complete with nozzle (see picture).

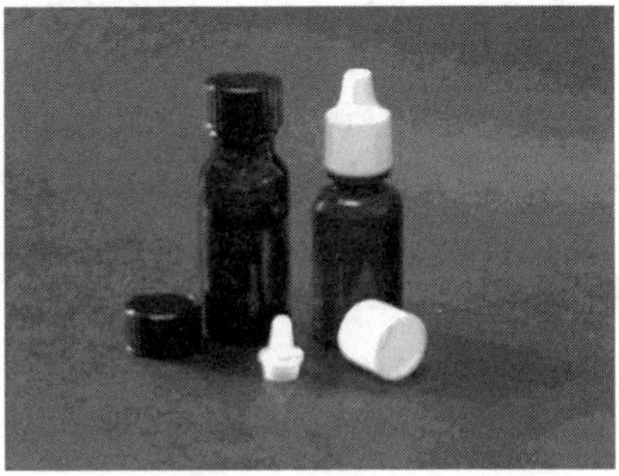

Fig. 62 Amber glass & polyethylene bottles and lids

DO'S and DON'TS

Do not switch bottle caps or nozzles. You may reuse a bottle if you rinse it 3 times with pure water and also rinse the nozzle and cap 3 times. Even one drop of a different frequency destroys a new bottle of drops. Since you have no way of testing whether a bottle is potent or blank, be extra careful not to confuse bottle parts. This is also the reason for taking drops one minute apart. New drops must not touch old drops in your mouth.

Do not combine bottles. Do keep bottles out of direct sunlight. Do not carry them in your pocket. Do not rubber band them. Do not touch them during copying. Do turn off the zapper before touching them to remove them. If you made a mistake or have some doubts, rinse everything and start over. You may reuse a bottle without rinsing if you are making the identical solution in it. Do not make drops out of zappicated water. Label water that has been zappicated.

Organ Drops

Each organ you take as drops will show activation of its WBCs specifically; no other organs are activated. The most important organs to activate are the kidneys. In fact they are so important you should always **take kidney drops first**, along with kidney white blood cells when beginning any drop-taking session.

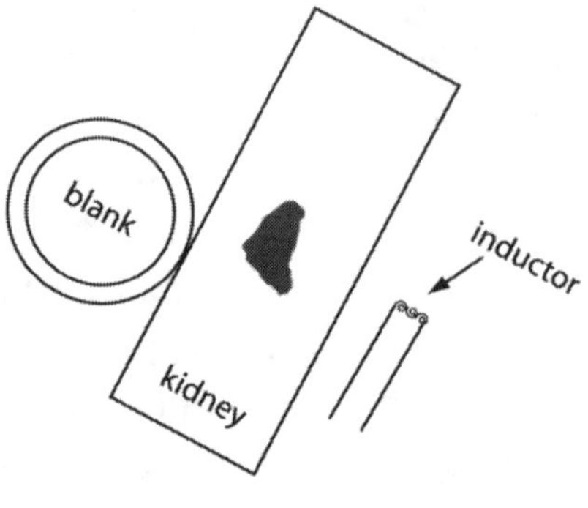

Fig. 63 Making a bottle of the Left kidney

To make your kidney protective set, to strengthen them, copy your slide or bottle of kidney tissue. Make a

Right kidney bottle and a Left kidney bottle. Then make Right kidney WBCs and Left kidney WBCs.

Making Dyes-Out-Of-Kidney

It is failure of the kidney white blood cells to keep the kidneys clean that "clogs" them and forces the toxins to accumulate somewhere else in the body, just where there is no immune power.

We will make *take-out* drops for each kidney and its WBCs to bring back normal kidney action.

The power in *take-out* drops is so huge that nobody should make them before reading this entire section on homeography. And nobody should take them if the source of their own dyes, heavy metals and wheel bearing grease have not been found and eliminated. In other words, you can't take out those things you are still taking in! That is why cleaning up water, diet, dentalware and cooking pots comes first. Nor can you clean large areas like the blood, the bones, the skin. It is meant for tiny amounts.

Take-Out Dyes From Right Kidney

Purchase a bottle of mixed azo dyes. Also purchase individual dyes: Fast Green, Fast Red, Fast Blue, Fast Red Violet, Fast Garnet, DAB, and Sudan Black. You may soon need them.

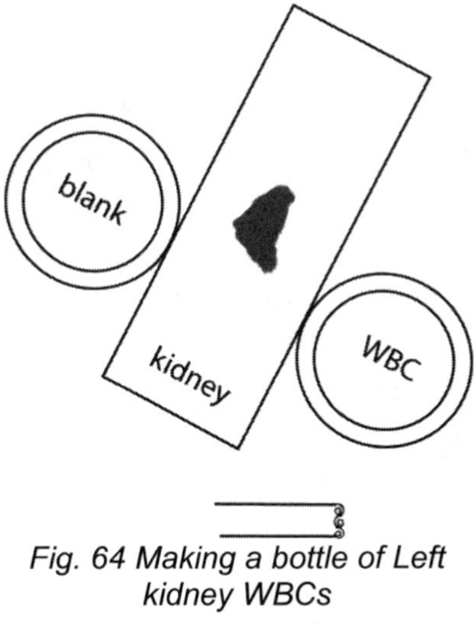

Fig. 64 Making a bottle of Left kidney WBCs

Place the dye sample on one side of the blank bottle, on the left by our convention. Place the organ to be cleared, namely kidney, on the opposite side, on the right by our convention*. Place metal tubes over all bottles. Add a 1 pF capacitor to the plate, not touching anything. Zap for 20 seconds with *Positive* offset voltage. Label your newly made bottle "*take-out* dyes from Right kidney".

Take-Out Dyes From Right Kidney White Blood Cells

Place blank at center. Place dyes on left side of blank. Place kidney slide on right side of blank, adding a 1 pF capacitor. Next, place white blood cells beside kidney, touching it. Use a WBC bottle or homemade slide, but not your own WBCs. *NOTE*: if you used a kidney bottle instead of slide and also a WBC bottle, the WBC frequency will have to pass through the kidney bottle to reach the blank and will remain there. The kidney bottle now has the WBC frequency in it. So relabel your kidney bottle "has WBC". You can avoid this by using a kidney slide or sample from meat shop (placed in zippered plastic bag). If you wish to use your kidney

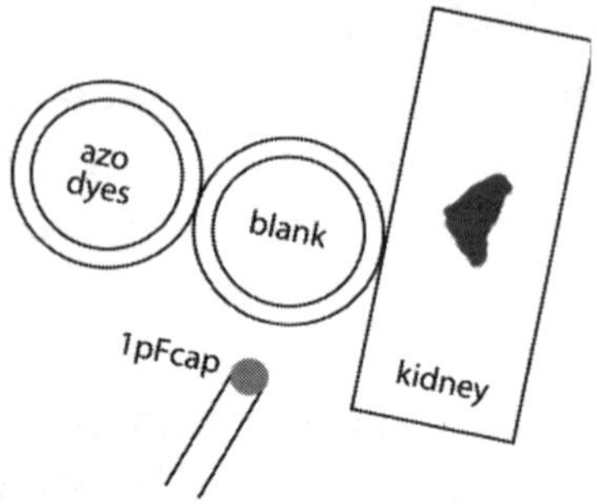

Fig. 66 Take-out dyes from Right kidney

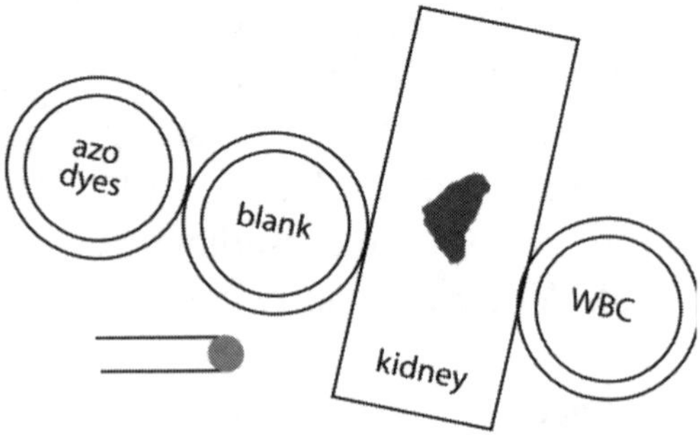

Fig. 65 Take-out dyes from Right kidney WBCs

* Testers, I no longer recommend making 2 take-out bottles at the same time. It is safer to make one and label it "master". Then copy the master into 2 bottles, one on each side.

bottle, make **a copy of it beforehand. This would keep one safe from accidental contamination, it is highly recommended for all your purchases**.

Take-Out Dyes From Left Kidney

Place blank at center. Place dyes on left side of blank. Place kidney slide on right side of blank. Place a 1 μH inductor loose on plate, not touching anything.

Take-Out Dyes From Left Kidney White Blood Cells

Place blank at center. Place dyes on left side of blank. Place kidney slide on right side and WBCs touching it. Add 1 μH loose on plate.

You now have a set of 4 *take-out* bottles for dyes from the kidney set. These can save your life when you are already on life support means with less than a week of life left for you. But they won't save your life if your very life support supplies dyes as they would if they were manufactured by a company that uses laundry bleach to disinfect its biologicals or if these supplies included colored plastic. Such dilemmas are common. Use your judgment. The rule is never broken that you cannot take out what you are putting in.

The whole *take-out* action is complete in 4 days, taking them 6 times daily for the first 2 days and 3 times daily for the next 2 days. Copy each bottle by cloning it before it is less than half full. Continue once a day for 2 more weeks. Store the remainder. If you are in a new emergency situation, take them all again, this time every hour the first day.

Making Heavy Metals-Out-of-Kidney

Purchase a bottle-copy of mixed heavy metals. Mine was made from a piece of unused amalgam plus cobalt, strontium, gold, antimony, uranium, chromium, radon, ruthenium and rubidium; these were missing in my piece of amalgam, so were added later.

Make your own with a chip of old amalgam from any, including your own, extracted tooth. Drop it into pure water in an amber ½ oz. bottle. To take all these out of your Right kidney, again place the blank in the center. Place the heavy metal bottle on the left side of the blank. Place the Right kidney on the Right side of the blank. Just before pressing the switch button, read the line-up as a final check, like this, from left to right, "Take heavy metals-out-of-Right kidney", and check each item as you read it. Ask yourself, "Am I contaminating any of my bottles?" If so, make a copy you can discard later. Then zap 20 seconds*. You may rinse the discard bottle and reuse.

Any piece of amalgam will be missing some heavy metals. Combine all the metal jewelry you were wearing, including watchband, earrings, necklaces, and dentalware you saved in one zippered plastic bag. Copy it all together. Then use this to make *take-out* drops for your kidney set.

Finish making and taking the heavy metals-out-of-Right kidney and Right kidney WBCs, Left kidney and Left kidney white blood cells.

Making Wheel Bearing Grease-Out-Of-Kidney

Since wheel bearing grease traps motor oil, dyes, metals, malonic acid and solvents and slowly releases them in your vital organs, this may be the most important *take-out* set. Be careful not to try to take this grease out of other locations before taking it out of the kidney set. It could relocate itself.

* ERRATUM NOTICE: This was wrongly stated as 20 minutes in the earlier book "*The Prevention Of All Cancers*".

Purchase a can of wheel bearing grease at any automotive supply store. Copy it into a bottle of water, placing a shield over the blank as usual. The large size of the can will make part of it hang over the edge. Copy it only into one bottle at a time (not several). Label it.

Make wheel bearing grease (WBGr)-out-of-Right kidney, WBGr-out-of-Right kidney WBCs, WBGr-out-of-Left kidney, WBGr-out-of-Left kidney WBCs. Also WBGr-out-of-lymph.

You now have 4 sets:

- a kidney set (and lymph) to help and protect them
- dyes-out-of kidney set and lymph
- heavy metals-out-of-kidney set and lymph
- wheel bearing grease-out-of-kidney set and lymph

Making Extra Drops

Copy the LYMPH bottle so you can take drops of lymph and *take-out* bottles from lymph as well as zapping lymph.

Copy the peripheral BLOOD slide so you can take drops as well. Label it CIRCULATION or BLOOD.

Copy the CD14s; take drops.

Copy the CD8s; take drops.

Make dyes-out-of LYMPH.

Make NICKEL-out-of CD8s.

Make NICKEL-out-of-CD14s.

Make heavy metals-out-of-LYMPH.

Make methyl malonate-out-of-kidney set, taking drops to rescue kidneys from failure.

Next, make DAB (dye)-out-of-WBCs. This is a single bottle. Having DAB in the white blood cells causes the alkaline phosphatase to be much too high. Having cobalt in them causes low alkaline phosphatase. Check yours. Hurry to take out DAB or cobalt or both. But where will they go after being taken out? They should go to the kidney WBCs. But if the kidneys have not yet been cleared of dyes or heavy metals, it will do no good. You must wait till you have taken the kidney drops for 4 days.

Next make Sudan Black (dye)-out-of-RBCs. Having Sudan Black in your RBCs causes the LDH to be much too high. If LDH is too low, there is cobalt in them. Make cobalt-out-of-RBCs.

Next make Fast Green (dye)-out-of-CD8s and Fast Garnet-out-of-CD4s.

If the globulin is too low, or too high, take all the wheel bearing grease, dyes and heavy metals out of the B-cells. B-cells are also called CD37 cells.

You can make your own RBCs and platelets by structuring them electronically like this:

RBCs = WBCs + 1 μH
platelets = WBCs + 2 μH
megakaryocytes = WBC + 4 pF

Gold —The King Of Take-Out-Drops

We have gold accumulations wherever there is a health problem. It seems more difficult for the body to excrete gold than other metals. Giving organic vitamin C helps most. But taking gold-out-of-male organs or female organs, as sets, can save an AIDS patient in 2 to 3 days. Gold-out-of-liver set or brain is equally powerful. Modern diseases where gold is involved respond surprisingly well when drained of gold.

Nickel —The Queen Of Mischief

Gold and nickel are placed together in your teeth as crowns, and together on your finger as a wedding band. The nickel reduces wear on the gold. But after removing gold with take-out-gold drops, the nickel is left behind. Unless it is removed, bacteria will be well fed here.

Make take-gold- and take-nickel-out drops for the kidney set and lymph first. This opens the pathway to excretion through the bladder.

If the throat can't swallow or lungs can't breathe, make Au and Ni out of the trachea, trachealis muscle, R. lung, L. lung, epiglottis, upper esophagus.

Wherever gold and nickel are deposited prions arrive to stop the flow of acetylcholine and epinephrine, our main neurotransmitters. The organ stops all action. But you can rescue it from death with these drops in 2 days.

If the total bilirubin is over the range given as normal on the blood test, take copper, cobalt, chromium and nickel out of all liver parts. Make separate bottles for each metal for a stronger effect than the heavy metal combination. (Follow the example on page 461.) Also make a bottle of heavy metals-out-of-each-liver part. There are at least 10 liver parts. You have only days to accomplish this before jaundice begins. After 2 days of such metal removal the fungus, Aspergillus, and its relative, Penicillium, will be in decline. You can now take aflatoxin-out-of-all-liver parts. After another 2 days you can take bilirubin-out-of-blood for 4 days. Make sure you are taking the 4 kidney cleaning sets at the same time. Then you are ready for a new blood test.

These are extra life-saving features of homeography. You can see that for jaundice you must find the sources of these 4 heavy metals; you must stop drinking and eating them or you will have your jaundice back very soon. Sources of these 4 heavy metals are few: food, drink, dentalware, dishes and supplements. Use extreme measures when a crisis is before you. (Eat only natural food, drink only rainwater, remove all synthetic dentalware, don't use dishes or cutlery, don't take any untested supplements.) Don't stop searching till you have found the source of metals.

Make and take drops of pyruvic aldehyde to correct the imbalance with thiourea and stop excess cell division.

Make and take drops of hematoxylin to remove lanthanide elements like cerium.

Make and take drops of hypothalamus gland to help avoid detox symptoms.

Make and take drops of Rhodanese enzymes for a week till your cancer-complex mutation is gone.

Prevent Mistakes

Because *take-out* drops are very powerful, consider the effect on you if you should make a mistake.

LABEL ALL BOTTLES YOU MAKE; put on details.

If you made protective drops (same as organ drops) that are accidentally blank or got mixed up they could never harm you.

Making Salmonella drops could hurt you. Never even make bacteria bottles or parasite bottles or virus bottles to prevent any such error. Don't make them for zapping either. Zapping them does no good! They might be gone for 15 minutes and then be back! Do not zap parasites, bacteria or viruses. Zap the location only. You have them because you are feeding them accidentally, while your WBCs aren't working (for lack of germanium, selenium and vitamin C).

Never make drops that take out bacteria, parasites or viruses. They could only be out for minutes anyway since they reproduce in the neighboring organs all the time. And, again, you are inadvertently feeding them while the WBCs are disabled. Make only the *take-out* varieties given.

Consider the hazard of making a mistake in a *take-out* bottle for dyes or heavy metals. If, by accident, your final bottle only had kidneys or WBC or RBCs in it, they would now be "organ drops", not harmful. But if your final bottle had only dyes in it or heavy metals, having missed the organ, I believe you could certainly harm yourself. It would be equivalent to taking the dyes or metals for about ½ hour. For this reason, do not purchase *take-out* bottles, ready-made. Make them yourself. Even you will occasionally make a mistake. But stopping each *take-out* bottle after 4 days gives a measure of safety. If you sense an error, rinse bottles and start over.

The Problem Organ

Next, make drops of organs with problems.

First make the organ with the tumor; for example, if you have cancer in the Right lung, the organ with the problem is the Right lung. Always make drops for both members of a set though, like Right and Left lung.

Lungs are quite large. It would be useful to reach bronchi, bronchioles, and alveoli, specifically.

Use these relationships:

lung/trachea = bronchus. The slash means these two test samples touch each other.

bronchus + 1 μH = bronchiole

bronchiole + 1 μH = alveolus

Make drops for all organs with any problem, like liver for jaundice (make the whole set), bone marrow for leukemia, adrenals for high blood pressure, and so on. Make drops for their WBCs, too.

Remember that zapping an organ at the same time as taking drops for it has an exceptionally powerful effect.

Always take the kidney drops first.

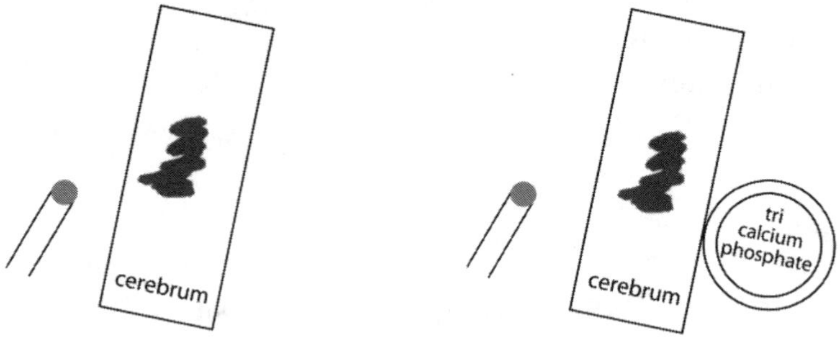

Zapping the Right cerebrum (at left) and Right brain tumor (at right).

Fig. 67 Zapping a brain tumor

No Drops for the Tumor

You will NOT be making tumor drops. It would be harmful, I believe. You do not want to strengthen the tumor.

But zapping it is supremely powerful. To single it out for zapping, attach a substance, **tricalcium phosphate**, to the organ slide (see page 176).

You do not need to make a bottle of the tumor since you can construct it easily on the plate for zapping. This adds a protection against ever taking drops of a tumor. Place your tricalcium phosphate sample touching the organ.

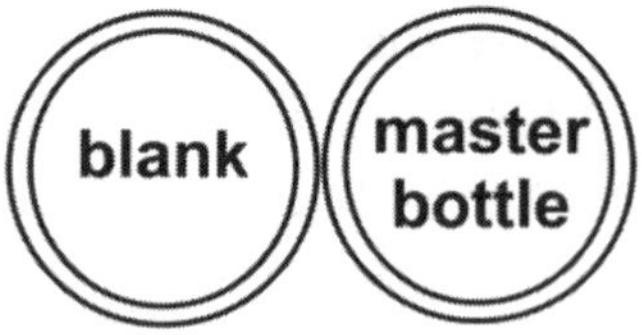

Fig. 68 To clone a sample, simply copy it

How often should you take drops? Whenever you start new drops, take them very often the first day, even every hour if possible. This increases the chance of treating it quickly because there is a cumulative action; 6 times a day is the minimum for a new organ.

Whenever intensive *take-out* treatment is planned, be sure you can take enough organic germanium, selenite and vitamin C (rose hips) too. Imagine if you could build a house in one day. It would be a very busy building site. You dare not run out of one frequently used supply, such as nails!

After two days of intensive treatment, most of the action is done. You should go down to 3 times daily for 2 more days. After this all *take-out* drops should be stopped but continue protective or *organ drops*. Continue these once a day. Hopefully you made copies and labeled all your bottles. So, if you had a new emergency, you could repeat it all, quickly.

Keep a daily log of zaps done and drops taken, along with a note about symptoms felt, if any, at each organ.

Next, make drops for every organ that is involved in your illness. For example, you may have:

- pain at right hip
- a new lump

Pain At Bones

Pain at bones is a very common experience. But how do you know which bone it is? How could you find exactly which bone to zap and make drops for? Chances are excellent that a chicken has such a bone. Its frequency pattern would be close to yours. Purchase chicken parts that include this bone. Cook till meat can be removed. It should not be completely removed; cartilage and attached tendons and gristle should be left on the bones. After removing meat, separate the large bones, but small bones can stay together. Place on paper towels to air dry, labeling them first, including left or right side. After 3 weeks in a warm place they should be fairly dry. (You do not need to dry them before using them.) Then put larger bones in their own zippered bags. Several smaller bones can share a bag. To find the bone that matches your painful bone, you would need a Syncrometer®*. But if you can guess which bones have your pain, you can copy them altogether into 2 bottles, one for zapping, and one for drops. Keep your real bones in the refrigerator.

A Lump

A lump visible under the skin often cannot be given an organ name using slides or specimens. Even a small lump on the face can be impossible to give a location for your plate.

To be able to zap these precisely, you can make a **paper skin copy** of them. The frequencies of energy coming from the body leave through the skin and can be caught in water placed there.

The copy will not be for drop-making since it is your own (not from a healthy rat or monkey). But it will serve for analysis by Syncrometer® and for zapping. Label it: ZAP ONLY.

Paper Body Wipe

By wiping over a skin area with a damp paper towel (folded 4 times to make a wad), you pick up the natural skin moisture and sweat. It will contain the frequency pattern of organs under it.

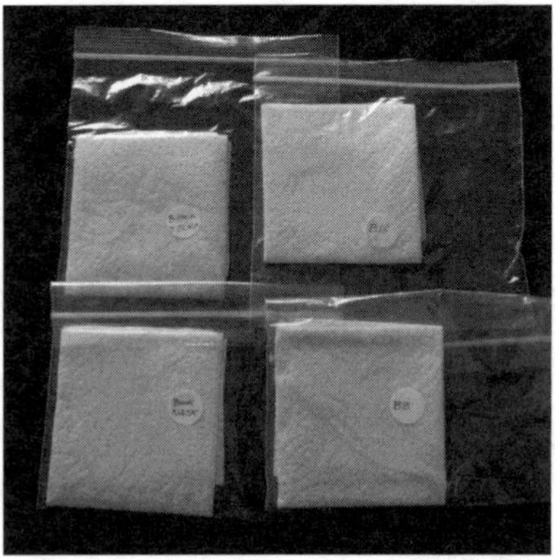

Body wipes made of damp paper towel pick up evidence of problems beneath skin at locations given.

Fig. 69 Radiation-free scan

* Testers, search for Streptococcus pneumoniae (pain) bacteria in bone locations, using chicken bones. Place bag of bones beside patient's saliva sample. Search for Strep pneu, OPT, etc. If *Positive*, test each bone.

You can use it directly for zapping. Do not make drops out of it; they would be "SICK" drops, coming from yourself.

Paper Skin Copy

Cut a circle out of white, unfragranced paper towel to fit over the lump. Carry a small amount of pure water with you to the couch where you can lie down for 10 minutes. Place the paper over the lump and pour enough water on yourself to hold the paper against the skin everywhere. Wait 10 minutes. Pick it up with your fingers inside a zippered bag. (Gloves could shed heavy metals.) The same way, stuff the paper into an empty amber glass test bottle or a plastic zippered bag. The damp paper should touch the bottom of the bottle. Shake it down till it reaches the bottom of the bottle. That is why you should use glass...to be able to see it. A zippered bag should be folded so the paper sample is only one plastic layer away from the plate. Do not add water. Close, label it; for example: Below Left Eye. Use this bottle or bag to zap. In this way you can zap and search any location on your body.

Zapper Alchemy

Freshly cracked apricot seeds and freshly picked Eucalyptus leaves are somewhat perishable—so just stuff them into a half-ounce glass bottle (no water used), or zippered plastic bag, and copy them for posterity! Label *master*. Taking drops of such copies gives you some of the effectiveness of the real thing; in general, about one-fourth.

Clone your *masters* for drop-taking and copy the copies before they are half consumed in order to continue getting strong copies.

Summary — Chapter 7

1. You can copy anything into a bottle of water and keep it intact for years.

2. Such a bottle-copy can be used to take "drops" that strengthen an organ or remove things from an organ.

3. Rain water collected an hour after rain has started is the safest water, provided you collect it in HDPE containers without filtering.

4. Copying into water is an extremely sensitive procedure. You must be extremely concerned over details.

5. Taking gold out of problem organ may become the most useful of all bottles. This is because gold has become attached, permanently, to many pathogens and because gold is found in chlorox bleach as well as many foods. At the same time it presents a special difficulty for the body to excrete it.

6. Making medicines and adding substances are logical applications that work. But it has its hazards. Medicines, supplements and herbs are extremely polluted with chlorox bleach, meaning polonium, and the whole list of carcinogens. Finding one without dyes, chlorox, heavy metals or radioactivity would be almost impossible unless they are unchlorinated. Taking the drops anyway would be taking magnified doses of the toxins, too. Copy only tested items. To protect yourself further, take them only 4 days.

CHAPTER 8

SHRINKING TUMORS

A tumor grows and a tumor accumulates. These are its most unique and destructive properties.

Just outside the tumor, only millimeters away, growth can be normal. We see this in liver tumors quite clearly. We could study the normal cells with a Syncrometer® and compare each detail with the tumor cells so close by. That is how the research for this chapter was done.

Normal organs regulate their own size. If the cells grow just a percentage too much the organ gets too big. Normally, a small percentage of cells is digesting itself; this makes the organ smaller. Imagine removing 1 brick out of every 100 in a large brick building; it would get smaller. To keep the same size, as our organs do, the cells that grow must equal the cells that get digested. Such self-digestion is called **apoptosis**.

Certain parasites and viruses slow down the speed of self digestion or apoptosis. This extends the life of tumor cells. These viruses are called oncoviruses, meaning tumor-promoting. The body's rules do not allow digestion at exactly the same time as growth is called for. That would be as inefficient as stepping on the brakes and accelerator at the same time in a car. We will search for about a dozen of the most important oncoviruses and destroy them by killing the parasites that bring them.

Accumulation Still Baffling

The accumulations inside tumors are more mysterious. Why thousands of toxins such as asbestos, azo dyes, heavy metals, and motor oil are coming to the tumor instead of to the kidneys for excretion has no satisfactory explanation yet.

Actually the toxins are not coming to the organ; they are coming to the tumor <u>in</u> this organ. The tumor is always south polarized. If the tumor is made of stem cells, this south polarization would be expected since stem cells' chief job is dividing in two to make growth. But why are they accumulating toxins instead of carefully screening them out?

The beginning tumor is inflamed and actively making PGE2. This makes the cells sticky so everything passing by sticks to them. Radioactive elements, lanthanide elements, bacteria, parasite stages such as eggs, and viruses all stick to the tiny tumor.

Why did these tumor cells and organ cells get inflamed? The Syncrometer® only finds 3 reasons. When these 3 reasons are gone the inflammation and PGE2 are gone, too. They are radioactivity, nickel, and an allergic food. The kidneys are constantly excreting radioactivity and nickel but the WBCs must capture them first. The nickel is stuck in very thick, sticky, wheel bearing grease. How can that get through the kidneys to the bladder?

In a cancer patient the kidneys are overworked by all the toxins in the chlorox bleach, and their WBCs are underfed.

They must wait for germanium, selenium and vitamin C to come along and feed their enzymes. But they can't wait too long, not more than a day. Then the toxins break loose and circulate again, this time finding the inflamed organ. They stick to it. The inflamed organ and its WBCs are south polarized and can't help at all. The organ cells fill up next, and all of them waiting for help from the WBCs, your immune systems' carriers.

That is why our program starts by feeding the WBCs their essential 3 nutrients. The kidneys' WBCs get fed first. Then they are stimulated with homeographic drops. This starts the whole detoxification process going.

Soon toxins will flow to the kidneys again and out of the body with urine excretion. The liver and other organs will follow this pattern next.

Other therapists have used the same strategy, using many kidney and liver stimulating techniques, and helping them with detoxifying supplements.

Nordenström[22], a radiologist, saw evidence of an electrical or magnetic force surrounding the tumor on the x-rays of tumors he took. My studies show south polarization, a magnetic force, at the tumor zone when north is normal. Fully understanding the implications of this must wait for the future.

We only need to keep feeding the kidney WBCs their ordinary "foods" to keep them excreting toxins for us. Extraordinary stimulation comes from the *"take-out"* drops. While the kidneys and their WBCs keep working we can turn to the task of stopping excess growth which will be there even after the malignancy is gone. We must learn to understand it.

Human Growth Hormone

Our pituitary gland, the very one involved in making the tumor nucleus, makes many hormones. One of them is human growth hormone, HGH. It is supremely important. The Syncrometer® sees that it is produced regularly for healing, especially at night. Then it is promptly excreted, even in the night. Maybe it is too dangerous to salvage or keep till morning. It is extremely powerful, so it is very carefully controlled—by the hypothalamus gland right above it. See page 82 and the drawing (next page). After all, we must not become eight feet tall or have extra long

[22] Björn Nordenström, radiologist www.ursus.se/ursus/publications.shtml

teeth or too short fingers. The pituitary gland is not allowed to release its HGH into the body until a **releasing hormone** arrives, made by the hypothalamus.

This is the case for other hormones, too. Each one must get its final permission, its releasing hormone, from the hypothalamus. It is like having both an accelerator and brake in a car. They are placed side by side to control speed. But it is the driver who will choose which one to use, not the foot.

It is the whole brain that decides which control the hypothalamus will choose. These are some of the hormones made by the pituitary gland:

- Human Growth Hormone (HGH)
- Thyroid Stimulating Hormone (TSH)
- Follicle Stimulating Hormone (FSH)
- Luteinizing Hormone (LH)
- Prolactin

These hormones are the accelerators for our organs.

Each hormone stimulates a particular organ, but not too much. The hypothalamus can put on the brakes by stopping releases and staying in charge.

These are the releasing hormones sent out by the hypothalamus to control the pituitary:

- Growth Hormone Releasing Factor (GHRF or GRF))
- Thyrotropin Releasing Hormone (TRH)
- LH/FSH Releasing Hormone (GnRH)
- Luteinizing Hormone Releasing Hormone (LHRH or LRH)
- Prolactin Releasing Factor (PRF)

Notice that each hormone has its matching releasing hormone.

This system works well for us. The brain surrounding these two glands <u>knows</u> whether more of a hormone is needed or not. Messages from our organs are constantly coming to the brain telling it what is needed next. These are our "master glands" because they work to respond to our most basic needs. Maybe it should not be so surprising that all cancers start right here. These organs are in charge of growth.

Hypothalamus cells that have left the parent organ during its micro-explosion are far away from the brain. They cannot receive messages from the brain. They keep right on making releasing factors, without a stop, some more, some less. The pituitary cells must receive them because they have become attached to the hypothalamus cells by fusing. In a duplex or triplet they are like Siamese twins, forced to do things together. They will be forced to make and release HGH without a stop. We will find high levels of HGH in the tumors of every cancer patient. They will be high enough to find in the saliva and urine day and night. What could be more abnormal and how can it be stopped?

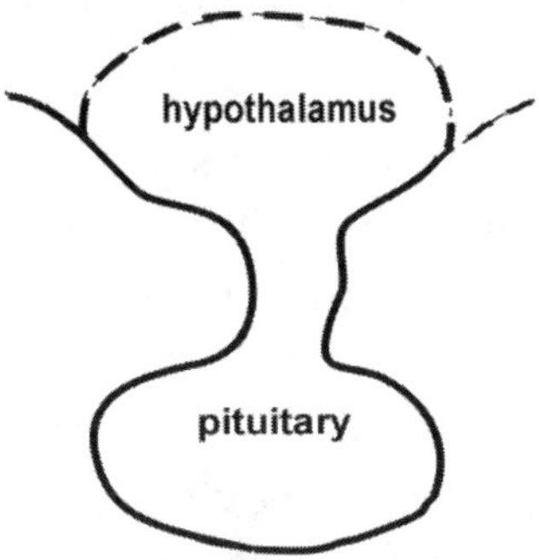

Fig. 70 The hypothalamus controls the pituitary gland

Just as mysterious, and vital to this picture, is **stem cell factor (SCF)**. The hypothalamus gland appears to make it, especially at night in healthy people. It, too, gets excreted at night. But again, it should be under tight brain control and it is not in cancer patients. It is being produced night and day without a stop.

Stem Cell Factor

How can a seed grow into a tree? How can a whole human being, made of some trillion cells grow from one male cell and one female cell, fused? What does fusion do? Is it more than just adding chromosomes?

Each original cell (egg and sperm) came packed with a little bit of a substance called stem cell factor. Plant seeds use the identical substance, as found by the Syncrometer®.

It is kept strictly where cell division is wanted, nowhere else. It also comes with a tiny bit of **iridium-complex**, perhaps a special product made to accompany SCF. We will learn more about this soon.

How An Organ Grows

An organ like your liver or prostate is made of very many tiny cells, easy to see under a microscope. They remind us of bricks used to build a wall and, actually, the whole building.

But cells are alive, connected to each other, and after a life of hard work, such as 10 days for some and months for others, they are aged and dying. Their cell voltage has run down. But just dying would be quite toxic to the rest of the body. Wounds give you this kind of toxicity. It would decay and be a burden to the body. You would get an extreme detoxification illness. You can't even allow a dead tooth to stay in the body without becoming toxic. Such a death is called **necrosis**. The aged cell is therefore not allowed to just die. It is carefully taken apart beforehand, dismantled in an orderly way, so that nothing toxic is produced and so useful things can be recycled. This is the process of apoptosis. Still, after this there is a hole in the organ structure where the old dead cell was. It needs to be filled. If such holes were not filled, the organ would soon get smaller and smaller. Does this happen as we age? We do seem to get smaller and smaller after middle age. Has this become unregulated in a cancerous tumor so the organ gets bigger and bigger instead?

It was thought until quite recently that any neighboring cell, where a hole had been left, could simply divide itself into two, then the one extra cell could fill the hole. This is not how it happens. To divide, a cell must stop its work schedule because chromosomes can't be duplicating themselves and working making proteins (being translated) at the same time. A cell has to prepare in an elaborate way for its own duplication. It must acquire more proteins and extra DNA first. It takes about a day to go through one cell division (bacteria can do it in 20 minutes). After this it must prepare again to go back to its normal work, called **metabolism**. It is inefficient to shift from metabolism to cell division and back again repeatedly.

The body, and plants too, have a different scheme. Each organ has a few cells set aside. They are spread throughout the organ. Their only job is to divide when called upon. There is no delay. They are always ready; they have what is needed. It does not interrupt the work schedule of others. These are called **stem cells***. How do they know when to divide and let the new cell slip into the hole? Stem cell factor reaches them to give them this important message. Stem cell factor is only sent when there is a need. It is only sent to southerly polarized locations.

It seems, from Syncrometer® studies, that only the hypothalamus makes stem cell factor; other organs, of the ones studied (most of the brain), did not. While the hypothalamus cells are in the brain, in their normal place, stem cell factor is made according to a demand from some damaged organ. This organ has a spot that has turned southerly. The damage itself has caused iron oxidation, this seems to be the way that magnetization switches to southerly. Oxidized iron is Fe_2O_3, common ferrite, and ferric substances. The brain learns about it immediately, in less than a second from the time you cut yourself. The

* Testers, search for placenta or umbilical cord, in any organ to identify the stem cells.

injured region, now being south polarized, invites stem cell factor.

SCF brings with it a "welcome wagon" of iridium and other trace minerals. Now new cells can be made. In a wound new cells are needed. But away from the brain, when hypothalamus and pituitary cells are afloat, it is not based on need; they continue to make SCF and HGH all the time. The Syncrometer® detects them all around the tumor and wherever a tumor nucleus has been "planted". They are even attached to bacteria and viruses!

SCF will surely reach some nearby stem cells in the organ where the tumor nucleus has landed*. Stem cells in the neighborhood could be expected to respond by dividing. I can still only speculate about how this happens. In fact, it may even be the stem cells themselves that are chosen for the fusions when runaway cells find each other. It may even be the stem cells that make the entire tumor. Recent Syncrometer® results show that the cancer-complex and the tumor nucleus both select the stem cells. This could even be the reason why tumor cells never mature (differentiate) into non-dividing, working cells. Electron microscope studies could make these details clear.

Cysts…Another Kind of Growth

Sometimes a mass can be seen on an ultrasound or scan that is not a malignant growing tumor. It appears to have grown for a while, then stopped and gotten encased by the body in a smooth thick coat. It is obvious to a radiologist that it is "only a cyst". What made it start and stop growing?

A cyst starts out the same way as a dangerous tumor. Bits of hypothalamus have come loose. They have fused

* Testers, construct "stem cells in an organ" by touching placenta to the organ slide. Umbilical cord slide works well, too. Search for SCF here.

with cells from the pituitary gland that were also loose and afloat. These duplexes swarmed about, free to join another organ. One such duplex has joined a third organ because Fasciolas and Ascaris stages are nearby. The Syncrometer® spots them easily. Lots of fibronectin and gluey threads are present to make the third organ a sticky trap. Now there is a tiny transplant of cells made of hypothalamus, pituitary and the third organ. But it is not the pancreas.

A cyst in the kidney has a "nucleus" made of hypothalamus, pituitary, and kidney cells. It is missing the pancreas portion. It does not have a true tumor nucleus.

The hypothalamus portion sends out its releasing factors, its SCF and iridium-complex. We will discuss this complex soon. The pituitary portion sends out HGH and its whole troop of hormones as demanded by the hypothalamus. The newly formed cyst begins to respond by dividing.

The organ also responds to the new hormones being poured into it. It may respond to **prolactin** if the cyst is developing in the breast. This makes the breast produce fluid. The kidney can respond to **vasopressin**, which would raise the blood pressure. The prostate can enlarge with excess male hormones in response to excess FSH. An organ, whether it is the ovary or prostate, always tries to make proper use of all hormones arriving there. All these responses can change the organ that received the tiny transplant, giving it too many "receptors" and even enlarging it.

In spite of all this, the newly growing mass does not grow endlessly in a runaway manner like a cancerous tumor. Just what force the body exerts or which chemical it produces to stop the growth of the cyst is a mystery. It should be studied. Apoptosis in a cyst is not totally blocked the way it is in a tumor. The numerous oncoviruses (viruses that start tumors) are missing in the cyst. Natural cell death by apoptosis can keep up with cell growth. But is that all? An endpoint is reached for the cyst when the body finally encases it, so no more toxins or bacteria can enter and accumulations must stop. It is undoubtedly meant to protect your body. It is now fairly harmless, but only fairly. A real tumor nucleus, complete with a pancreas portion could still be formed, could easily land in the same location and change everything.

SV40 stands for simian virus #40.

The difference in the cyst is the absence of the pancreas cells and a virus that comes with pancreas cells. It is called SV40.

The Secret Of Pancreas Cells

The presence of pancreas cells in the tumor nucleus makes the difference between forming a cyst or forming an ever growing tumor. Does the pancreas cell provide something unique that makes the body powerless to restrain the growing force in the tumor nucleus? In stem cell factor? In HGH? In the iridium-complex? Does the pancreas cell bring something that removes the limit on cell division that every human cell should have? Does it bring a block on apoptosis so cells can never terminate and digest themselves as normal aged cells do? These were things the Syncrometer® searched for and did not find. What it found in the pancreas cells were merely SV40 viruses! But they were not alone. Attached to its "coat tails" were a series of oncoviruses, much like skaters holding hands, pulling each other along. And all of them, the whole troop, were outside the pancreas cells, too, trying to get into the cells. But only the organ with the tumor could let them in, not others. Nearly all bacteria, which are also cells, would let them in. Some attachments are even to other regular viruses, like Flu and mumps, all sticking together. They formed a gang. Small gangs of viruses are arriving in the organ where the tumor nucleus has attached itself, and in all the local bacteria. Their leader is SV40.

The Secret Of SV40

This virus has already been researched extensively. It is called an oncovirus because it can start tumors when it is given to animals; *onco* means *tumor*. How can it do this? We will soon see.

The Syncrometer® sees that the virus arrives in the body with the pancreatic fluke and escapes quickly to infect our pancreas*. Then it enters our blood. Once in the blood it can reach any organ quickly. Soon SV40 can be detected all over the body. But it does not start tumors in all these locations. Nor does it bring a special symptom. It seemingly can't get into most places. The body cells are keeping it out. It can only get in at one site, besides at bacteria. It will be the primary tumor site. Why there?

Our special immune cells, **lymphocytes**, normally eat and kill viruses. They are ready for these SV40's. They can all be eaten very quickly. But, again, to kill them the lymphocytes need organic germanium, organic selenium (or selenite) and vitamin C. The minerals make up their killing-enzymes. The vitamin C (preferably organic, as in rose hips) has an unknown action and some actions that are known, but my speculation is that it does much more. A cancer patient's lymphocytes are deficient in germanium, selenium and vitamin C, being full of azo dyes, wheel bearing grease, mercury, and nickel instead.

* Testers, search for pancreas / SV40 in the lymph; and SV40 in the pancreas organ.

The cancer patients' minerals become oxidized by these heavy metals and by chlorine, as have the iron molecules inside the lymphocytes. The killing enzymes don't work. The Syncrometer® finds no peroxidase, for instance. The iron in this enzyme was oxidized. Plain germanium, plain selenium, plain ferrite (Fe_2O_3), plain ferric phosphate, are all quite toxic to these same enzymes.

Oxidized minerals become plain metals.

When the deficient lymphocytes cannot kill the SV40 oncoviruses which they have eaten, the viruses break free again, to continue their body invasion. They invade quickly and multiply quickly.

The Syncrometer® detects SV40 wherever there are pancreatic flukes in cancer patients. Yet, other people (and cows!) may have innumerable pancreatic flukes, in diabetes for example, without showing the SV40 virus! What is the difference between cancer patients and others? We will soon see.

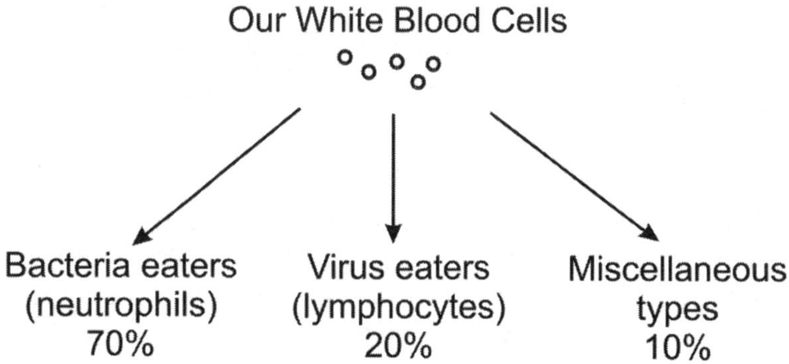

Fig. 71 Our white blood cells are specialized into classes

SV40 is believed to come to us from certain monkeys in Africa and from contamination of polio vaccine given to us years ago. These may indeed have been sources. But the Syncrometer® detects an ongoing source, the common pancreatic fluke. Possibly these monkeys had pancreatic flukes then, as many animals do now. Parasitism must be millions of years old. **Horses**, **dogs** and **cats** that have contracted cancer today, have the pancreatic fluke with its SV40 viruses just as we do. Chickens in the market place (in USA) have them, although we do not pronounce them cancerous, or even dangerous!

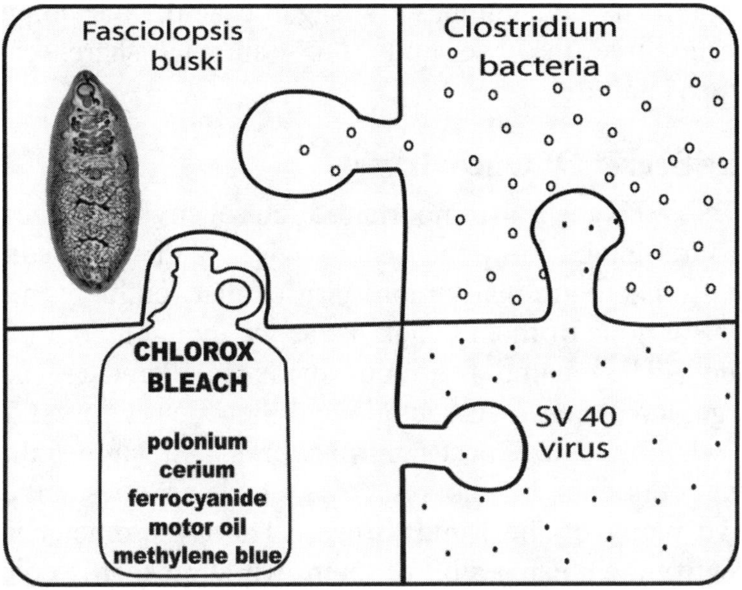

A cancer parasite, cancer bacteria and cancer virus are three living actors that play essential roles in the cancer drama. Chlorox bleach is the immunity depressor that also brings the polonium-cerium-ferrocyanide-motor oil and methylene blue alkylators to the patient. Chlorox disinfected water gets direct access to our DNA.

Fig. 72 The cancer puzzle

SV40 viruses, like other viruses, must be triggered to emerge. In animals or in humans they can be triggered by one food phenolic substance, gallic acid. This is the same substance that acted like an allergen and inflamed the pancreas to make roaming cells. It can do two things: inflame the pancreas, and trigger the SV40 virus out of the pancreatic fluke. Diabetics are not full of gallic acid as cancer patients are. Chickens used as human food in the market place (in USA) are full of gallic acid. Other animals with cancer are full of gallic acid, like human cancer patients. This conclusion is based on small numbers of horses, cats, dogs and chickens (not like the hundreds upon hundreds of humans tested) but there were no exceptions. It seems very probable that the trigger for releasing SV40 viruses from pancreatic flukes is the same for animals and humans. It is gallic acid…the common preservative that we and "our" animals share, called **propyl gallate**!

The Secret Of Oncoviruses

SV40 is the most important of our oncoviruses because it starts gangs forming. That is why I call it the **cancer virus**. There are many more viruses that routinely invade us. But none of them attack us, as we thought, "out of the blue". They come from our parasites. Parasites, being large, have their own bacteria and their own viruses! That is why biological pest-control works. All large animals that get tumors, like horses, cows, chickens, dogs and cats, have many of the same viruses. The Syncrometer® can identify them using a bit of their own DNA that is unique. If the Syncrometer® finds a bit of a virus gene in a parasite or in us, I might assume the virus is there, not just the gene. And when the gene has spread throughout the body I might, again, assume the virus is present and spreading, not just a gene. That is how the Syncrometer® research was done—with oncogenes. But my research leads to the conclusion that they represent real viruses, spawned by specific parasites.

Common oncoviruses in humans besides SV40 are RAS, FOS, MYC, JUN, SRC, and NEU (also called ERB). Besides these we have Flu, mumps, CMV, hepatitis B, EBV, and Adenovirus, which may not be true oncoviruses but which frequently participate in a cancer patient's illness.

The Syncrometer® shows that each oncovirus enters us from a parasite or other invader that actually lives in us. In the following table are listed the oncoviruses seen in all cancer patients, some more, some less, all more frequent in the organ involved in the cancer because that is where the parasite also lives.

Together, the oncovirus gang keeps cancer cells growing endlessly (immortalized) and makes bacteria appear resistant to anything we use against them (also immortalized), such as antibiotics. It makes them appear to be drug resistant by gene-decree!

In the following table the name of the parasite is given that brings each oncovirus and the trigger required to activate the virus genes. This lets you stop triggering it immediately.

Parasites Bring Oncoviruses Table

Parasite	**Oncovirus* it carries**	**Virus trigger**	**Kill parasite with**
Ascaris	measles	linolenic oil	ginkgo leaf, chrysanthemum
Ascaris lumbricoides	NEU measles Adenovirus 16	linolenic acid (food oil), quercitin	starvation¤[¤], cysteine, levamisole, ripe jalapeño seeds, BQ & RZ
Ascaris megalocephala	NEU	linolenic acid (food oil)	
Ascaris megalocephala	mumps papilloma warts	casein (dairy food), ASA	
Ascaris mixed	Adenovirus (common cold) Adenovirus 16	myristic oil, linoleic oil, quercitin	
chicken & eggs**	MYC		avoid unless tested

*Oncovirus genes are underlined.

¤ This means not eating the food required by the parasite.

**Not parasites, of course, but playing the role of parasites when we eat them. MYC is not killed by ordinary cooking, baking or frying. But 3 hydrochloric acid drops kills it.

Parasite	Oncovirus* it carries	Virus trigger	Kill parasite with
Clonorchis (human liver fluke)	Hepatitis B	umbelliferone (carrots)	starvation, BWT ***, 6 fresh seed recipe
Dirofilaria (dog heartworm)	FOS	oleic acid (olive oil, other oils)	starvation, levamisole, BWT
Echinoporyphium recurvatum	EBV papilloma warts, Adenovirus 16	rutin, hesperidin, vitamin D3	starvation, cilantro, chaparral
Echinostoma revolutum	Adenovirus 36 (obesity virus)		starvation
Eurytrema pancreaticum (pancreatic fluke)	SV40	gallic acid	starvation, BWT, 6 fresh seed recipe, cactus ****
F. buski (intestinal fluke)	MYC		starvation, BWT, spices, 6 fresh seed recipe
F. buski (intestinal fluke)	Flu	death of parasite host	
F. buski (intestinal fluke)	HIV	benzene	
Onchocerca	JUN	strontium	BWT, burdock root, starvation, levamisole
Plasmodium (malaria)	SV40-HIV		6 fresh seed recipe, Eucalyptus, starvation
Strongyloides	CMV (Cytomegalo virus)	lauric acid (lard, food oils)	starvation, levamisole
Strongyloides	EBV (Epstein Barre virus)	linolenic and palmitic food oils	
Strongyloides	SRC	lauric acid (food oil)	
yeast (bread)	RAS	asparagine	turmeric, chromium deprivation

Fig. 73 Parasites, their oncoviruses and triggers

If we have 10 oncoviruses, should we expect to have about 10 parasites as their sources? Yes. At first, a newly

***BWT refers to the whole green Black Walnut tincture recipe, including wormwood and cloves.

****This is prickly pear cactus, an ethnic food in Mexico.

diagnosed cancer patient might only have 5 or 6, but as the disease advances the numbers and varieties go up. The body becomes the host for a teeming population of bacteria, yeast and parasite stages, trading their oncoviruses with each other and adding to their total number.

Meanwhile, the bacteria have changed, too; they are not acting like themselves anymore because of their multiple viruses. Our tumor cells are now full of these infected bacteria besides oncoviruses. They might look glassy, waxy, pink, and bumpy, not at all normal. Skin with tumor cells is rough and hard, not smooth and soft. In the past, these places were called "proud flesh" or "cancer" (meaning crab-like). They might grow "roots" or tangles or wrap-around sheaths, not normal cell behavior. The genes inside the tumor cells seem to be adulterated with those from viruses, bacteria, and even bread yeast. All these must be killed and stopped from multiplying before the tumor can shrink. But they are protected!

> Radioactivity protects parasites! Polonium protects F. buski specifically.

It also protects E. revolutum. Since uranium produces polonium, the parasite actually has 2 protectors. E. revolutum is also protected by thorium.

Remember, shrinking a tumor requires 3 processes: apoptosis, ordinary digestion, and white blood cell phagocytosis. This means self-digestion, digestion by our own enzymes, and being eaten by CD8 and CD14 white blood cells. First, we will stop its growth by removing SCF, HGH and radioactivity. Then we will start its apoptosis by removing Ascaris and all other parasites that bring us oncoviruses. Digestion by our stomach and pancreas enzymes will follow and we will also supplement it. Then we will dispose of the remains with CD8 and CD14 white blood cells whose immune power is restored. When all 3 processes are started, it only takes days to see shrinkage visibly or feel it internally. If you do not, search for the missing process using the *Testers Guide* or *Flow Sheet*.

Growth itself always occurs in 2 parts: the accelerators and decelerators (brakes). The main accelerators are SCF and HGH, but contributors are DNA suppliers, ribonucleotide reductase suppliers, thiourea producers, carcinoembryonic antigen (CEA) makers, Human Chorionic Gonadotropin (HCG) makers, and south pole forces. The decelerators are our longevity-limiter gene, our pyruvic aldehyde, and north pole forces. We will soon get to know all of these and regain control.

Stopping making SCF and HGH is quite easy by stopping the erosion of the hypothalamus and pituitary glands, namely with diet. By now you may already have done this. Stopping overproduction of DNA, RRase and thiourea is quite easy, too, by killing Clostridium bacteria. Stopping HCG is easy, by killing Fasciolopsis cercaria, so they can't become part of the cancer-complex. CEA, DNA polymerase, and AFP (alpha feto protein) will be removed by killing bread yeast. Switching south pole to north pole forces is instantly accomplished by removing nickel, even though it is buried in wheel bearing grease and will return many times before the whole body is degreased.

Cleaning and feeding the WBCs is quite easy. Supplying extra enzymes is quite easy. Supplying pyruvic aldehyde is easy with homeographic drops. North pole forces can be brought in with zapping. The pair of substances, thiourea and pyruvic aldehyde can be regulated by killing most bacteria; see discussion in the earlier book, *The Cure For All Advanced Cancers*.

We will soon be in control of the tumor's growth and shrinkage and can follow our progress if we can test with a Syncrometer®.

The miracle in our lives is that even at this late stage we can fix this desperate situation.

Only radioactivity is still to be conquered. There are many kinds, each element being unique. Each turns on your DNA at a slightly different time in the course of one minute. Turning on your DNA can make the tissue grow. The body can remove the radioactive elements itself with the help of chelators, but not if they are locked into the teeth. Finding them first with a dental probe, any dentist can remove them as we will see.

Summary — Chapter 8

1. In order to shrink, a tumor must stop growing and start being digested.

2. There are 2 kinds of digestion: self digestion, called apoptosis and ordinary digestion by your own enzymes.

3. A tumor will shrink much faster if your 2 kinds of lymphocytes start to eat it. They are the CD8s and CD14s. These are the only cells allowed to eat your cells. But they can't eat anything if they themselves are full of nickel. Nickel also turns them southerly.

4. The reason that toxins and other refuse accumulate in our tumors is not clear yet, but seems to be due to blockage of the kidneys and underfeeding the WBCs. The WBCs require organic germanium, selenium, and vitamin C.

5. Cancerous tumors are full of HGH and stem cell factor, being forced to produce these by the tumor nucleus.

6. Stem cells may be the chosen cells to receive the tumor nucleus and for the attachment of the cancer-complex, perhaps even for the whole tumor. This would explain the absence of differentiation in tumor cells.

7. Stem cell factor brings to the stem cells packets of ultra trace minerals including the iridium-complex, evidently to get the new healing points supplied with them.

8. Cysts are missing the pancreas part of the tumor nucleus so they never get infected with SV40.

9. The pituitary part of the tumor nucleus makes many hormones. These stimulate the organ with the tumor nucleus.

10. Parasites bring oncoviruses, which bring immortality to cancer cells.

11. Growth is increased by any radioactive element. When radioactive elements are locked into your tooth fillings you cannot get away from the constant stimulation of your tumor's growth.

CHAPTER 9

OUR COSMIC CONNECTIONS

Healing

The body must heal itself every day from the damage done by living. It seems to do this at night. We may go to bed with aches and pains but wake up good as new…at least in childhood. But nighttime is a difficult time to study anything with a Syncrometer® so more research is badly needed on the subject of body repair.

The body must also heal special places if big traumas occurred, like burning, cutting, smashing. These places get healed day and night. This is the kind of healing I studied for this chapter. It is a subtle, quiet process, as astounding as the nature of stars and the cosmos. Maybe we should not be so surprised since we are a part of it.

Falling down from the sky, as gently as miniscule feathers, is the cosmic dust. Day and night, night and day, sometimes more, sometimes less, cosmic dust and bits of meteorite land on everything…the grass, the ponds, the fur of animals…everything except human beings. Only we humans have sheltered ourselves from the cosmic dust most of the time, especially in the last century.

It comes down in larger amounts during a rain. Every wild animal gets some dust when the dust isn't even 1 minute old. Animals lick it off their fur. They drink it from the ponds, rivers and tiny trickles that run through the ground. Even plants drink it up through their roots. Only humans do not. We "purify" it out of our water. First, we filter it through gravel, aluminum and sand. Then we add a very strong oxidizing disinfectant, such as chlorine. We do not eat or drink the tiny flakes of cosmic dust, or at least very little. We have given up a precious natural resource, the cosmic dust, and with it the life-supporting element, iridium.

We should think about our lost cosmic connections in our own quiet moments. There is no evidence favoring or for discarding such notions. But until we can study them we should surely preserve more of our animal heritage.

What Is Iridium?

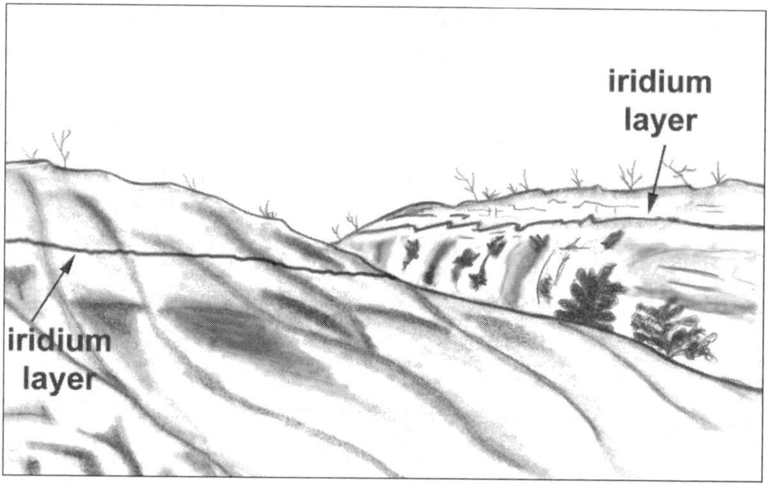

All around our planet a thin (¼") line of black sediment is the iridium dust that landed 65 million years ago. It marks the end of the dinosaur age. Read more about this K-T boundary on the Internet.

Fig. 74 Drawing of earth's iridium layer

A black layer of dust landed on our planet 65 million years ago. Now it is only ¼ inch thick, compacted under all the layers of sediment that has since been added. This thin layer contains large amounts of iridium. It fell to earth with the meteor that landed swiftly and suddenly at that time, digging a huge crater in the soil and raising a dust cloud that circled the earth. Dust loaded with iridium would fall for 100 years afterwards, and then stop, leaving only the gently falling cosmic dust again. What is on a cosmic dust particle?

Catching The Cosmic Dust

If you set out a new zippered plastic bag, unopened, on a dinner plate, you can catch a sample of cosmic dust anywhere outdoors. Other kinds of plastic or a bare plate might seep and contribute its own elements. (The bag should not test *Positive* for chlorox bleach, either, or it will contribute many more elements. You can find a good plastic bag with a conductivity indicator, see page 614). Let the covered plate stand outside for 10 minutes only. Cut a 2" x 2" square of paper towel, dampen it slightly with tap water and take a swipe across the bag (well water has more elements that could be confusing). Hurry indoors to test it by Syncrometer®*. You will find an iridium compound, a cobalt compound, a selenium compound made of selenite, a chromium and a germanium compound, a vanadium compound, a rubidium compound, but most of all, iron. It is magnetic iron, Fe_3O_4, also called magnetite. Remember to test the tap water alone, too, as well as the paper and a part of the plastic bag (bottom side) to serve as "controls", in case these elements come from them (they will not).

Now carry it all indoors. After 20 minutes take another swipe from the same plastic bag right beside the first swipe and notice that some "chemistry" has happened. What was coming down earlier was **tetra iridium dodecacarbonyl**. Each molecule of this compound is made of 4 atoms (tetra) of iridium surrounded by 12 (dodeca) carbonyl groups. Carbonyls are just carbon and oxygen held together with a double bond (C = O), also called carbon monoxide. Altogether, it is 4 iridium atoms inside a cluster of 12 carbon monoxide molecules.

---

* Place it in a zippered plastic bag for testing; later, test the controls for those things you find in the dust.

There was tetra cobalt dodecacarbonyl, and triiron dodecacarbonyl and similar other minerals. But soon these are all gone. In 20 minutes they have become much more oxidized. Now we see some plain iron, plain selenium, plain cobalt and chromium, plain vanadium, plain rubidium, and even some plain iridium powder, like the ¼ inch earth layer.

If the cosmic dust is wet, the minerals oxidize much faster. Fresh raindrops develop these oxidized elements in less than 10 minutes. And if the sun is shining on them (not so common while it's raining) they switch their polarization!

The falling dust is north polarized as long as it contains Fe_3O_4 (magnetite). But in 10 minutes Fe_2O_3 is being formed which is south polarized. Polarized does not mean simply having a "pole". It means it shows the <u>influence</u> of a magnetic pole.*

All the raindrops and rainwater collected is north polarized when it lands on earth (in Italy, Spain, Mexico and USA). All living creatures drink it in this state. Again, only humans waste it. Humans drink municipally supplied water, which has no predictable polarization. All the chlorox bleach waters were south polarized! NSF bleach water was often north polarized.

What Is Polarization?

We are familiar with the north and south poles of a magnet. Many kinds of iron, even nails and tin cans of food have a north and south pole in them, showing us the strength of the earth's magnetic field, which produced

* Testers, use a sample of very pure water, in an amber glass bottle that has been placed on a large ceramic magnet labeled north for 3 to 5 minutes. The large magnet size ensures that you won't be near an edge where some flux lines of the other (south) side might trespass. Label this sample *north*. Also make a *south* water test bottle.

them. Less than ½ gauss, which is the approximate strength of the earth's field in USA, sounds small but it had the strength to produce these magnetized items! That is not polarization, though. It is **polarity**. All magnets have a south and north pole, called polarity. Often many poles lie like a pile of logs, not neatly aligned, in metal objects. Going around the rim of a tin can with a compass even shows reversals that identify where the pole's axis is switched. Each axis has poles at the ends.

There is never a south pole without a north pole and, actually, all molecules whether made of iron or not have some polarity. To produce a polarity, all that is needed is a moving charge such as moving electrons and these are possessed by all molecules. But sometimes the polarity of a molecule is very strong and sometimes very weak. Strong polarity can reach out to neighboring molecules and align whole blocs of molecules into domains so that the crystal structure of a piece of metal is affected by them. Iron molecules are especially capable of this, so iron makes strong magnets.

If you have a rather long magnet, such as a 6 inch nail, the influence of each of the poles can be seen separately. One end is north and the other south. These forces are not the same, or merely in opposite directions. Water is influenced differently by the north and south pole of a magnet. Water is our most important substance. It is part of the very Nature of life, present everywhere in our bodies.

When a small bottle of water taken from the kitchen faucet is placed on the north pole of a magnet (actually standing right on it) something happens. It can easily be identified by the Syncrometer® later. After a few minutes the water will resonate with the north pole of a magnet and not with a south pole. A tiny 10 gauss ceramic magnet held 3" above the Syncrometer® plate with the north side down resonates the circuit when the north pole water is placed on the sister plate. Water placed on a south pole magnet will resonate with the south pole of a magnet held above the plate. Notice that the water develops the same polarization as the magnet it is placed on. It resonates with the same magnetic field that created it. This is opposite to the behavior of a metal like iron. If a piece of iron is placed near one pole of a magnet, the opposite pole is produced in the iron. And as surely as one pole is produced in iron, there is another pole produced farther away so that in reality both poles are produced.

Water behaves differently. It has been influenced by the magnet to produce the same pole-like behavior. Living tissue behaves like water. Only the same polarization is produced as the pole that made it. No equal and opposite polarization has ever been measured by Syncrometer®.

When rainwater falls into a plastic bag and is immediately tested with a Syncrometer® it is north polarized. It always contains Fe_30_4, which acts like a north pole. It is the same for the southern hemisphere. But its chemistry soon changes to more oxidized forms of minerals, and from Fe_3O_4 to Fe_2O_3, from magnetite to ferrite. When this has happened the water switches to south polarized. It now resonates with the south pole end of a real magnet or any sample of water that was placed on a south pole.

Water is called **diamagnetic**, maybe for similar reasons. Water without any iron is unpolarized. Water with both varieties of iron shows bipolarization, both north and south.

Should we be drinking water that is north polarized, namely, bringing minute amounts of Fe_30_4? Or should we be drinking south polarized, unpolarized, or bipolarized water? The water that induced cancer in all our cancer patients was south polarized. Remember that stem cell factor is attracted to south polarized regions. Cell division only occurs in south polarized places, according to Syncrometer® tests. Asbestos in water makes it south polarized.

Water is never pure in Nature. It has innumerable elements and compounds dissolved in it or floating about in it. Water from your tap has many more chemicals besides. They were added without regard for polarization. I believe it does matter, judging by these Syncrometer® observations.

Food, too, in its natural state is north polarized, except for the seed, which is south. Cell divisions will begin in the seed after water enters. The seed grows in water; all life takes place in water. Is the south pole a villain? Does it represent all that's bad? Not at all! Plant matter and animals are only north polarized by daytime! They switch in the night to south polarized. The switch back comes in the early morning with the first rays of sunlight, and repeats the cycle in the early evening, before sunset. South polarization must have vital importance, too.

Plants reproduce at some location within themselves. These locations are south polarized, just as they are in the human body. And the entire south polarized region, but never north, has stem cell factor present in it.

Back To Stem Cell Factor

Surprisingly, stem cell factor does not come alone when it arrives from the hypothalamus gland at a south polarized organ. It brings a gift to the healing zone. Stem cell factor as it comes in pure form from a manufacturer is just a bit of protein. But in the body it has company. Clustered together with SCF are these unusual substances:

- tetra iridium dodecacarbonyl
- tetra cobalt dodecacarbonyl
- triiron dodecacarbonyl

- Fe_3O_4 (magnetite)
- a selenium compound (not identified)
- tetra ruthenium dodecacarbonyl
- tetra rubidium dodecacarbonyl
- a germanium compound (not identified)
- a chromium compound (not identified)

Are these not surprisingly similar to the cosmic dust particles?

There was nothing else, though not exhaustively tested.

Do these represent elements needed by the body?

Should a sick body be given rainwater, iridium supplements, cosmic dust, compounds of minerals found in cosmic dust, Fe_3O_4, food that is perfectly fresh? All these questions must wait till more research can be done on them. But rainwater and fresh food need not wait. Fresh vegetables are the preference, in fact, the requirement, for many animals, and rainwater is all they drink. Rainwater is the true elixir of animals and plants. It tastes full-bodied and very good. Collect it after the rain has been coming down for an hour or so, after all smog and industrial chemicals have been washed down out of the sky in cities (this is very important). Wait 30 minutes in open countryside. Test it by Syncrometer® for its quality in your area. Test for beryllium (jet fuel), strontium (firecrackers), vanadium (fossil fuel), and chromium. Do not drink such polluted water. Do not let your rainwater stand in sunlight (it switches polarization). Do not let it stand open. It absorbs so much carbon dioxide from the air it soon tastes "sharp", like carbonation. Do not filter it if there are no particles in it (see *Rain Filter* page 202).

Catch snow in a stainless steel container or plastic zippered bag and treat it similarly after melting. It is all north polarized and rich in iridium and the ultra trace minerals of life. There was no lead, aluminum, cadmium, mercury, or other toxic metal, not even nickel, though these were not exhaustively studied, either.

There was a time some decades ago when rainwater or snowmelt was shunned, due to the need for storing it in cisterns. We were taught and knew instinctively that we should not drink standing, namely stagnant, water. It was a cardinal principle, taught in grade school, to drink only flowing water.

But such common sense gave way to the bottled water industry. We have been drinking "stagnant" water from bottles for several decades already. Drink your rainwater fresh, storing only enough to get you to the next rainfall.

Drink it in small amounts, daily, at first. Add nothing to it. It is one of Nature's perfect foods.

Don't expect miracles from this. We must not "judge" it until we know what to judge. The Syncrometer® sees that the body shares the iridium it gets with all the organs that have low levels instead of letting it go first to the most needy organ. To see a result and actually measure effectiveness of rainwater, a homeopathic or immunologic system of measurement could be created. When this is done, the youngest and the healthiest of people are seen to have the highest, most "potentized" levels of iridium substances. All animals have iridium, but very few plants do, that is, in measurable amounts by Syncrometry. The legume family and many herbs do. Water from municipal sources that have no heavy metals from its bleach treatment often does! Spas do, and natural springs do, those known for their health-giving properties.

Later, we will see what iridium actually does; how it combats the power of nickel to change our iron atoms to south pole. We need iridium to heal our battered, sick bodies.

Research is needed to explore the biosphere's reliance on cosmic dust for life's ultra trace minerals and perhaps even for life itself.

We will be able to heal ourselves again, using iridium from herbs and good water. We will be able to control growth again, when we can take back our escaped stem cell factor and HGH. We had been flooded with growth promoters brought in by our invaders: bacteria carrying radioactivity, viruses bringing immortality to our tumors, and the radioactive or lanthanide elements themselves. We will challenge all these invaders who have stolen our strength and brought us illness. First we will view the oncoviruses. Who, exactly, are they?

CHAPTER 10

SICKNESS BE GONE

In the early stages of cancer we can easily be motivated to search for new ways to survive for ourselves: an old recipe we have faith in, a successful therapist we heard about, inspirational reading. Our will to live is strong. We are determined to keep a good attitude. We are eager to comply and do our best to stay with our loved ones, right here on planet Earth.

But in the advanced stages of cancer we can be persuaded that it is hopeless, that there is nowhere to turn, that our doctor knows best after all, and we desire nothing as much as relief from pain and symptoms, not survival.

Your doctor is beginning to advise "setting your affairs in order", "there is nothing more that can be done", that "palliative care is all there is", that you should not "waste your money on unproven, unscientific" treatments. Alternative treatments are seldom if ever mentioned, as if loyalty to their own professional principles came before life. I am suggesting that there are still many ways to extend your life and some that could cure. It makes little sense to give your life's savings to a cancer research group when you could do the research yourself, and stand some chance of success.

Your doctors, nurses, and loving family and friends have no way of knowing extraordinary principles of healing and curing. They give up much too soon.

Cancer Be Gone

If your doctor sympathetically prescribes morphine or codeine for you, say NO. Just say NO. Offering morphine is the subtle message of hopelessness. If you listen to it, it will terminate your life in its own way. That is how the doctor tells you he/she does not believe you can survive much longer. It is well meant.

If only we knew the truth; that people in most ancient of times knew how to cure cancer…just as the Iroquois tribe of American Indians knew how to cure scurvy. They did it without microbiology, without computers, without anything modern. Science, as a discipline was not even born.

If only we knew what those truths were! But we do! The answers are in the storage bins of our herbal supply companies. The chemistry and science in our world of plants is unexplored and endless. It is in the weeds growing along the downtown boulevards, surviving all the herbicides. It is in our own gardens and spice racks.

But which one of these is it? Which one for constant back pain, shoulder pain, headache, and so on? And which one would work for you and agree with your digestion and be compatible with your handful of drugs? Such a study is now possible with a Syncrometer®. We need to start before health has completely vanished.

It seems impossible that people 1000 years ago knew more than we do. But they did. The Syncrometer® today is discovering the same herbs they knew about then! And we have them before us the way they never did. They could not travel or communicate with others as we do. The Peruvians had the bark of a tree. The Egyptians had a flower. The Amerindians of the southwest had a bush…it is still growing wild everywhere in the desert. Other Amerindians had flowers and trees. There are many cures, not just a few.

When western Europeans came to the Americas they pried open all the native secret cures, to plunder and squander them. The medical professionals, scientifically trained, were not interested in how they might work, and perhaps learn more about the disease. So nothing remains of the vast knowledge our professionals scorned. We must rethink our philosophy of living, our "reason" to live and try to salvage what is left of the vast treasure.

The ancients knew there was a difference between early and advanced cancers…that different treatments were needed to cure different symptoms like bloating, headache, constipation, insomnia. All these could be cured because they were treated like the different problems they are, without knowing about different bacteria, viruses, and microscopic parasites. And not as if they were all "just cancer".

In present day ignorance they all get lumped together as if they were "cancer". Nothing is further from the truth. Your bloating may be due to E. coli, diarrhea to Salmonella, loss of appetite to Flu, fever, fatigue and nausea to different combinations of these, sweating in the night to Mycobacterium avium, dizziness to prions, pink skin areas to Staph aureus and pain in many places to Strep pneumoniae in all these places, and so on…rough glassy skin to Yeast, horrible coughing to Strep G…and a bone abscess to Strep pyogenes in your teeth, and so forth.

In ancient times they were confronted with the same complexity in each person as we see now. They gathered as many curative items as they could and combined them! Therein lies the magic. And we can do the same.

The longer the recipe, the more successful you will be. What doesn't work for somebody will for someone else, because it is in a different organ. What doesn't work for the brain may work for the eyes. By combining 10 or so curative items we can reach difficult places and get a much broader spectrum of action. At the same time much less of any one herb is needed than could possibly give you a side-effect. That

is why, no doubt, there are no side-effects to any of these lists.

> Use the modern magic in the recipes below to cure yourself of E. coli, Salmonella, Flu, Strep G, and a few more that are responsible for nearly all cancer-related illness.

The most important caution with herbs today, as with all other foods and medicines is to test for chlorox bleach disinfectant and avoid these. This will come to about ¾ of everything you test. A single one will hurt you. Also test for thallium, a common pesticide in imported herbs. It will make your shins ache and give you red spots on the skin.

The second most important caution is to sterilize them, each one, as you do your food. It is even more important than sterilizing your food because they have not been cooked; all the more potency for you. Freeze all of them at -20° F or colder for 24 hours exactly. Always write the time on a label or bit of tape so you could make no mistake. Be sure to mark those that have been frozen.

If you can't disinfect your herbs with freezing, ozonating, sonicating or Lugol's, use them only cooked into the traditional teas, about 20 minutes.

One-Day Cancer-Fighting Recipes

This title means you can cure yourself of these cancer-associated bacteria in one day. The hindrance is eating them again. Learn to avoid that by disinfecting everything except homeographic drops.

For all these recipes the dose is given in the first number. The number of times a day is given in the second number. The number of milligrams is not as important as spreading them through the day.

Do not wait to assemble the whole recipe. Use whatever you have.

To kill Salmonellas of many kinds

- **Lugol's iodine**, 6 drops X 4 in about 1/2 cup water (not if allergic to iodine) This means 4 times daily. There is no need to wait for a particular time. But there is a burning need not to eat the food with Salmonella again. Throw out all the food you had been eating earlier that day or put it back in the freezer for sterilizing. Refreeze your supplements and products, such as toothbrush, floss, salt, flour.
- If you have a diluted iodine solution (Veggie Wash) use 10 drops instead of 6.
- acetic acid (vinegar), 1-2 tsp. before any food (<u>not in colon or prostate cancer</u>) (see *Sources*).
- hydrochloric acid, 5%, 10 drops in a glass of water before the meal. You still need your other 5 drops with your meal, stirred into the food.
- digestive enzymes (DE), 2 before any food – the exact composition of the enzymes is not so important. Using one capsule of several kinds is more helpful than one kind only.
- ginkgo leaf, 1 X 6
- pantothenic acid, 2 X 4
- bromelain, 2 X 4
- burdock, 1 X 6
- epazote, 1 X 6
- chrysanthemum, 1 X 6
- elecampane, 1 X 6
- cleavers, 1 X 6
- birch bark tea, 1/4 cup X 4
- anise oil, 6 drops X 1 (for 3 days only)
- cardamom oil, 6 drops X 1 (for 3 days only)
- basil oil, 6 drops X 1 (for 3 days only)
- Reishi mushroom, 1 X 4
- rose hips, 1 X 6
- hydrangea root, 1 X 6
- eucalyptus, 1 X 6
- citric acid, 1 X 6

Take oils for only 3 days. Do not increase dosage.

Oils are much more potent than dried plant parts. Pour your oils into a ½ oz. HDPE dropper bottle and count drops accurately. Put them into an empty capsule, combining about 4 varieties. Swallow quickly. Do not take with food for best results. Freeze or sonicate them.

Cancer patients can assume they have **Salmonella** invasion even without symptoms. Bacteria in your body acquire the same radioactivity and lanthanide invasion that your body cells do. It changes their nature, too, and hides them from your immune system. Their favorite congregating place is in your pancreas; then it cannot make all its digestive juices as it should. It can still make trypsin and lipase, but not cellulase to digest yeast walls, nor arginase nor chitinase. All cancer patients have a pancreas that barely digests half their food. All the more is left to feed bacteria and parasites.

Salmonella is a detox-bacterium, so it jumps at you from within, as well as from your food and hands. It will jump again and again, as often as you succeed in killing a F. buski parasite. There are 3 common varieties of Salmonellas; the Syncrometer® can test for them together. Which symptoms you get depends on which variety you have and where it is attacking you.

The world is full of Salmonellas. We all eat and drink them with every mouthful, though we think our food is essentially sterile and clean.

Salmonella is in most canned food and in cooked food. It is in supplements, drugs, even in empty gelatin capsules. Other people don't seem to get sick; they only challenge their immune systems. But yours is not working; you are made sick even when you don't feel it. You will recover much faster if you stop the constant Salmonella invasions. Simply sterilize every food and beverage, everything that goes into your mouth, even if not food. It will be quite easy if you purchase a new chest freezer with a temperature of at least -20° F (see *Sources*). Freeze your dishes, salt, flour, beans, contact lenses, condiments, spices, supplements, supplements in liquid form, empty gelatin capsules…everything. It only needs to be done once. Dead bacteria do not revive.

Salmonella does not tolerate acid, nor iodine, but just using these is not enough to eliminate them.

Why has Salmonella become such a widespread pest? There is no scientific answer, but we must come up with some possible answers and speculate on the mechanisms. Without some creative speculation and learning how to reduce them, other bacteria will follow the same path. My speculations are:

1. Gold has begun to substitute for other metals in Salmonella's enzyme requirements. Withholding gold reduces the bacteria.
2. The spread of radioactivity with bleach disinfection and dental supplies gives them protection.
3. Human hygiene has deteriorated.
4. We eat with our fingers in restaurants without being able to wash them first. We eat other people's cooking much too often.
5. To wash our hands we go to the filthiest room in the house, the bathroom. On our way out we pick up more Salmonellas than we had before. Washing before eating should be arranged for in building plans. It should be separate from toileting, such as in the kitchen where parents can watch children and each other.
6. Killing certain parasites results in Salmonella being set free, for example, F. buski, Fasciola, E. recurvatum.
7. Our flush toilets splash filthy water on our buttocks and body openings.
8. Our toilets should open and close and flush automatically to avoid touching anything.

The Syncrometer® finds gold in all the bread that I tested in the USA. Eating gold daily gives it a constant presence for Salmonella's environment inside us. The gold in people's jewelry and dentalware raises the amount substantially. Salmonella must adapt to the competition of its minerals with gold. This competition by gold will be greatly promoted when a radioactive element, like polonium or uranium, attaches itself to Salmonella bacteria as they ride around our lymph and in our intestines. The opportunity for mutation is much increased, while the gold competitor is right there, making an option for its enzymes. We have seen that other pathogens have acquired gold as an option for their minerals, too. They include SV40 virus, HIV, reverse transcriptase enzyme, prions, and the new Avian Flu. These are all modern pathogens. To avoid further evolution of our commonest bacteria we need to study them (as scientists already are) but to apply much more speculative creativity than before. Lay persons' ideas seem especially promising.

Gold, in the form of jewelry and dental supplies is hardened with nickel because by itself it is too soft to resist wear. This creates another problem, nickel.

The Syncrometer® has found that the common denominators for all allergies making PGE2, are only 2: nickel and radioactivity. Eating the allergenic food prolongs the PGE2 effect so the allergic organ can never heal, and technically becomes a third cause of allergies, but is, of course, under your control. You could free yourself of allergies with this simplified approach!

As soon as one day has passed where you are not accidentally eating Salmonella any longer, your feeling of illness will improve. Be patient with your own mistakes. Aim to sterilize every item that touches you or enters you. You will have several choices in sterilization techniques. Provide yourself with several.

More One-Day Cancer Fighting Recipes

To kill E. coli

- turmeric, 6 X 3
- fennel, 6 X 3
- eucalyptus, 1 X 6
- peppermint leaf, 1 X 6

- wormwood, 1 X 6
- burdock, 1 X 6
- nutmeg, 1 X 3
- cloves, 1 X 6
- olive leaf powder, 1 X 6
- cilantro, 1 X 6
- slippery elm (moose elm), 1 X 6
- thyme leaf, 1 X 6
- milk thistle seed, 1 X 3
- boneset, 1 X 6
- cleavers, 1 X 6

The second most common bacterium that makes you feel sick is **E. coli**. It gives you gas, bloating, headache, insomnia, loss of appetite, a bad mood, constipation, diarrhea.

These are very similar to the symptoms of Salmonella. Cancer patients always have both Salmonella and E. coli widespread in the body. That is why they feel so sick and miserable. E. coli is found where human hands have touched food, or in pills, supplements, as for Salmonella. It will be on your hands from bathroom visits. Make an alcohol hand cleanser for yourself and spray it on your hands anytime you have touched the door knob, the faucet handle or the flushing handle. There are several hand cleanser recipes in older books. Don't put your E. coli-fingers to your lips to flip pages! Spray with alcohol first! Don't eat anything with your hands until they have been alcohol-cleansed or Lugol's-cleansed. Lugol's cleanser is made in seconds with:

- 2 to 5 drops Lugol's
- 1 cup water in a non-breakable jar.

Dip one hand in after the other and wash them vigorously.

How can only 2 bacteria, Salmonella and E. coli, make you so miserable there is no interest in even staying alive? Combine the 2 recipes for total success. Your zest for life can come right back. Be sure each item was itself first sterilized or you could give it right back to yourself.

A good way to kill both Salmonella and E. coli bacteria together is to line up all the herbs along a table edge. Choose even hours or odd ones to give yourself one of each and set the kitchen alarm. On the hour-mark take one of each from the X 6 row. Then one of each from the X 4 row. Then those taken X 3. The time of day does not matter.

Remember that all plant (and animal) material has Salmonella and E. coli. You may be killing one "bug" with the recipe while giving yourself another one from the pills you just took. Very accurate freezing seems the easiest way to disinfect many items with a fail safe method. Electronic ways discussed in past books are not quantitative yet so we cannot rely on them for absolute protection.

You may empty any of the capsules and combine them in a boiling tea, but expect to lose some potency.

You can see there are many herbs that are good for both illnesses. In fact, they are good for <u>many</u> illnesses. How they work should lead to some fascinating new concepts.

Choose the common denominators for both recipes if you are forced to economize. You will still have a good recipe, but will need to take it longer.

Do not put faith into any assurance that ultra-pasteurizing, drying, adding salt or being "straight from the manufacturer", or having GMP rating, or having "never been opened", would mean free of all bacteria. The bacterial official test may be *Negative*, but yet there are so many bacteria left that you, and not others, will get sick from them. Only sterilizing with ozone, Lugol's or UV light is reliable, besides sonicating or deep-freezing at -20° F for 24 hours. You should feel no symptoms from any herb. As soon as you are better (hopefully in 1 day) reduce the number of doses by one, then 2 each day. When you have not eaten the bacteria for one full day, your body can kill those remaining in 24 hours.

To kill Strep pyogenes (abscess bacteria)

- nocephalosporin (copy of cephalosporin, tested free of chlorox bleach) drops
- nogaramycin (copy of garamycin, tested free of chlorox bleach) drops
- noampicillin (copy of ampicillin, tested free of chlorox bleach) drops
- hydrochloric acid, 5%, 10 drops in water before any food
- chrysanthemum, 1 X 6
- pantothenic acid, 1 X 6
- epazote, 1 X 6
- boneset, 1 X 6
- burdock, 1 X 6
- rose hips, 2 X 6

Strep pyogenes is a very serious abscess "bug", and might be hidden in an ear or a bone or some other rather special place. Since it is a "strep", we know it requires chromium and must be getting it somehow (see table on page 328). An inside source like metal teeth is most likely, but metal glasses frames, earrings, and watches always contribute. Any cooking pan is suspect, as are, of course, any ground herbs or supplements. You do not get this bug from food or water. It seems to get its start in a tooth. Whenever an abscess is found in the body, the Syncrometer® also finds it in a tooth while the chromium is widespread in the body. The tooth infection is often "silent", meaning there is no pain. That happens when the abscess is not under pressure, meaning it is draining *into you*. It is draining into one of your organs, preferring bones or brain for its next home. By the time it has spread to a bone, it requires antibiotics in addition to herbs. But unless chromium is removed to starve the bacteria, and the tooth cleaned and repaired in a metal-free way, they reestablish themselves. If it spreads to the brain it will reach the spine and bring you into a wheel chair. If you are already in a wheelchair search for S. pyogenes in the brain, spinal cord, and teeth.

As soon as Strep pyogenes is gone from the saliva, lymph, and organ (1 to 3 days) reduce all herbs to 1 X 4. After 4 more days test again for Strep pyogenes. If it has stayed away you may reduce the herbs to twice a day. At this point, if the bone abscesses have also been cleared but the tooth not yet found, hurry to remove metal, plastic that covers metal, radioactivity (porcelain), and root canals. Leave teeth "open" (unfilled) for 1 day, while cleaning them with *Dental Bleach*. This lets you test for leftover metals before "closing" them by replacing with composite.

To kill Strep G

- nocephalosporin (copy of cephalosporin) drops
- nogaramycin (copy of garamycin) drops
- noampicillin (copy of ampicillin) drops
- hydrochloric acid, 10 drops before any meal or snack
- sheep sorrel, 1 X 2 plus 1 vitamin B_6
- Reishi mushroom, 1 X 3
- pantothenic acid, 2 X 4
- epazote, 1 X 6
- eucalyptus, 1 X 6
- burdock, 1 X 6
- boneset, 1 X 6
- rose hips, 1 X 6

Strep G is another very serious "bug" that prefers lungs, joints, and special hidden places. In fact, it can be so well hidden, you never do find it before you have killed it. It can cause fever, extreme fatigue that puts you to bed, failure of a whole organ, severe weight loss and no appetite. You must force the victim to eat, preceded by hydrochloric acid in water with the WBC supplements on the side, along with pantothenate and 1 vitamin B_6 of any size. To prevent weight loss blend each food, till it can be drunk. The vitamin B_6 will counteract stone forming from the oxalic acid in some herbs. The oxalic acid may be part of the herb's action, very important for its success, but any excess will be removed.

For unexplained reasons clinical doctors do not find any of these 4 bacteria although they are the chief cause of illness in cancer patients.

I suspect this is due to outdated clinical assumptions. The clinical goal is to find <u>one</u> major infection that can be targeted and treated, not multiple infections with contributing symptoms. This is taught in bacteriology courses, because as a practical matter finding 20 bacteria makes it impossible to find "the culprit" and treat the correct one. The student is expected to somehow reduce the varieties to <u>one</u> and learn to guess right or use the most broadly acting antibiotic.

As soon as Strep G is gone from the saliva, lymph and organ (1 to 3 days) reduce all herbs to 1 X 4. After 4 more days, test again for Strep G. If it has stayed away, use this window of time to search for its true origin. You may still uncover a flaring infection in some faraway place that gives no symptoms. This is likely to be the true source. After treating till this location is cleared up too, you may reduce the herbal potions to twice a day. **Be sure to come back to all streps in a few days to check on them**. Infections that do not clear in about 5 days will be seen to be fed (with chromium or other necessity) see page 328.

Clostridium is our silent stalker, with nothing to be seen or felt. But it is much more dangerous than others. There are 4 common kinds. C. botulinum makes you weep. Even a grown man will openly weep when "C. bot." overruns the hypothalamus. This only happens when you have killed very many liver flukes. Clostridium tetani causes muscle stiffness as in your neck ligaments when you may believe you "slept the wrong way".

Clostridium perfringens and C. septicum are two more varieties.

The whole Clostridium family are "undertakers". Each serves its own parasite and is already stationed where access will be the best, like vultures over a dying animal. They tolerate no oxygen, so are called anaerobes. The poisons they make can be deadly. So, **throughout the parasite-killing program, we treat for Clostridium bacteria**. As soon as they appear you know you have killed something large. They are the undertakers for Fasciolopsis. When C. bot. arrives at a nerve or the brain its poison blocks the production of **acetylcholine**, one of our chief neurotransmitters. Acetylcholine keeps our muscles working, our digestive juices being made, our lungs breathing, our brains sending messages. To tamper with acetylcholine means tampering with life itself. For example, people in wheelchairs are not sending acetyl choline to their muscles. Wherever any of the Clostridiums appear, they must be killed immediately, without any higher priority.

Clostridium does not tolerate oregano oil. Even 10 drops is lethal to them. But your mouth and eyes do not tolerate oregano oil, either, in an equally severe way. NEVER put even 1 drop in your mouth, or on your lip, or anywhere near your eyes. But your stomach tolerates 20 drops! The challenge is to get it past your mouth. Put the 10 drop dose into a capsule and swallow it quickly. Three such small doses a day can keep up with all the Clostridium varieties that are produced in you by killing parasites.

Although it is silent where it grows, it leaves a very obvious "calling card" in your blood test results. If your uric acid level is too low you will find yourself "swimming" in Clostridium, even in your blood.

Start to kill them immediately without waiting to identify the species or location or amount. Then you can enjoy knowing you killed a thriving population of liver flukes instead of shedding tears as if you were depressed.

Every parasite of considerable size also has its "friendly companion" bacteria. They are inseparable. Fasciolopsis and **Bacillus cereus** are inseparable. But Bacillus cereus can buzz all about the body while buski adults must stay put. Bacillus cereus can cruise around in the blood up to 3 days after its "big brother" is killed, but then they disappear. They seem to have a dependency on buski, too.

Bacillus cereus goes quietly about its own business, there are no pains or appearances that give it away. And yet it might carry the deepest mystery of all locked inside itself. It seems to go about, changing north polarization to south. Polarization seems to follow a path leading through L- and D-tyramine and l- and d-thyroxine, our thyroid hormone. One by one, our amino acids follow the trend of change in structure and polarization at the same time, when Bacillus is present. Bacillus cereus has its own companions, too. They are **mycoplasma arthriditis**, and **papilloma** viruses, found in joints and warts respectively.

To kill Bacillus cereus

It is impossible to kill Bacillus cereus with herbs alone, probably because they are sheltered by "big brother", F. buski. The best solution is to kill buski. The recipe for this is the cancer-curing program. But it helps to add these herbs, especially if allergies are numerous.

- cumin, 1 X 3
- periwinkle, 1 X 3
- Oregon grape root, 1 X 3
- chrysanthemum, 1 X 5
- nutmeg, 1 X 3
- olive leaf powder, 1 X 5

Bacillus cereus lives only 3 days after its buski host has been killed. It does very little good to kill it though when the neighboring buski is streaming them out into your body, soon occupying you from top to toe again.

B. cereus also comes from a most unexpected source—a plant. The black line along the center of bananas has B. cereus. That could explain why bananas have tyramine, the cause of many headaches. We should **never** eat the black center of bananas.

To kill Streptococcus pneumoniae

(Strep pneu [pronounced noo])

There has never been a "pain" recipe" to my knowledge. But since a single bacterium is responsible for pain, it should be possible to assemble a recipe for it. It often works after a single dose of each item. You could free yourself from narcotic painkillers and come back into the land of hope again! It is "worth more than rubies and diamonds". For this reason it is worthwhile to be persistent in acquiring these herbs.

- sheep sorrel, 1 X 2, plus 1 vitamin B_6 each time
- EDTA, 500 mg., 1 X 2
- Notobramicin (drops)
- Noampicillin (drops)
- cardamom, 1 X 6
- ginger, 1 X 6
- marshmallow root, 1 X 6
- elecampane, 1 X 6
- nutmeg, 1 X 6
- rose hips, 2 X 6
- milk thistle seed, 1 X 6
- birch bark, ¼ cup tea X 3
- bromelain, 1 X 6
- catnip, 1 X 4
- thioctic, 1 X 5
- olive leaf, 1 X 6
- ginkgo leaf, 1 X 6
- cloves, 1 X 3
- wild lettuce, 1 X 6
- vitamin E, 1 X 6

The most relentless of all bacteria is our pain-causer. It is always present in the liver, without causing pain, but ready to pounce on the tiniest bit of blood available anywhere. It seems to eat blood. We constantly bleed in very tiny amounts. Our platelets are our patchers, going about from bleed to bleed, patching everything. But if they are not quick enough, the pain-causers, waiting behind the scene, have their meal and begin to grow. They are the **Strep pneumoniae** "bugs". From small pains to big pains, a broken bone, a twisted ankle, joint pain and muscle pain, and chronic pain of unknown origin follow this path. But I have not studied all kinds of pain, such as headaches, pressure from a slammed door on your fingers and gas pain in the intestines, or childbirth. Cancer pain and pain of chronic disease is always due to Strep pneumoniae.

How fortunate that the mightiest pain, requiring 3 narcotics to control it is just as dependent on chromium as other streps. Our approach will be effective in 2 to 3 days, namely, no pain. But the Strep pneumoniae will not all be gone from your body; they are back in hiding in the liver. This is a good time to remove all the chromium metal from the liver and hiding places so that pain cannot suddenly come back from a single mistake you might make.

Starving Strep pneumoniae requires metal removal, specifically chromium[23]. It can come from any kind of cooking pans or utensils, any metal in your teeth, any jewelry, or glasses, watch or ornament worn around the neck or wrist. There could be metal in your bra, or cap, or belt. These are the obstacles in the path of curing pain.

Plastic is not safe, either. It can seep huge amounts of metals! The only safe plastic is "cooked" plastic that you have hardened not to seep. The only safe cookware is tested cookware (see page 366 #5). The only safe glass,

[23] Recently, some Strep. pn. with gold attached were found in extreme-pain cancer cases. After removing gold from the mouth and draining gold out of kidneys and lymph, the Streps become manageable without narcotics.

ceramic, Teflon, enamel, polypropylene, and other new materials or coatings are tested ones. The industry has changed greatly for such materials. Old rules or generalizations do not apply anymore. When going shopping for appliances, take a number of zippered plastic bags with you, each holding a square of damp paper towel. Make a rubbing of the blades, or sidewalls of appliances to take home for testing. Explain your "sensitivity" to the clerks to get their cooperation.

> The only safe, non-seeping material that can be relied on without testing is high density polyethylene (HDPE), of the opaque kind, usually used for milk and gallons of water.

Cut dishes from HDPE water bottles. Use a conductivity indicator (see *Sources*) to test your pans, although it is not perfect. Cook your plastic cutlery for ½ hour. Remove everything else from personal contact including contact lenses. After this you will be ready to use the recipe to kill Strep pneumoniae—and by extra good fortune, staph, other streps, and yeast. All these are present together in many cancers including breast, skin, and bone, and all are dependent on chromium.

To stop bleeding diseases use the same list as for Strep pneumoniae. They may not cause the bleeding but somehow prevent it from stopping.

You may be tempted to leave out the 2 antibiotics, but when 2 or 3 narcotics are being used for pain relief it is important to take everything that could replace them. Making drops will save your original prescription and avoid side-effects.

You may empty any of the supplement capsules into a beverage or into food, provided you drink it at once. Do not use molasses or syrup or honey because these feed the bacteria particularly; wait at least 5 days before allowing yourself any sweets.

When the cause of bleeding is a very big one, like malaria or hemorrhages you should not stop the recipe till the malaria or hemorrhages are reduced.

Prions increase when Salmonella has just been killed and a great deal of gold is suddenly available. They also increase when the parasite Macracanthorhynchus increases. This parasite normally uses **ruthenium** in its enzymes, but gold can substitute and sticks to the ruthenium as a "dual-mineral". Are prions companions for Macracanthorhynchus (Macra for short)? They quickly invade the brain and peripheral nerves. Soon you feel dizzy but not sick. In fact, you could be in rather a good mood.

For an elderly person particularly, it is important to stop killing Salmonella or "Macra" and start removing gold as quickly as possible. Make *take-out* drops for gold from kidneys and lymph first, then from hypothalamus and pancreas. Then test for left over gold in liver, throat region, genital organs or wherever the main problems are. Results can be seen in two days. The true gold source is usually in tooth fillings and gums, jewelry, bread, and honey, Teflon and glass dishes, besides chlorox-bleached water.

Alzheimer's patients often have prions as part of the problem. They should remove all gold from their teeth, their jewelry and wedding ring. All baked goods should be homemade because store-bought breads have gold. Glass and Teflon pans and dishes seep gold. Symptoms can disappear as suddenly as they came but the experience should not be forgotten. Never wear gold or eat gold again. The next prion symptoms are difficulty in swallowing and breathing!

To kill Prions

- Reishi, 1 X 2
- cardamom, 2 X 4
- Shiitake, 1 X 3
- chaparral, 1 X 4
- birch bark, ¼ cup X 5
- periwinkle, 1 X 3

Do not try to kill prions or Macra till all the gold is drained from the body, so none is seen in the urine.

Staphylococcus aureus is not very common in cancer, but is present in every breast cancer. Staph is a "skin and bone" pathogen and I believe, though this is not yet proved, that it all starts with tooth infection. The lymph nodes in the neck try to catch the staph bugs before they spread to the rest of the body, but when they spill over (during sugar binges) the lymph nodes in the armpits and around the collar bones and above the breast join the battle (to save your body). The sweating in the armpits is meant to remove toxins and oils that otherwise might help the staphs; do not use sweat-stoppers nor shave here. Use scissors and deodorizers like MSM. Do not wear a bra that lifts the breast; it puts back pressure on the lymph flow under the breast to handicap your body. At the same time the bacteria invade the breast, often finding an old trauma like a breast abscess that was formed in baby-nursing times. This may have left a small fibrous mat that did not get completely healed and removed. Such a history of a breast cancer does not have enough evidence to be considered a fact, but such epidemiological data is very important and should be gathered by women themselves. Keep a history of breast bruises, traumas, abscesses, hormones taken to enlarge or reduce them, and other notable practices. It would be wise for women to take their health into their own hands and forge new paths for themselves, instead of waiting for "science" and committees.

Staph brings inflammation and tenderness to the breast but not actual pain. The breast may look red and feel hot as the body tries to burn up the bacteria with fresh arterial blood. Staph does not start the inflammation, though. A food allergen, apiol is the breast's "enemy". It comes from soybeans but contaminates essentially all other oils on the market. Do not use oils unless tested for apiol. Natural food oils as in peanuts or avocados and fish, in moderate amounts, are sufficient. For the ducts of the breast, phenylalanine is the food allergen, namely, cows' milk.

Staph will keep invading the breast skin while the streps prefer the deeper breast tissues. When Strep pneumoniae joins the others, the breast lump becomes painful and now has considerable internal bleeding. Fortunately there is overlap between all the bacterial needs so they can be killed all together. Be sure you give each "bug" the correct herbs to kill it. But first of all, repair the tooth.

Ozonating the breast while doing the program brings the fastest relief and results. Tape a plastic shopping bag around the whole breast using only masking tape. Do not remove the tape later. Only add tape where needed, so no skin is eroded. Place the ozone tube inside the bag. You should see the bag bulging out so you know there is a slight pressure and the ozone will penetrate deeply. Ozonate for 30 minutes, 4 times a day till the breast is completely well.

To kill Staphylococcus aureus

- noampicillin (test for chlorox bleach and chromium) drops
- nocephalosporin (test for chlorox, chromium) drops
- hydrochloric acid, 10 drops in a glass of water before any food
- eucalyptus, 1 X 6
- boneset, 1 X 6
- cardamom, 1 X 6
- elecampane, 1 X 6

- epazote, 1 X 6
- cloves, 1 X 6
- nutmeg, 1 X 6
- burdock, 1 X 6
- peppermint leaf, 1 X 6
- thyme, 1 X 6
- mullein leaf, 1 X 6

slippery elm bark (moose elm)

Staph travels very quickly through the skin, seeming to form an alliance with YEAST. Together they give the skin a rough, bumpy, texture with a glassy redness, though not pain.

This alliance may actually be a shared need for chromium. Recently, a gold-requiring Staph aureus and a nickel-requiring YEAST have been found. Draining both the gold and nickel brings fastest relief.

Yeast of the bread and alcohol variety is the dangerous kind in cancer, not the vaginal or mouth variety. Its scientific name is **Saccharomyces cereviscia**e. It can push its growing "hairs" into our cells, acting like roots to suck up our cell juices. It is quite destructive, but not truly killing our cells. It thrives on our blood sugar and our body temperature. We must not let it get a strong foothold at the breast because it can blaze through the rest of our skin without causing a disturbance until it is too late. Then it draws up all the blood sugar while the patient becomes emaciated in the last few weeks. Even then, this herbal method works by stopping the YEAST if you do the starving and killing at lightning speed.

To kill Yeast (S. cereviscia**e**)

- zinc, 1 X 2
- bromelain, 1 X 2
- cardamom, 1 X 6
- rose hips, 2 X 6
- ginger, 1 X 6
- vitamin A, 5000 units X 3
- epazote, 1 X 6
- burdock, 1 X 6
- milk thistle seed, 1 X 6
- eucalyptus, 1 X 6
- folic acid, 1 X 3
- turmeric, 1 X 6
- pantothenate, 1 X 6

Remove all chromium, gold, nickel and cobalt, namely, amalgam, to starve yeast. Then start the yeast killing recipe as soon as every item has been properly frozen.

Yeast is responsible for producing CEA, the well known clinical cancer marker. It also brings RAS the oncovirus and AFP, another cancer marker. It seems to be able to turn on the ribonucleotide reductase enzyme by itself to make DNA. This is a preliminary finding.

Although staph and yeast do not cause pain they quietly steal your food (blood sugar). They don't make you feel sick although extreme fatigue, loss of appetite and weight loss gives you and your family the hint that the end is near. You must rebel at such a notion and find help quickly that can go from one problem to the next, solving each one at lightning speed.

Shigellas do not cause pain either, but give quite distressing symptoms.

Two shigellas are very fierce in cancer patients or anyone. They are Shigella dysenteriae and Shigella sonnei. They come from Onchocerca parasites. Shigella dys (for short) causes severe diarrhea. Shigella son (for short) adds depression to the diarrhea. They can give you extreme headache. If nothing stops them they will continue to invade, preferring the nervous system, as in brain cancer or the spine. The body has to give up quite soon to the Shigellas, yet they are easy to prevent, and to stop, just with stomach acid, hydrochloric acid. Take 10 drops in a cup of water before meals. Even vinegar stops them; take tested vinegar in water with meals. Vinegar should not be used in prostate or colon cancer.

Clinically, a drug that slows the intestine is given to stop the diarrhea. This causes the bacteria to become chronic since nothing is done to remove them or kill them.

To kill both Shigellas

- pantothenate, 1 X 6
- burdock, 1 X 6
- epazote, 1 X 6
- boneset, 1 X 6
- cardamom, 1 X 6
- ginger, 1 X 6
- rose hips, 1 X 6
- milk thistle seed, 1 X 6
- bromelain, 1 X 6
- hydrochloric acid, 10 drops X 6
- vinegar (not in colon, prostate cancer)

There is only one **virus** that makes you feel sick but not very sick if it is by itself. It is Flu. **Influenza A and B** together are commonly called Flu.

Viruses in general are quite sensitive to your body temperature. Maybe this is why our bodies have learned to start a fever as soon as they arrive. That slows them down and buys time for your immune system to make antibodies. We may be uncomfortable, but we should put up with Nature's intent to make strong antibodies for the present and for your future. It does not seem wise to take a temperature-lowering drug before it has reached 101 ½° F.

To kill Flu (Influenza A and B)

- Oscillococcinum, 1 at bedtime (not useful for avian variety)
- boneset, 2 X 6
- epazote, 2 X 6
- burdock, 2 X 6
- eucalyptus, 2 X 6

Keeping the body warm is an instinct we all have. We should wear enough clothing to keep the body at 99.0° F for a cancer victim. Temperatures much higher than that have often been used by therapists in the past. Now this therapy is called hyperthermia.

The flu can give other uncomfortable symptoms like aching all over, aching in the joints, nausea, lack of appetite, vomiting, diarrhea, intense fatigue, headache, and more. Unwittingly, it is considered part of your cancer. This belief keeps you and your doctors unwilling to treat it. The only treatments known are homeopathic and herbal, not in the doctors' interest. This attitude is defended by saying the flu virus changes genetically too often to make a medicine worth its cost in research.

The flu virus in cancer patients is often chronic because they carry your radioactivity on themselves, similar to bacteria. This makes it much harder for your WBCs to catch them, eat them, process them and deliver the remains to other WBCs for shipping to the bladder. It uses up vitamin C so that soon all the WBCs are deficient in vitamin C and, therefore, disabled. The whole immune system is soon stalled by the radioactive intrusion. You can see the necessity of taking vitamin C continually, throughout your cancer, a point stressed by Dr. Linus Pauling years ago.

Bird Flu or **Avian Flu** is a new Flu variety that has recently changed its enzymes. It can use gold as a mineral instead of the ordinary minerals. This is not yet proved and needs research. The herbs that can kill Flu should be learned by everybody.

The eucalyptus tree is so useful everybody should grow one! Fresh eucalyptus leaves are <u>much more potent</u> than dried ones, as in capsules.

To kill Bird Flu (Avian)

- remove gold from teeth, jewelry, bread
- stop using glass or Teflon cook ware
- take drops of *take-out* gold from kidneys and lymph
- boneset, 2 X 6
- burdock, 2 X 6
- epazote, 2 X 6
- eucalyptus, 2 X 6

Adenovirus, the common cold, is seldom a perilous illness, but some scientists consider it an oncovirus.

There are usually no cold symptoms in a cancer patient, although the common cold can make anyone miserable. This virus often attacks quietly during a flu attack. The homeopathic Oscillococcinum is just as useful to prevent colds as the flu.

To kill Adenovirus

- eucalyptus, 2 X 2
- Reishi mushroom, 1 X 2
- epazote, 2 X 2
- boneset, 2 X 2
- elecampane, 2 X 2
- cleavers, 2 X 2
- pancreatin-lipase, 2 X 4
- 2 tsp. lipase to remove all oil accumulations, once a day

> The average cancer patient has only 4 of this list of infections: Salmonellas, E. coli, Flu and one other. These give the most symptoms, and are quite easily conquered. But they will keep returning since they are your own bowel bacteria and because all food and objects are contaminated with them. Our habit of licking our fingers and not washing hands, even before eating, makes us easy targets.

Cancer Fatigue

The fatigue of cancer seems to be mainly due to the high level of free cyanide in the body, enough to poison metabolism chronically. There is almost no cytochrome C detectable in the saliva, possibly because most of the iron in the cytochrome oxidase enzymes is combined with the cyanide. The enzyme is blocked from oxidizing your food to make energy.

> We give oxygen in the form of ozone in water for cyanide toxicity and get immediate relief.

Terbium Fatigue

This is a new term, pointing to the lanthanide metals, as a group, in our diseases. If your body doesn't have free

ATP, which is our body fuel, then life must shrink into itself and keep you bedridden.

Search for terbium or yerbium, lanthanides that easily attach to your ATP. It's best to move away from a lanthanide-loaded geographic area. Other lanthanides can do this too. Search all 15 for ATP, ADP, and even AMP attachments in your body.

Lanthanides may be the main cause, but there is another more sudden cause: a very shrunk Krebs cycle.

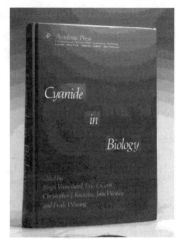

The enzyme rhodanese can detoxify organic cyanides as in food. But the water additives, ferricyanides, are not organic and accumulate to bring us free cyanide, the real poison in chronic doses.

Fig. 75 Cyanide in Biology

Chronic Cyanide Fatigue

If you can't find cytochrome C in your saliva, you are missing enzymes or are full of enzyme inhibitors like sodium cyanide. Hurry to stop poisoning yourself. The enzymes, peroxidase, and Rhodanese might be missing, due to mutations caused by the polonium-cerium duplexes as in the cancer-complex. The mutations are caused by different parasites linked to ferricyanide in your drinking water. Without these enzymes you can't detoxify the ferricyanide. It is normally changed to **thiocyanate** by rhodanese. When this does not take place, any acid-forming tendency will make plain cyanide out of it. Plain cyanide is attracted to iron and to iron enzymes like the **cytochrome oxidases**. These oxidases will now be poisoned so you can't oxidize your food into energy…ATP energy. Hurry to get oxygen from ozonated water. Hurry to drink and cook with unchlorinated water.

Do not risk well water that you think is unchlorinated. Use a *Total Chlorine* test paper; it should test zero. Do not risk bottled water with its radon daughters. Do not risk "spring water straight from the rocks" or ground. Only rainwater is under your control. Drink this. Hurry to kill the parasites that bring you these mutations. In a week, test again. There should be no free cyanide in your saliva. There should be cytochrome C and rhodanese present instead. Never go back to chlorinated water.

Of course there are other causes of extreme fatigue, like thyroid and liver diseases that should get quick attention. But if nothing helps, find a Syncrometer® tester who can help you investigate the cyanide and lanthanide problem.

Summary — Chapter 10

1. Being offered morphine is the low-key warning given by doctors that you are soon to be a terminal case. Refuse it.

2. Feeling sick is not due to your cancer. It is due to untreated bacteria, viruses, and parasites, besides the toxins from chlorox bleach that have accumulated in you.

3. You can give yourself *One-Day Cancer Fighting Recipes* to kill your tiny invaders in one to two days. The longer the recipe, the faster it acts, but hazards of non-sterility increase.

4. Some infections are very serious and require antibiotics; but we will use the copied variety in the form of drops. This will avoid side-effects and bring no toxicity, cost or addiction.

CHAPTER 11

THE MALARIA CONNECTION

The association of malaria and cancer was first noticed about 2003. Since then I have tested nearly every cancer patient for malaria by Syncrometer®. The association becomes much stronger as the cancer becomes more advanced. Is the association a new development or does it go far deeper into the past?

Is one parasite the carrier for the other, or does one predispose to the other, or do they share a food source?

Malaria is another parasite-caused disease. But it is much more complex in its stages and behavior than Fasciolopsis buski. Malaria has more than 20 stages, and all much tinier than Fasciolopsis. Malaria stages could easily enter Fasciolopsis stages and be sheltered from the immune system's WBCs or from malaria-killing drugs. It could even appear like a case of drug resistance in malaria when it might not be.

As soon as a patient starts the cancer-curing program, their malaria subsides, too, along with the cancer. This has been the case for every patient and is responsible, no doubt, for its very late discovery. They get worse together and better together. The responsible factor seems to be benzene. Benzene is one of the chlorox bleach toxins. How the benzene assists malaria is not yet known. It may make the cell's membranes more fluid and easier to penetrate.

HIV/AIDS, too, is associated with malaria. In this case, the dependence on benzene is already known from other books (see *The Cure For HIV and AIDS* by this author).

All our cases would be considered subclinical malaria. The definition is based on quantities. A sample of blood is smeared on a glass slide and the parasites viewed as tiny granules in the red blood cells. Another criterion used is 20 or more malaria parasites for 200 WBCs counted. This issue does not concern us as much as the scarcity of study materials. The different stages are not available. Another concern is the implied acceptance of this infestation of the human species by the use of the term "subclinical".

Finding samples of stages could lead to finding their food requirements and ways to starve or kill them. But first, of course, should be the clearing of the water from benzene by adhering stringently to the regulations for its bleach antiseptic quality.

As soon as we have detected malaria in a cancer patient, on their second day, we give a set of 6 anti-malarial drugs in copy (drops) form called **quinones**. The response is immediate (a few days). No measurements of side-effects have been recorded. The results are anecdotal and very much in need of further research. The effect of removing chlorox from the drinking water on their first day may be the strongest of the variables that improves malaria. The response may also be immediate because the quinone medicines are strong oxidizers. They also do precisely what is needed to disable the <u>ferro</u>cyanide part of the cancer-complex, at the same time as killing malaria parasites.

We have seen no drug resistance in 2 years of use. In fact, out of 6 quinones chosen, all were effective in our setting of benzene removal.

By oxidizing ferro to ferricyanide, the cancer-complex no longer makes OPT. Cancer markers disappear.

By treating the malaria, based on Syncrometer® identification, the very advanced cancer patient improves much more quickly than expected. The symptoms improve dramatically in 2 days. Flu, Salmonella, and E. coli, besides malaria (falciparum), will test *Negative* and a sense of well being returns.

The anti-malarials chosen are common quinine-like substances. We wait to give them until the patient has stopped drinking chlorox-treated water and started the first set of kidney cleaning drops. There are no side-effects except fatigue.

Malaria parasites roam from organ to organ, depending on which one is inflamed. They only seem to enter those exposed to radioactivity or benzene or the food antigen of that organ.

The primary organs to be attacked are your red blood cells and your liver. The parasites' requirement is iron and they will get it from you! They will burrow through the RBC walls (membranes) to reach the hemoglobin inside. They dismantle it all to get the iron atoms in the hemoglobin. But they don't choose the most perfect and the best RBCs. They choose the inflamed ones with benzene and **fructose** in them. Maybe the membrane is thinner or more fluid here, making it easier to dig a hole. The source of the benzene is the chlorox bleach these patients were drinking in their water, similar to cancer patients, so when the program is started with a change in water, the malaria immediately improves, too.

Another source of benzene is a fungus, **Potato Ring Rot**. It produces a **mycotoxin**, **zearalenone**, which interferes with reproduction by causing feminization in animals. Zearalenone is detoxified by the body to benzene and finally to formic acid. Potato Ring Rot grows in the dead remains of the parasite Macracanthorhynchus, both requiring gold. Macracanthorhynchus is always accompanied by prions which surround the parasite. Prions compete for the gold possessed by the parasite and its fungus. When the parasites are killed there is an immediate large increase in prions, to the point of causing symptoms. It is unwise to kill this parasite until your body has been drained of gold.

Syncrometer® results show Macracanthorhynchus to be an AIDS parasite which leads to attrition and wasting as well as loss of neurological function and finally death.

Macracanthorhynchus appears to be the most likely cause of AIDS together with its prions and gold.

Fructose is the allergen for the RBCs, making the cell channels stand open and causing PGE2 to be made.

> It is important for the malaria patient to avoid honey, aspirin, and lemons because these contain the main malaria allergens; fructose, ASA, and limonene.

We could easily think there was only 1 disease (cancer) for any one person when actually there is a **cluster of 4 diseases, coexisting: cancer, malaria, HIV and AIDS**.

How could all these patients get malaria and when did they get it? The existence of some subclinical malaria is to be expected from past generations that were parasitized and transmitted the stages through blood contact during pregnancy. But this should be waning over the years and it is gradually increasing. The most direct explanation is the increase of chlorox use in food and water.

It could also be explained by a huge increase in consumption of potatoes, mechanically prepared as for potato chips and French fries. Moldy areas would not be recognized by the machines. This would lead to benzene increase and immune lowering.

There is a large literature on subclinical malaria on the Internet. Others have speculated on different causes of the malaria increase. Very many people have had their blood examined in the fresh unpreserved state by a "Live Blood Analysis" test. Here they find a few malaria stages in nearly everybody, it is stated. It is due to inheritance, they claim, which allows a tiny bit of bleeding from the mother to the unborn child, especially when aspirin is being used. Malaria in our ancestors is not remote, being perhaps only a few generations in the past. The southern USA was malaria-ridden even in the 1800's. As swamps were drained, DDT sprayed everywhere, the chief carrier, a mosquito, declined in population. But some stages got transmitted with every birth so a few remain today. This past century saw an increase in benzene pollution of the global environment through spread of one brand of laundry bleach, bringing with it uranium, polonium, benzene, potassium ferrocyanide, and automotive products. Benzene's accidental entry into the food chain has done great harm, but should have been expected with development of the gasoline engine. Actually, carelessness with gasoline is not the cause. Carelessness with bleach quality, as it gets into the drinking water from use of filters and softeners attached by homeowners, besides the water departments' additions seem to be the actual causes.

My preliminary data from Syncrometer® testing shows that a somewhat similar complex as the cancer-complex is formed in malaria. For cancer the cerium part of the complex bonds loosely to the Fasciolopsis' DNA to produce some of the cancer-related mutations. It also bonds to the DNA of an inflamed organ which will become the primary cancer.

In malaria the cerium part of a similar complex, the malaria-mutagen-complex, bonds to the DNA of malaria parasites.

Remember that the trigger that activates the HIV virus to come out of F. buski is benzene (read *The Cure For HIV and Aids*).

> Benzene appears to activate malaria and to trigger the HIV virus.

As health deteriorates, the condition called AIDS is reached.

Checking back over several years of HIV and AIDS patients the MALARIA CONNECTION became visible here, too. Making homeographic copies of their saliva samples made a "library" of cases possible. Examining them for **Plasmodium falciparum** showed an astounding 90% had both malaria and HIV!

HIV and AIDS patients all are drinking benzenated water produced by adding chlorox bleach to the water. Any test of chlorox bleach using a Syncrometer® reveals it.

In HIV patients a similar mutagen-complex has been made as in malaria and cancer. But in this case the cerium part of the complex bonds to the CD4 lymphocyte's DNA and also to the malaria parasite. The CD8 lymphocytes' DNA is similarly involved, but this time to the ferrocyanide, much like the cancer-complex. In fact the CD8 complex does yield OPT as a mutation and could be expected to increase their numbers. A variety of cancer-like mutations are produced from the 2 kinds of complexes, while other mutations are malaria-like.

In gay men with HIV disease, the cerium part of the complex also bonds to the medulla, an organ in the brain. The medulla now produces 3 kinds of female hormones: estradiol. estriole and estrone. The latter two are normally produced by the adrenal glands in menopausal women. I assume they are mutations produced by the medulla as a result of a similar mutagen-complex there. Gay women, with or without HIV, have not been studied; nor have gay men without HIV. But women with HIV and AIDS had 8 hormones being produced in the wrong organs, including the medulla. This could contribute to the wasting disease seen in advanced illness, besides prions.

It seems then that the 4 diseases, cancer, malaria, HIV and AIDS belong in a set, all derived through a family of mutagens that can only attach to the DNA at a particular place. The mutations will be somewhat alike and somewhat different. It can all be expected when a preformed carcinogen is found in a popular product or food. In the case of chlorox bleach, the "nitrogen MUSTARDS" and "sulfur MUSTARDS" are there. The "allyl sulfur" compounds are there, all together comprising a group of alkylating agents. They are also present in all motor oil and wheel bearing greases. Finding these automotive greases contaminating our water, even in the minutest traces, brings in these very dangerous mutagens. Undoubtedly they are the animal residues of dinosaurs that collected in the pools of crude oil that we now pump to the surface. The alkylating agents are linked to cerium through potassium ferrocyanide and ferricyanide. The common laundry bleach called chlorox contains ferrocyanide whereas NSF bleaches contain ferricyanide. Ferrocyanide links to the parasite F. buski while ferricyanide links to most other parasites. The iron cyanides are used to protect the pipes with their anti-scale and anticorrosion action. Small polonium-cerium duplexes are present in both bleaches, as they are everywhere in the environment, but the addition of iron cyanide and alkylating agents makes them particularly dangerous. It is inevitable that they should form a larger complex considering the high reactivity of cerium with DNA and with the iron cyanides. This was already known in 1953 when a book on the ferrocyanides was published (see photo). There is an abundance of active DNA in parasite stages, bacteria, and regions of high growth in animals. This makes it inevitable that the few sites that allow the carcinogen-complex to bind tightly will be found. The family of mutations representing the parasite and the iron cyanide will be produced again and again.

It is important to stop this. The cerium end of the polonium-cerium duplex could react with any active DNA. No animal (and perhaps plant) would be spared these site-specific mutations that lead to cancer, HIV, AIDS, and malaria from water with chlorox bleach. Other diseases, particularly genetic diseases, would result from water with NSF bleach.

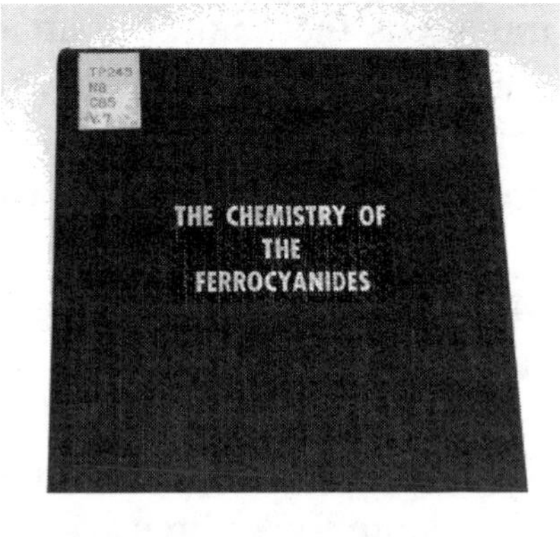

Fig. 76 "The Chemistry Of The Ferrocyanides" by American Cyanamid Co.

Our water-protecting agencies should be required to implement their original responsibility—to test and disclose all chemicals added to the drinking water. This includes the liquid bleach, the filter disinfectants, and water "conditioning" chemicals, in fact, everything.

Our agencies should provide a testing service for all substances that touch the drinking water. It is my belief that the public would be eager to use them, even at personal cost. Or give references to labs that do such tests. The tests should include filters, softener salts, buffers, anti-scalants, anti-corrosives, popular dyes such as methylene blue, and automotive products.

Just requesting the avoidance of all cyanide compounds in water treatment would already remove the cause of most of our diseases, I believe. It could be tried in ½ of a city where economic and social differences are lower than average. The other half could act as a control. If the population is large, corrections should not be necessary for smoking, cyanides in food, vitamin B_{12} status and other fairly large influences on cyanide exposure.

It could be tried in Africa where the improvement in health would be most visible.

Such an experiment in Africa would be quite low cost since the use of boilers and huge heating systems is minimal due to the warm climate. Adding anti-corrosives to reduce boiler scale might not even be needed. Switching water pipes to plastic to avoid corrosion problems might be the biggest expense. Perhaps a city could be found that already has plastic pipes and where the experiment could be done. An analysis of new cases of all 4 diseases should already be significant in 1 year, I believe. Perhaps Africa will be teacher to our world as it once was cradle.

Our cancer, HIV and AIDS, and malaria epidemics arose due to carelessness, allowing water softeners and filters to be applied to personal water pipes, not knowing they were contaminated with serious mutagens. And to negligence, thinking that no harm could come from adding a scale-reducing and corrosion-reducing chemical in regulated and very small amounts but that would eventually turn into cyanide, a most unthinkable poison in a special group of people.

Perhaps we could put into place several university departments of chemistry to act as regulatory advisors for the EPA and FDA. Perhaps it is not too late to turn our health debacle around.

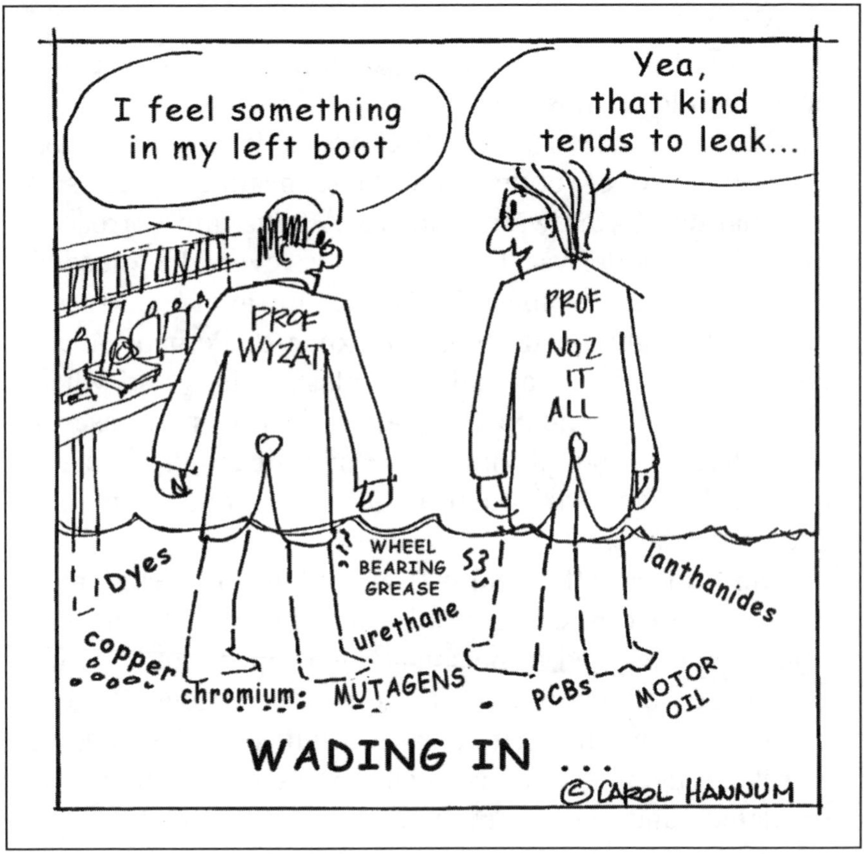
I feel something in my left boot
Yea, that kind tends to leak...
PROF WYZAT
PROF NOZ IT ALL
Dyes
WHEEL BEARING GREASE
lanthanides
urethane
copper
chromium
MUTAGENS
PCBs
MOTOR OIL
WADING IN ...
©CAROL HANNUM

CHAPTER 12

STOPPING METASTASES

Many are unreal! Seeing numerous tumors in the form of lumps under the skin or throughout the lungs or liver may be overwhelming when you first look at your CT scan or actually feel them. But it need not be so daunting when you realize they are not true metastases at all. They are merely more of the same kind you already have. You are simply making more and more. If you can get rid of one you can get rid of all. Obviously more and more tumor nuclei are making a successful fusion with the primary organ, be it skin or lung or lymph nodes.

Why are they getting so numerous? The fact that the fusions are occurring in the same organ is your clue. The inflammation in the skin or the lung or lymph nodes is spreading, so the tumor nuclei can fuse with more and more cells. You must ask: Am I still accidentally eating the food antigen for this (the primary) organ? Find the food antigen in the *Cancer Location Table* (page 292); then check the *Food Table* (page 97) to see which foods have this antigen. For the skin the food antigen would be **acetaldehyde**. In the lungs this would be **coumarin**, and in lymph nodes it would be **SHRIMP**. Find yours as soon as you read this.

You may feel quite certain that you are not eating the food that has this antigen. Yet your recovery depends on finding it. Try to find a Syncrometer® tester to help you find the allergy indicator (PGE2) in the organ with the tumor. Then find the antigen there and even the foods you should not be eating. It is not necessary to be physically present for the tester*. The ability to make a homeopathic or homeographic copy of your saliva sample lets the tester receive it by mail to search for your antigens. The saliva itself is considered a biological waste and hazardous to ship. Instructions are on page 619.

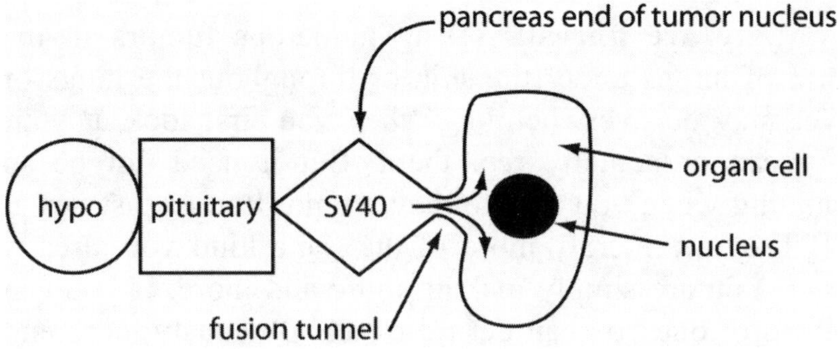

Fig. 77 Diagram of fusion to body cell by tumor nucleus

When tiny tumorlets have started everywhere in one organ or type of tissue it is because the food allergen has caused "inflammations" everywhere, and that resulted in PGE2 being made everywhere (see page 124). Prostaglandin E2 is a substance made by your tissues when they are irritated by an antigen. As soon as the pancreas end of a tumor nucleus fuses to your skin or lungs or lymph nodes, a tumor growth is started there. And if the pancreas end is bringing the SV40 virus, it can slip into your skin or lung or lymph node cells through the fusion site. See the diagram, as interpreted from Syncrometer® data.

---

*Testers, if you find acetaldehyde in the skin, search next for yeast (any package of dry yeast) in the skin, which makes acetaldehyde. Then search for asparagine which feeds this yeast. Search for chromium and cobalt deposits which are also necessary for yeast to grow. Then search dishes and food for the presence of chromium or cobalt. Search in powdered food supplements, herbs, spices, cooking pans. Search in plastic, glass, Teflon, ceramic, enamel cookware and cutlery. But most often they come from artificial teeth and jewelry.

There are many free-swimming SV40 viruses too. But they only enter the cells of an inflamed organ that is making PGE2 because of an allergic reaction.

> Check the *Cancer Location Table*, then check the *Food Table*, then analyze your diet. Eat nothing that isn't listed and found safe. Use no "loopholes", like cooking the banned food.

Suspect the foods you have "always" eaten. Obviously, you are eating a lot of the culprit food. If there are no clues or no time, change it all. Eat nothing that you were eating before. Eat Thai food, Korean food, Chinese food, Japanese food, Mexican food—anything but the daily foods you were accustomed to.

Such a diet switch can't guarantee that you won't get the same allergen in one of the new foods. But chances are excellent that your switch will work. Learn to do food testing yourself with a Syncrometer®. It will give you the freedom to be a connoisseur in spite of deprivations in whatever land you live.

You can cure all the hundred lumps I call **pseudometastases** and start them shrinking in days. Lymphomas are an example. Stopping eating SHRIMP and fish puts them on hold immediately.

Real Metastases

When a new organ gets involved in your cancer it is a true metastasis but it is much easier to stop or cure than the original cancer. In reality you have acquired a new allergy of the PGE2 kind. Nickel and radioactivity are the only 2 suspects that cause this. They are increasing in your body. They are actually coming from your radioactive tooth fillings since these are constantly eroding.

Link To Teeth

A tiny chip of polonium or a miniscule crumb of uranium is stuck in a tooth location such as a filling. The uranium has a tiny bit of polonium right beside it, representing its radioactive decay. They let loose tiny bits of themselves constantly.

The very small nerve that leaves from the tip of the root is jammed with Po. Is it the radiation or a frequency pattern or the actual element that really travels along the nerve? At the end of this nerve a buski parasite will be reached. A permanent pathway is established between the buski and the polonium source in the tooth filling since neither of them can move away. The link between tooth-polonium and the buski parasite is NOT through an artery or vein or lymph vessel, only these tiny nerves.

A New Allergy

How does the new allergy develop? All food has phenolic substances. They give the food its color, its flavor, its fragrance. You may have put yourself on a diet rich in cabbage, broccoli and other members of the "cabbage-family". These will bring the substance PIT*. Or on a diet of carrot juice! This brings the substance **umbelliferone**. The intention to eat much more of these fine natural foods was good, but you can be misled. Your metabolism, the body's quiet chemistry, has been disturbed by many parasites and bacteria. The liver and pancreas can no longer digest and detoxify your food efficiently. The food phenolics become allergies at the organ that is attacked.

The Syncrometer® has shown us some of the details how the allergy happens. One small part of your body was

* Testers, purchase phenylisothiocyanate, or improvise with a cabbage leaf, copied, and labeled CABBAGE (RAW).

turned southerly by the heavy metals that entered, particularly nickel and radioactivity. If that part also acquires a Fasciolopsis stage, it and its own partner bacteria will be very stimulated to multiply in this south polarized zone. Its partner bacteria are *Bacillus cereus*, ordinary soil bacteria. But they produce tyramine in a steady stream. Tyramine formed in a southerly region becomes d-tyramine, not the kind your body can work with. Soon its closest relatives, l-tyrosine, l-thyroxine, and l-phenyl alanine will all become d-forms, too. These cannot be used by your body either. Your ever-alert immune system will notice this immediately because having no useful thyroid hormone (only d-thyroxine) is an emergency. Your body will start to destroy them. It will destroy any "wrong form" amino acid anywhere in your body and those that you eat, too. Examples are coumarin in the lung, menadione in the blood, d-histidine and any other d-forms at other organs. You may call it a mere allergy when you have symptoms like cramps, rashes, and swelling, but the Syncrometer® detects that your white blood cells are hard at work in an allergic tissue. They are eating and getting rid of these wrong forms.

Only 2 Causes Of Allergy

We have been taught that allergies are caused by cats or pollen or a thousand other possibilities. How exciting it was to find only 2 common denominators for all organs with allergies. These are nickel and radioactivity.

In previous books I included Salmonella as a third allergy cause. Since then I have seen radioactive particles stuck to these Salmonellas so that radiation could still be the real cause.

As our search for a true cure for allergies continues we may soon come upon the cure for metastases. Meanwhile, we can learn which allergies belong to particular organs.

Cancer Location Table

Every organ has its own allergy, sometimes more than one. When your liver can't detoxify the allergic substance after you eat it, it circulates. Soon it passes through the organ that is inflamed with nickel or radioactivity. The allergic compound can enter the cells because they are open with inflammation. They make PGE2. This is what invites the tumor nucleus to start a cancer there.

Below is a list of organs and their food allergies. The list is not complete. Many, in *italic*, need further verification. Foods given in capital letters have not been analyzed yet to find the true phenolic allergen. Testers are encouraged to find more and share results, especially for other diseases. To use this table find the location of your problem first. Copy the name of the phenolic that is its food allergen. Next, find the foods with this allergen in the *Food Table*, page 97. That is all.

I do not know which of these events comes first. But by stopping eating this food the cell doorways close. PGE2 goes away. It only takes days. Stopping the allergic food is the first step to take to cure metastasis.

Cancer Location Table

Cancer Location	Food Allergen (antigen)
abdominal mass (Onchocerca & lymph node)	CORN, SHRIMP
adrenal gland	mandelonitrile (almonds), *aldosterone*
alveoli	D-mannitol (sugar variety)
aorta	menadione (raw greens & grains)
artery	hippuric acid (dairy products)
B-cells	*CORN*, D-malic acid (malonic family)
bile duct	acetic acid (vinegar)
bladder	cinnamic acid (cinnamon)
bone	PIT* (cabbage)
bone marrow	limonene (lemon)

* phenylisothiocyanate

Cancer Location	Food Allergen (antigen)
brain & spinal cord	caffeic acid (fruit, coffee)
breast	apiol (soy products, oils)
capillaries	hippuric acid, *pyrrole, benzoic acid*
cardiac (upper) stomach	*phenol* (derived from benzene)
cartilage	wheat
CD4's (T4 lymphocytes)	ASA (aspirin)
cervix	ASA (aspirin)
chest mass (Dirofilaria & lymph node)	lactose (milk sugar), SHRIMP
choroid plexus (brain)	alphaketoglutaric acid
cochlea (ear)	cinnamic
colon	acetic acid, pyrrole (blood, smoked food)
crista (ear)	malvin (red & blue fruits)
diaphragm	NGF (nerve growth factor), sardines, mannitol
epiglottis (throat)	naringenin (oranges), retinol (synthetic vitamin A)
esophagus	menadione
esophagus, upper	menadione, *acetic acid, caffeic acid*
Eustachian tube	butter, *beef*
eye	lily family (ONION, GARLIC, asparagus)
eye, iris	galacturonic acid (dairy products)
Fallopian tube	umbelliferone (carrots)
fimbria	*chlorophyll*
gallbladder	acetic acid
heart	tryptophane, tryptamine
heart (pacemaker, purkinje)	lactose (cow's milk)
Hodgkin's lymphoma	lactose, SHRIMP, *acetaldehyde*
hypothalamus	chlorogenic acid
ileocaecal valve	*PIT, naringenin*
Islets of Langerhans in • head region of pancreas • tail region of pancreas	 quercitin phloridzin
To find these, touch insulin sample to pancreas sample and add 1pF or 1μH for head region, and 2 or more μH for tail region.	
kidney	albumin, casein (dairy food, cheese)
ligamentum nuchae	limonene
liver	umbelliferone (carrots)
lumbar spine	caffeic acid
lung	coumarin (vanilla, rice, clover honey)
lung lymph nodes	tryptophane (milk)

Cancer Location	Food Allergen (antigen)
lymph node	SHRIMP (fish, seafood), *D-mannitol*
lymph vessel valve	lactose
malignant melanoma	phenyl alanine plus mercury
medullated nerve	*apple* (not phloridzin), *caffeic acid*
medulla + 1pF	*galacturonic acid* (dairy foods), allyl methyl sulfide, diallyl sulfide (ONION)
medulla	*apiol*, ONION
medulla, left	*tryptophane*, *piperine*, *gallic acid*
megakaryocytes	ASA, cinnamic (A.M. Leukemia)
nipple and ducts of breast	Phenyl alanine
non-Hodgkin's lymphoma	SHRIMP, CORN
nose, tip (nasal epithelium)	hippuric, sodium pyruvate(red apple)
omentum	limonene
osteomyelitis	umbelliferone (carrot)
optic nerve	caffeic
ovary	phenyl alanine, apiol (milk, oils)
pancreas	gallic acid (preservative in oil, grain)
parathyroid	guanidine (not guanidine HCl)
parotid gland (cheek)	hippuric acid
penis	ASA (aspirin)
peripheral nerve	apiol, *caffeic acid*
pineal gland (brain)	*caffeic acid*
pituitary	phloridzin
platelets	limonene, D-malic acid
prostate	acetic acid, naringenin
RBC (red blood cells)	fructose (sugar in honey, corn syrup)
rectum	NGF (nerve growth factor), D-mannitol
salivary glands	casein
seminal vesicle	ASA (aspirin)
skeletal muscle	melon (not cantaloupe), *lemon*
skin	acetaldehyde, nuts, *NGF, apiol*
sperm	glycine (amino acid)
spermatic cord	quercitin (squash)
spleen	peanut
stomach (all parts)	*phenol*
sublingual gland	citric acid
submaxillary gland	eugenol (cloves)
tendons	*D-mannitol, rice*
testis	phenylalanine, D-tyramine, glycine

Cancer Location	Food Allergen (antigen)
thymus	naringenin
thyroid	d-tyramine, chlorine, fluorine, bromine
tongue, filiform	naringenin, MSG (monosodium glutamate), retinol, beta carotene
tongue, fungiform	ASA, naringenin, MSG, menadione, benzoic, retinol
tonsil	ASA, naringenin, MSG, retinol, D-tyramine
trachea	*phenol*, *phloridzin*
ureter	*D-mannitol,* avocado
urethra	caffeic acid
uterus	phenyl alanine (milk)
vagina	acetaldehyde, nuts, ASA (aspirin), *banana*
vas deferens	estrone (estrogenic)
veins	*menadione*
vein valves	*CORN*

Food allergies invite the cancer to a new organ.

Fig. 78 Cancer locations and allergens

How Metastases Happen

To make the primary tumor, the tumor nucleus fused itself to one of your organs to make a 4-tissue combination. We can also call it a quad-tumor or just a "quad", perhaps a quad-breast or quad-prostate (see diagram). Quads can be seen floating in your body fluids everywhere. These quads can fuse to another new organ to make a quint-tumor if the new organ is inflamed. This could be a quint-breast-lung or quint-prostate-bone. The quint combination is the first true metastasis. Certain combinations are more likely than others because the organs are nearby and share their toxins and parasites. If you have 4 or 5 metastases, you might have very many different combinations of organ cells. For example, you could have octets of hypothalamus, pituitary, pancreas, breast, bone (rib), skin, lung, lymph node (neck location). Or you could have octet-tumors of hypothalamus, pituitary, pancreas, breast, lung, bone (collar bone), lymph node (at collar bone), and bone marrow. There does not seem to be a limit on the number or the order of new organs involved. Only the first three organs and their order stay constant for all cancers. They were the tumor nucleus.

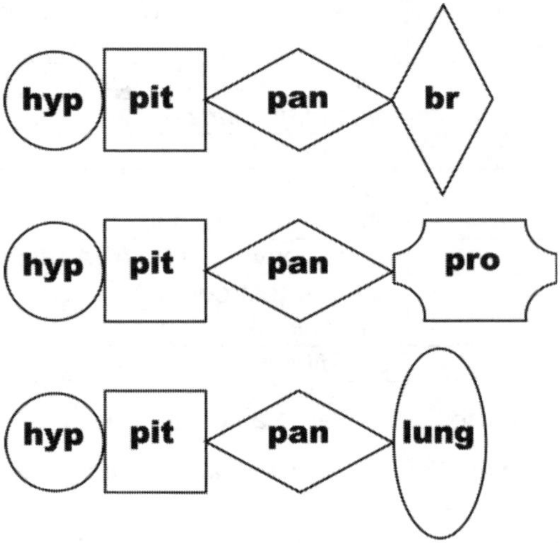

Top: primary breast tumor; Middle: primary prostate tumor; Bottom: primary lung tumor. The 3 organs at the left of each are the tumor nucleus.

Fig. 79 The primary tumor

Organ combinations without the hypothalamus, pituitary, or pancreas exist, but they do not form tumors or cysts.

Combinations of organs with one of these three exist, too, but do not form malignant tumors. Different combinations with pancreas cells exist, but have not been studied.

Even if you have tumors everywhere, quite uncountable, and the picture looks completely hopeless, these metastases and pseudometastases can be stopped as suddenly as they came. The principles are the same as for the primary tumor. Only now it is much more urgent. You must find what you are eating that has the allergens.

What becomes more and more difficult is finding safe food for yourself. Yet, the splendid variety of local and imported foods in our food stores makes it easier than it ever was in the past. Find a tester to help find polonium-free and uranium-free foods (namely, chlorox-free). Learn to cook new foods! Get help cooking and shopping. You should not lose weight.

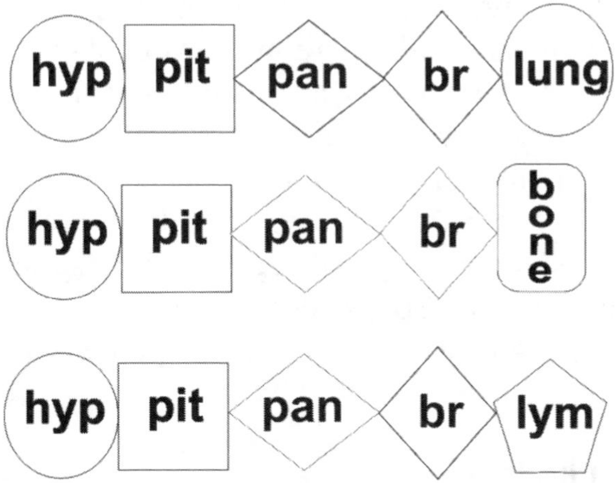

Top: breast cancer metastasized to lung; Middle: breast cancer metastasized to bone; Bottom: breast cancer spreading to lymph nodes.

Fig. 80 Quint tumors become the first metastases

You have already stopped the primary tumor's growth and now you have stopped your metastases, too. You are even preventing metastases from forming by washing the cancer-complex out of your body and removing all polonium and uranium from your teeth*.

Real Metastases...From The Outside

You can ABSORB the cancer-complex from your own house, from the chair you sit in, the bed you sleep in and the carpet you walk on barefoot. Your skin is very

* Testers, because polonium is part of the decay series of uranium, you will always find a tiny bit of polonium situated right beside uranium. To see these extra small amounts, amplify your results by placing regular shielding tubes (as used to make copies) over all bottles. Place uranium and polonium test bottles touching each other on the opposite plate from organ or saliva.

absorptive. If you touch the tip of your little finger to an apple that is sprayed with chlorox bleach and then touch it to a sheet of thin plastic or paper you will transfer it. It acts like poison ivy oil or wet paint that never dries. The Syncrometer® easily finds it. And if you touch your finger to your skin anywhere, the skin absorbs it. You could make a malignancy right there under your skin where you absorbed it or wherever it was carried by your circulation, similar to poison ivy. You must not allow yourself to absorb polonium from your contaminated house. Imagine a houseful of poison ivy…carpets, furniture, bedding, floors, dishes, towels, everything. Carefully scrub it away using polonium-free soaps, detergents, water and strong cleaning agents (see *Sources*) before you even start the program.

…From The Inside

If your teeth were filled with dental supplies that had been disinfected with chlorox bleach the polonium in the bleach is trapped in the filling. It can be detected years later! It is constantly diffusing out of the tooth and reaches your tumors. It is a game of Russian roulette when the new malignancy will happen. It can never stop trying to happen, even if you radiate, "chemo" or surgically remove the tumor. Its path from the tooth has already been laid down. It can make new paths from the tooth to new tumors. The only solution is to remove the polonium from your mouth by extracting these teeth. Drilling into polonium-teeth spreads the polonium…all the more metastases! We will see how to identify them later.

Summary — Chapter 12

1. You can stop making new tumors in the same organ by finding the allergic food you are eating.

2. You can stop making new tumors in a new organ (real metastases) by removing the polonium from your teeth, and from your surroundings.

3. You routinely absorb polonium from furniture, carpets, clothing that was washed in chlorox bleach. It acts like poison ivy or wet paint, never going away. That is why you must clean the house before starting the program. That is why moving to a house that never had chlorox contamination is so helpful. That is why the curing program has a special recipe for laundry and shampoo.

4. The cancer location table tells you which food to avoid to stop the allergy for the organ with cancer.

WANTED DEAD—OR DEADER

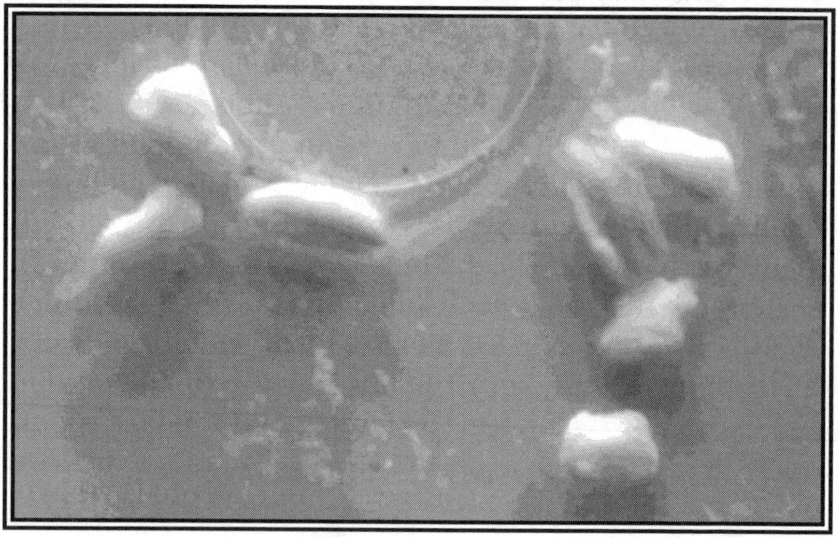

Looking like inanimate tiny particles of styrofoam "dust", these snow white larval stages betray the presence of Macracanthorhyncus. Macra's companions will be prions, derived from hypothalamus "free cells".

CHAPTER 13

OUR AMAZING IMMUNE SYSTEM

Our immune system was only discovered about 100 years ago by Metchnikov and others*.

Our white blood cells **are** our immune system.

The immune system in each organ takes care of its own organ. It is made of special "soldier" cells that guard this organ. These white blood cells call this organ their home. They may, though, leave this organ to visit ("communicate") with others in other organs. Most of this is done in your **lymph nodes**, their communication centers. It reminds us of beehives with their elaborate communication systems, all meant to keep the hive unified and thriving. Our white blood cells have the same purpose and for this reason they have special powers.

They can "sense" an enemy of ours from far away, for example, lead molecules or SV40 viruses. For this they need their "skins". Their outer membranes are their skins. Special sensors are imbedded in them. The rest of the membrane is made of a double-layered "fence" of fat molecules that keeps out intruders and toxic molecules.

The white blood cells can tell the difference between friends and enemies from a long way off. When a macrophage senses an enemy it moves toward it. Its big clumsy feet are called pseudopods but they can make long thin pseudopods, too. It reminds us of an armored tank when we watch it move in a live blood sample. White

---

* www.nobelprize.org

blood cells have a number of ways they can attack our enemies. Large enemies must be attacked and killed before they can be nibbled away. Smaller enemies like bacteria and viruses can be eaten whole just by engulfing them and then killed after they are inside. They are easily picked up with long thin pseudopods sent after them. Even prions are eaten.

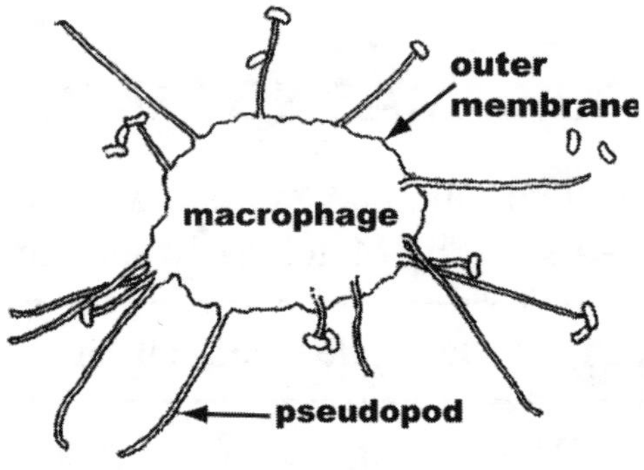

Fig. 81 Macrophage eating Salmonellas

White blood cells can make powerful chemicals called **cytokines** and **leukokines**. They include **interleukins** and **interferons**.

The Syncrometer® has detected many more such chemicals, also in very minute amounts. I have called them <u>weapons</u> (see page 194). Weapons are used to destroy the larger parasites so our digestive enzymes can digest them and our white blood cells can eat them. All available weapons are used in times of heavy parasitism.

DMSO is one such weapon that was discussed in earlier books. Due to its unavailability in USA, substitutes were found. MSM (methyl sulfonyl methane), another weapon we make, destroys **diallyl sulfide** and **allyl methyl sulfide**, ONION-chemicals that take part in the cancer-complex. Benzoquinone, another weapon, is made in very minute amounts. It destroys dozens of toxins such as these as well as many parasites including malaria. Rhodizonic acid in tiny amounts destroys Ascaris megalocephala.

Complement is another very important part of the immune system. It is part of a family of molecules used as spears! It is a way of spearing our tiny enemies so the white blood cells can eat them.

Different white blood cells are given different jobs to do and stay very organized.

Using the Syncrometer®, I have distinguished ten kinds of white blood cells. They are CD4 and CD8 lymphocytes, CD37 B cells, CD14 macrophages, and six more varieties that eat dyes and motor oil. The CD4s eat and kill viruses. The CD8s include our natural killers. They are even seen killing CD4s when these are not able to kill the viruses they have eaten. The CD14s eat everything, except you. Both CD8s and CD14s are flesh eaters; only these can eat tumor cells and large parasite pieces. We can also distinguish, electronically, the red blood cells (RBCs), platelets, eosinophils and megakaryocytes, all of them floating in the blood. Platelets are just tiny chips, not even cells, too small to hold a nucleus. Their job is to fill in the tiny tears and holes that are always developing in our arteries and veins. This job is called blood clotting. Eosinophils are white blood cells that can spit histamine at enemies especially Ascaris.

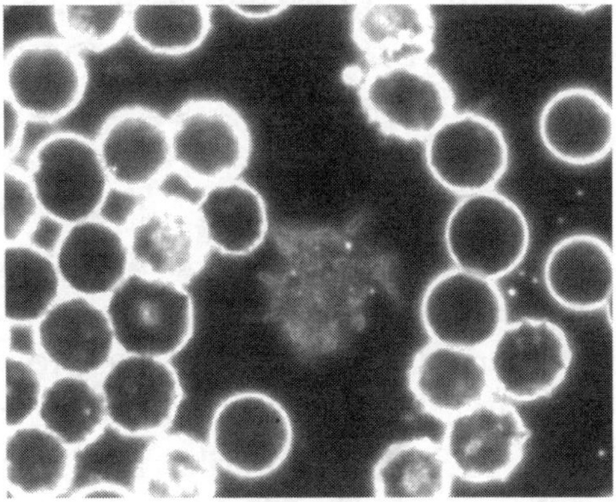

A macrophage, CD14, is at the center. The rest are RBCs.

Fig. 82 Live blood analysis

During the growing period of a tumor thousands of things are brought into the organ that has the tumor. They should have been brought to the liver or kidneys but, instead, they were deposited at the tumor site. Why didn't the white blood cells kill or remove all of these undesirables and bits of trash? That was their job. Why couldn't they keep up? They, too, along with the tumor cells and kidneys, became south polarized by the cargo they had to carry. PCBs, benzene, asbestos, dozens of heavy metals, including polonium and cerium, malonic acid, isopropyl alcohol, motor oil that included ONION, GARLIC, and MUSTARD oil, and hundreds of dyes as well as wheel bearing grease that had nickel imbedded in it, all arrived together from the drinking water. This kept them south polarized constantly. They could not cycle from north to south and back again to do their work. They were meant to pick up a southerly cargo, which temporarily turns them south, process it, expel it, and turn themselves back to north again for the next cargo. Northerly is their normal state for making a pick-up. But it takes work and living energy to process the cargo and turn itself back to northerly. This system of cycling can fail when the white blood cells are overwhelmed with too much ferrite iron or nickel and other heavy metals that are south. We will help them recover by stopping to burden them and by feeding them. Their biggest burden was chlorox bleach.

Removing The Burden

It is a common belief that we should boost our immunity, but it is much more effective to remove its destroyers. My emphasis will be on removing our biggest immunity inhibitors, those we were drinking in chlorox bleach water, before becoming aware of it.

PCBs

PCBs are toxins that get trapped in white blood cells' membranes. Since the membranes are made of fat, and PCBs dissolve in fat, it is understandable why the white cells lose their special powers. That is where their special sensors are located.

The main source of PCBs is the chlorox bleach added to about half the population's drinking water. Food manufacturers use this same water to prepare processed food. Because all the produce in the market has been washed several times, and moved through different water zones, most of it acquires PCBs.

Read about the actions of PCBs on the Internet.

Benzene Everywhere

Benzene is another immunity destroyer. It would be quite unwise to start taking immune boosters when benzene is in your water supply from an attached filter or softener.

Our agencies, FDA and EPA, have been vigilant over benzene in air, household chemicals and even gasoline but were never in a position to test food or water correctly. Using antiquated tests that can only find benzene in parts per billion (ppb) would never protect American citizens. Although the legal limit set by our agencies was 5 ppb, I never detected such huge amounts. If I had, such families would be languishing in hospitals. Our immunodepression comes from much smaller amounts. We must be protected from parts per trillion (ppt) amounts, a thousand-fold smaller. This is what I routinely find in processed foods. The entry of benzene into the food chain was not noticed because of this technical problem. Now it is in and on our food in such large amounts, most private testing labs can detect it.

Benzene has become a huge food problem, due to contamination with food spray and chlorox bleach water. Benzene comes right from your favorite supermarket and organic food store. You must stop using or eating everything that has it. Your food must be tested for it to be safe.

The body does not have a "safe amount" of benzene. But, as more and more benzene gets discovered in food, the public agencies will give up and shift their focus to higher "undetectable harm" amounts to spare the food industry. Beware of such shifts in wording, as "significant risk level" or "no detectable harm level". This is a deception, not science-based. It is meant to lead us to complacency over our failure to keep benzene out of food. Our children's health will be sacrificed for this. It will raise our cancer, malaria, HIV and AIDS incidence even higher. The focus should stay on <u>zero</u> amounts as it presently is, and, science-based.

Benzene also enters our food with flavors, colors and fragrance. It enters with pills, whether they are over the counter drugs, food supplements, or prescriptions. Flavors and colors were extracted and manufactured with solvents that came from the petroleum industry, including benzene. It was falsely believed that you could easily evaporate it out of the product. And certainly, enough came off to allow the product to come under the "limit" of detection for the measuring device. But it only gave us false security.

There are more ways that petroleum products come in contact with food. For example, the grain* that will make your bread is doused with "mineral oil" to keep the dust down. It has traces of benzene. And wherever petroleum grease is used—like in baking pans under cookies and breads!—benzene rides along. It may be surprising to find benzene in so many places where the temperature was raised above its boiling point; that is no safeguard. It was evidently trapped or it recondensed.

* Search "Grain Dust Explosions" on Internet.

The attitude of manufacturers and producers is: "You can expect benzene to be everywhere. It's even in the air and the blacktop in your driveway. It's negligible. As long as we meet FDA & EPA requirements, where's the problem?" This reminds me of an event in history, about 350 years ago.

In 1665, the worst year of the bubonic plague in England, the grain that was used to make peoples' bread was contaminated with rat feces and rat urine. But the merchants did not want to throw it out. If they ground it all up into tiny specks it would not be seen or tasted. It was everywhere in small amounts. You could not smell it or see it because the grain was ground finely into flour. It was not suspected to bring the bubonic disease since the sick and the healthy people all ate it. From this terrible tragedy we should have learned one lesson: When widespread illness comes to people we should examine our staple foods first, our bread and water, milk and meat. Bacteria and viruses certainly play their roles, but the vermin bringing them into our homes and our household habits supporting them should be analyzed in food before air and driveways. Private agencies, even independent scientists could quickly and easily find the causes of our diseases! It is the highly trained, professional investigators that cannot. Their hands are tied by contract and technology.

Benzene has been known to cause cancer for decades, especially the leukemias. That is why our agencies were given the important task of monitoring it. Yet they have failed to protect us, setting and raising legal levels instead. We have more leukemia than ever before. Why should benzene be legally permitted in beer when half the men are getting cancer? Regulations should not be based on tests done solely on the food later on, when the concentration will, of course, be less, making it all the more difficult to detect. It should be based on knowledge of "what goes in". It is evidence of a lack of concern for the public's well being. Communities should not depend on government agencies.

In a desperate England in 1665, rats were so numerous they crawled the streets openly. How could tiny bits of rat filth in the bread matter? It was everywhere. Besides, bread was baked, that should make it safe. The same "logic" was used then as now. We see people with and without cancer all around us drinking the same water. And it is all chlorinated, that should make it safe. The concepts are very flawed. Eventually, instead of killing rats, dogs and cats were removed in England, precisely those animals that could reduce disease by killing rats, an easy mistake to make when you're just guessing. We should not be guessing. We have scientists. We should be using them. We are only using medical professionals now who are not trained as scientists and who must give an attentive ear to all their vendors. We need physiologists, biologists, parasitologists, cytologists, entomologists, epidemiologists, ecologists, when studying a difficult problem. Instead, physiology departments at universities were closed in the 1960's on the pretext of saving expense! Only medical physiology departments were left open, paid for largely by the pharmaceutical industry. In the present day USA we are increasing and emphasizing the chlorination method of sanitizing water...the very treatment that is inadvertently doing the most harm.

We should be testing our food and water with the best equipment, of research quality. But we can't expect industry to create high standards for itself. Society must create them independently. There are very many retired doctors, scientists and individuals with a proactive attitude to disease prevention and societal welfare. Besides, we should not trust corporate testing nor agency testing when their personnel frequently "trade jobs". We must solve the problem of conflicts of interest. We must put renewed energy into parents' and society's responsibility to provide safe food and water for our children—children are most affected by leukemia.

Our white blood cells are forced to stop eating our enemies after they get benzene onto their membranes. One of benzene's actions is to let viruses into our genome. A special enzyme called **viral integrase** allows this whenever benzene is present.

Benzene activates malaria, triggers the HIV virus, causes immune deficiency in AIDS and causes cancer indirectly. There is even one route in our bodies that leads to benzene production by a fungus—Potato Ring Rot. Benzene must certainly be our worst scourge.

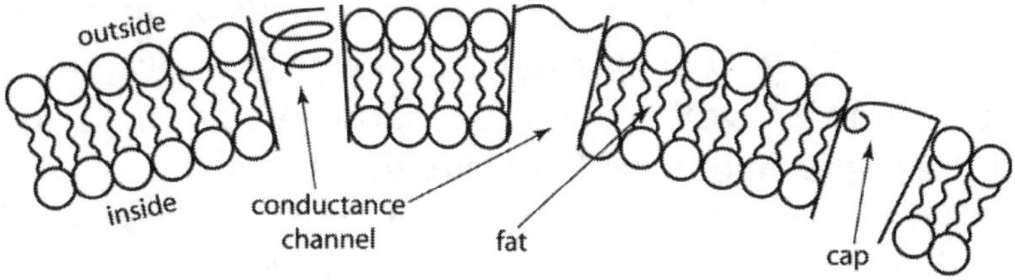

Fig. 83 A section of the cell's membrane

Your body has a moderate ability to get rid of benzene without help. It has a natural detoxification pathway. But it leads to pain and bleeding before it is all gone. Learn how to prevent this (see page 455).

Asbestos in our Food and Water

We have been so focused on asbestos in walls and ceilings that we missed the most obvious places, food and water. Not being able to detect the smaller fibers (under 10 μm), while these are actually the most harmful and numerous, made the agencies' regulations almost useless. A microscope should have been used and developed into an automated technique.

When the tiniest bit of asbestos is put in water, all the water around it becomes southerly polarized. This is because asbestos has iron molecules made of ferrite (Fe_2O_3), which is south polarized. When a tiny bit gets stuck in your tissue, the surrounding fluid, blood, and tissue become southerly. This is the trigger felt by the hypothalamus in the brain, telling it to release its stem cell factor. The message received could be imagined as "*Iron has been oxidized to south pole; this organ is surely traumatized and open to air, it will be in need of growth to repair the trauma*". Your body cannot be expected to know this is a false alarm. We did not evolve with asbestos in our food or water to make it wary.

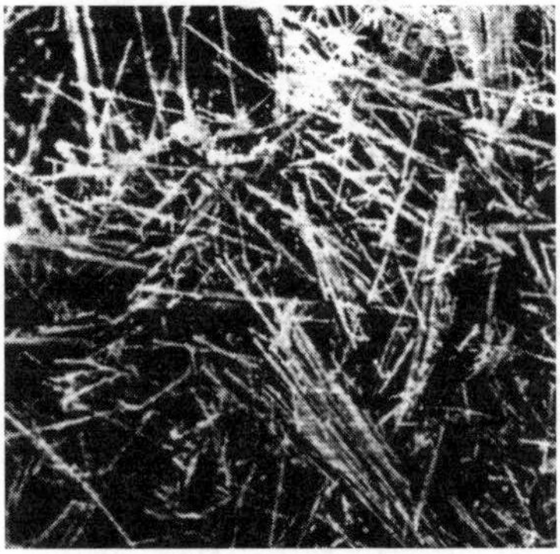

Fig. 84 Asbestos spears magnified

But at the same time, your white blood cells sense the truth: "there is a strange intruder; something needs to be eaten; it is not a mere trauma", and begin to eat the flood of tiny asbestos spears that are arriving. It is followed by drastically unhappy results! Asbestos spears each have built-in iron! When these tiny spears are eaten by a white blood cell, a lot of iron, of the south pole kind, has entered the white cells. A gene is triggered by this to produce **ferritin** because ferritin is the storage molecule for iron. It is the body's way to safely store such iron. Soon an excessive amount of ferritin is produced; so much, it oozes out of the white blood cells and coats their outside membrane. This ferritin coating acts like an oil slick over the immune cells and stops them immediately from eating more asbestos or anything else. They can't see. They can't sense.

Fortunately, we can wash the asbestos off our food if we use special hot-washes as we also do for PCBs and benzene. After this we can take a special supplement, **levamisole**, to remove the ferritin coating from the white blood cells. The enzyme, papain, can remove it, too, but is unbearably smelly.

The asbestos in water has not gone undetected. Water is said to have asbestos in it from old clay pipes used to bring it from the water reservoir. Read the pamphlet you get from your water department about asbestos. This could make anyone despair. But the Syncrometer® shows it never comes from the reservoir, even with these old clay pipes. It comes from the same pumping station or from a filter or softener salt where the wrongful bleach is added! The bleach itself had it. Perhaps gaskets from the pumps there had it, too. However, bleach of the correct kind (NSF stamped) does not have asbestos. Nor does water that is treated with NSF bleach.

There are huge amounts of asbestos on our food, both fruits and vegetables. Being sprayed with bleach water (laundry bleach) is a common practice to guarantee safety from bacteria. This brings asbestos with it and also wets the food as it rolls along conveyor belts. Conveyor belts are made with asbestos. Old frayed belts add huge amounts to the food, all to be tightly stuck as the produce dries under hot-air blowers. That is why 2 hot-washes are needed to remove it.

When asbestos has left your organs, along with nickel and radioactive elements they become north polarized again.

Remember that south polarization is not to be demonized. It is reserved for the nervous system by day and the body's <u>growing and healing points</u> at all times. The blood, though, swings from northerly to southerly and back again, minute by minute. Work is being done here that is still quite mysterious. It is an exchange of iron status, using iridium. And the white blood cells cycle from northerly to southerly and back again, too, with every toxic load they process and shed. You will get back these normal rhythms, and get back to a normal life when the polarizations are correct.

Dyes Stick Fast

Why are young children eating colored candy, colored drinks, colored cakes, and colored pieces of ornamental sugar on their food? Why are we so complacent about this?

Even the most primitive cook knows, and has always known, that food is off limits to tampering. Food is not a frivolous part of life. And paint may go on the body, temporarily, for dances, but not in the body. Such instincts are especially applied to children. Parents, throughout the ages, have seen to it that young children got no tampering.

Why have our instincts gone astray? Did we all feel safe in the care of our government agencies the way children feel safe with their parents while they take risks? Did we believe that enough scientific experiments would have been done and long-term tests required, preventing any catastrophe from ever happening? As food dyes, one by one, were removed from the food market in the 1960s, after a big increase in the cancer rate, we should have become suspicious of other dyes taking their place and of agencies in general. But as a nation of eager consumers, we did not.

Agencies are not all the same. Cautious agents who put the people's health first can be followed by agents who put other motives first. It will take people's groups, who are made up of real parents, not government agencies, to take back control over food and water safety. Agencies have too many conflicting interests. When any piece of meat, chicken or fish has azo dyes, and even the colored produce is dyed, food tampering is at an extreme. It is no wonder that every tumor tested showed the presence of a multitude of dyes. When a cancer patient's blood test shows an LDH or alkaline phosphatase level that is too high, they have succumbed to dyes in the laundry bleach, even though they are at an invisible level. The implication is quite grim…that we have hundreds and more dyes accumulated in all of us. One dye is always present in cancer patients—Fast Green #3 (also called Food Green)*. The Syncrometer® detects that it lengthens the life of cells that absorb it, although they become non-functional. Life is extended up to 15 times! It is acting just like the gang of oncoviruses! Cancer cells that would have, at least, died at their usual time, are now not able to turn on their own apoptosis. We have already seen oncoviruses doing exactly that. The longevity gene, bcl-2, is much too active. This gene is a major controller of apoptosis and is one of the mutations produced by the cancer-complex.

Normal Longevity

Two genes, bcl-2 and bax, have a big role in deciding how long each one of our cells may live. They keep a balance between living too long or not long enough. The longevity gene is bcl-2, while bax shortens life by triggering apoptosis. We could have suspected dyes to unbalance these two genes since they were found to mimic mutations in the past. Why haven't dye-caused mutations been found in regular research? Research choices are partly economically and partly politically made. Parents would make different choices. The Syncrometer® sees Fast Green dye concentrated in our CD8 natural killer cells. The cells remain quite alive after this, in increased

* This is Fast Green FCF with color index (CI)-42053. Search Fast Green, FCF on Internet.

numbers, but not able to kill anything. Food Green has accumulated in every USA cancer patient I tested. In the *2-Week Program* we will get the dye out with homeography after the dye sources, mainly chlorox bleach in food and water, have been removed.

Chlorox bleached water contains many dyes, although they can't be seen. Hundreds of dyes are contained in sprays and essentially all food is sprayed. Dyes are even on undyed food because laundry bleach disinfectant is used in washing it. It is even on freshly caught fish if the knives and cutting boards are disinfected with laundry bleach. I recently visited a fisherman's booth near a beach in Mexico. The freshly caught fish were whole and lay on ice. We saw the fisherman take his knife from a bucket of "water" and swish his table with a jug of "water". In a corner, on the floor, was a gallon of chlorox bleach. I bought a filleted fish and an unrinsed whole fish off the ice. I tested each. The fillets were full of dyes and hypochlorite (the telltale sign of chlorination). A piece of washed fish, not filleted, was full of dyes, too. Only the unwashed whole fish was safe to eat. There is evidently no safe fish in the market place. The Syncrometer® showed that canned fish, frozen fish and fresh fish were all processed with chlorox bleach. This food cannot be cleaned up. We must search for unbleached fish.

Wherever there is organic matter, dyes are absorbed deeply, the same way as in your tumor cells. They were invented to do exactly that—to stick fast (not fade).

Dyes do very damaging things. DAB is 4-dimethylaminoazobenzene. This dye raises the **alkaline phosphatase** level. Check yours on your blood test results. When it is too high DAB has filled the white blood cells. When it is too low, threatening organ failure, it is due to cobalt. When dyes are in your B-lymphocytes the globulin level is disturbed. Sudan Black B and Fast green can raise your LDH. Check yours. It will be in the red blood cells, stuck there, sometimes with vanadium. High LDH and alkaline phosphatase are drastic events in terminal cancer patients. When LDH and alkaline phosphatase levels have gone over 500 or even 1000 it has been speculated about in clinical science but no true cause found or pursued. Fast Red and Fast Red Violet cause edema and effusates to develop in the lungs or brain or abdomen. This is a common cause of death from these cancers! Fast Red Violet blocks the body's ability to detoxify **maleic anhydride**. It has been known for decades that this substance causes "leakage and effusions" (see *The Merck Index*, 10th edition). The maleic anhydride comes from the malonic acid in food sprays, in cooking oils, and tooth fillings, and from plastic from your dishes, but mostly from chlorox in your water. The body has a route for detoxifying it, but not if a dye blocks this (see page 476).

I have studied only seven of many dyes in our food. They need to be studied in all our diseases.

Another dye that is suspect for causing disease is common *methylene blue*. It is considered so safe, it is used to stamp meat and fruits and to add to laundry. The Syncrometer® sees that it goes to the DNA, like any other alkylator, thereby transporting parasites, bacteria and viruses into our chromosomes. All these living things are dyed by it, making a tight connection between parasite DNA and our DNA. Electron transfer, life's driving force, must happen between them. Our genes could get activated by theirs.

The extent of pollution with dyes is almost unimaginable. Here is a real example. Recently a one-mile stretch of ocean beach was being prepared for a beach festival in California. Regular ocean water samples were taken and found to have some E. coli bacteria, not uncommon in these waters. The Navy forces were called in to make the beach safe. Soon the ocean was pink! The Syncrometer® detected chlorox laundry bleach and many dyes in it. Apparently the Navy poured in bleach, but also added red dye to mark the area that was treated—we tested the pink water. It looked intensely pink for about ½ mile offshore, and lasted for about one week. The public was informed that it was due to "red tide", certain algae! All the azo dyes in my test kit (18) were in the water, including Fast Green, no doubt a pollutant of the red dye and in the laundry bleach. The dye did not go away; it sank to the bottom of the ocean and could be seen for 2 years afterwards in shallow areas. It will bring immunodepression and growth of tumors to fish, sea mammals and shore birds. (See page 475 for the eventual outcome.)

Modern enamel cookware seeps huge amounts of dyes. Your toothbrush seeps copious dyes. Your plastic glasses and wristwatch seep. Your plastic teeth seep dyes even when they are white!

After stopping drinking them in chloroxed water we can begin to pull the dyes out of your tumors. We will use 2 supplements (vitamin B_2 and coenzyme Q10), round after round of zapping, and finally homeography. We will use drops of **propylene carbonate** to pull methylene blue off your DNA. But the fear is that the dyes will get stuck again in your kidneys or liver along the exit path. Be sure to keep the bowels moving and the bladder emptying.

Heavy Metals in Water and Food

Nowhere in the plant or animal world do we see shiny metals taking part in the growth of an organ or even just being present. Yet these same shiny metals can be changed by chemistry to another form, called **organic**. Atoms of the metal can be tightly held by special proteins to make **enzymes**. Now they are called **minerals**, not metals, although the elements are the same. Some metals are never changed into minerals: uranium, palladium, and the lanthanides, for example. Find these in the *Periodic Table* on page 36. Lead, antimony, cadmium, bromine, fluorine, aluminum are further examples. The lanthanides were called "rare earths" until recently. There are 15 of them in a group specially marked on the chemical table. They are more magnetic than other metals, though not as magnetic as iron. They always occur together and can hardly be separated, so there are no "pure" preparations. Thulium, gadolinium and lanthanum are all lanthanides. There must be some very important reason for Mother Nature to keep certain metals and the lanthanides out of our bodies. Are they too oxidizing? Would they compete with other minerals? Would they disturb our magnetic polarization? The real reasons will not be known till biologists have uncovered many more secrets of life, including electronic and magnetic properties. Till then, Mother Nature gave us instinct. Metal does not taste good or feel good; the implication is that we should not eat it or wear it on our skin even though we don't drop dead when we do. Nature's rules have millions of years of wisdom behind them. But she could not anticipate "civilization", which should perhaps be labeled "regression", quite often. Metal did look good, with its sparkle and its shine. We fell in love with them, too, as we did with dyes.

Although metals are safe deep in the earth, far away from us, we have dug them up, thrown them in the air just for thrills (firecrackers on the 4th of July in the USA fill the air with strontium). We have puffed them into the air as car exhaust, wrapped them around ourselves to wear, stuck them inside ourselves as rings, cooked in them and, finally, put them right in our food. We wallow in metal. Aluminum, an unthinkable "food", found nowhere in

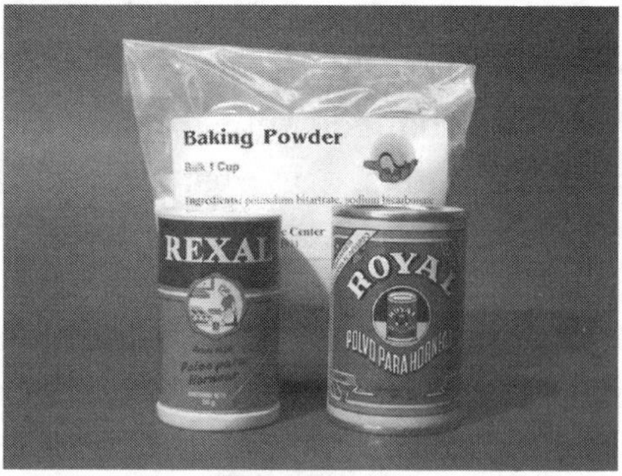

Fig. 85 Aluminum-free baking powder

living things, was actually dumped into our food in the 1880s and has been there ever since. The "invention", called baking powder, was none other than adding aluminum to a liquid; it bubbled! That is how non-yeast-rising breads were born. Now that Alzheimer's disease is rampant, with its accumulation of aluminum in the brain, and Herpes and EBV (chronic fatigue) very common, this practice should be stopped as well as the practice of adding aluminum to all drinking water before it is disinfected!

We wallow in chromium and nickel in our food. Anything finely ground or blended with steel blades that get hot (powdered supplements, smooth peanut butter) brings them. We must test each jar.

Choosing plastic, ceramic or glass cookware gives us even more! These seep mercury, nickel, thallium(!), gold and malonic acid, besides.

Teflon and glass seep copious amounts of thallium and gold.

Gold, The Curse?

Gold is much more difficult to detoxify than other metals. So it becomes the job of our WBCs to eat it and remove it. But if radioactivity is present the WBCs lose their vitamin C and can't work. Our organs gradually fill up with gold. This feeds prions and attracts Macracanthorhyncus. The organ is now marked for failure and death. Gold has been considered a curse in the past and for good reason. Replace it with "precious non-metal".

Yet, what could be worse than eating metals from our plastic dishes, and copper water pipes? One thing! Sucking metals straight, like lollipops, in your mouth day and night in the form of tooth fillings. The dissolved metal sweeps into your tonsils, your thyroid gland, parathyroids, thymus, and directly into your tumors. If we see a child sucking on pennies or other change we quickly snatch it away…we instinctively know it is harmful. There are about 40 metals in each such tooth-lollipop (see page 37). How could we blunder so badly as adults? Your body is barely able to keep up with the heavy metals left behind by <u>its own enzymes</u>, let alone added ones from tooth fillings. Those from enzymes of all sorts are copper, cobalt, chromium, vanadium, gold, germanium, molybdenum, ruthenium, rubidium, selenium, manganese, zinc, iron, nickel, and iridium. They are not necessarily from our <u>own</u> enzymes. They are left in us by fungus and bacteria. This will give us some astonishing insights. These metals steal our youth, our health, and our destiny (longevity) as they slowly accumulate with age. If they accumulate suddenly, we are in a crisis—a disease like liver failure. If they accumulate slowly, we believe we are aging and accept it meekly. They are our "natural" heavy metals, coming from living matter (living in us!). Obviously, we should not <u>eat</u> more of them to hasten our end.

Copper from water pipes often brings lead, too, from the solder joints. If lead and copper are detected by a Syncrometer® tester or a water lab, change your pipes to PVC or have them epoxy coated on the inside (see *Sources*).

Nickel turns us southerly.

Just by the very act of harboring other creatures in us, we become a repository of all their metals. The harm that is done by nickel alone, besides inviting infection, is major. It consumes our iridium and it turns us southerly! Iridium levels fall very low wherever nickel deposits are seen. A tumor, due to its stockpile of nickel from Clostridium bacteria, cannot salvage its own iron deposits and make it usable again. There is an iridium shortage. Yet, the iron ferrite (Fe_2O_3) deposits must be cleared away somehow to get the tumor zone back to a northerly polarization.

Healing cannot go forward because of low iridium levels. A very low level of 29 is reached for iridium (in homeopathic units of 1 in 5 dilution) in advanced cancer. Levels in the 80's are normal, and a level of 120 is seen in young children.

Aging

Each of us, whether sick or healthy, is full of heavy metals by the time we are old. But it is not a random assortment of heavy metals. It is always these:

- chromium
- copper
- cobalt
- germanium
- lanthanides
- nickel
- radioactive elements
- selenium
- vanadium

Is it not astonishing that these are the same metals described in earlier books to be the common denominators of tumors?

The body's metals in cancer, in disease, and in aging are the same ones, having become oxidized, left behind by dead enzymes of our own and from our invaders. The tumor cells are unable to reverse the process to make organic minerals again and reclaim them. Nor can healthy bodies do this as we age. We just can't keep up with this part of our housekeeping (body maintenance) chores. Copper turns us brown in spots, cobalt gives us heart disease, vanadium disturbs our globulin (antibody) production and RBC formation, oxidized germanium gives us WBC deficiencies, chromium gives us blood sugar problems and pain, gold gives us ovary disease, diabetes, prion disease and obesity, nickel brings us more and more infection, baldness, and allergies. Yet, none of this seems necessary! It should be avoidable!

The same metals are used by our parasites, bacteria, and even viruses and prions. These fuel our diseases.

> Illness, including cancer, is metal disease. We should fall out of love with metals.

Ruthenium belongs to many leaves, stems, and branches of bushes. No free ruthenium can be found, though, for 20 seconds after picking the leaves. I presume it has oxidized in this time so the ruthenium metal is no longer attached to its enzyme. Then we can detect it. Coconut shells have much ruthenium. Charcoal filters are steeped in it. It gets into all the water that is poured through them. Is it harmful or harmless? At least one parasite, Macracanthorhynchus uses it. Malaria uses it, too. Certainly drinking large amounts of it as we would if we drank filtered water, would accumulate to toxic levels. Such an ultra trace element was meant to be present only in the tiniest amounts.

That is why I recommend prewashing the coconut charcoal filter in hot water…to wash out the ruthenium and the over abundant oils.

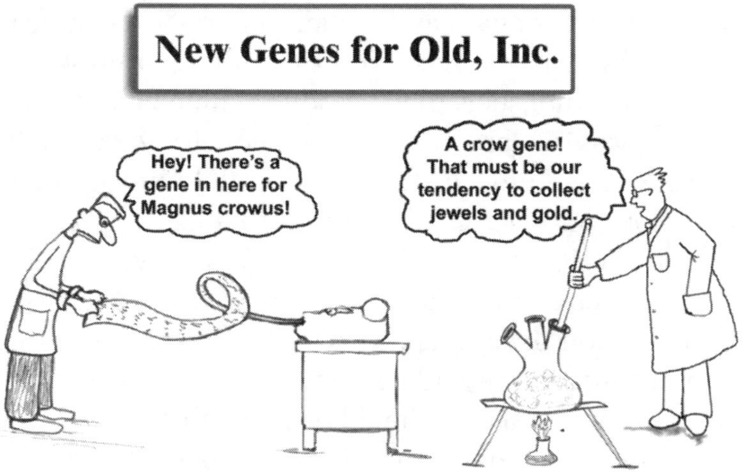
New Genes for Old, Inc.
Hey! There's a gene in here for Magnus crowus!
A crow gene! That must be our tendency to collect jewels and gold.

Radioactive Elements

We had no idea until recently that we are surrounded by radioactive elements. Some come from bomb testing a few decades ago but many are frivolous and come from an attitude that scorns caution. The attitude is one of "finding a use" for them. And so uranium, leftover from making bombs and stockpiled for many years, was turned into dental replacements to make them sparkle and glow on x-ray film (easier to spot).

Radioactivity was only discovered about 100 years ago, so ignorance and lack of wisdom must take its toll but the older and parental generation should do its part to protect the young. The discoverer of radium died from merely handling it a number of years. How could we be so bold as to let our children suck on it for years by putting uranium, which always turns into some radium and polonium, right in their mouths?

Radioactive elements come up from the ground under us if we are living over shallow phosphate rocks. Uranium is combined with the phosphates. Uranium keeps breaking apart into lighter and lighter elements. Uranium leads to thorium, which is thought to heat our planet from within. It also leads to radon, which is a gas and bubbles up under our houses and lakes. We must be quite careful to avoid radon because it breaks up further into radioactive **lead**, **bismuth**, **thorium** and **polonium**. Polonium does more harm than others because of its **alpha radiation**. Alpha can do more harm in 1 mm of travel through us than other kinds of radiation do even in many inches. The Syncrometer® has found that polonium causes all our cancers.

> Polonium causes all our cancers, not just lung cancers, by starting the cancer-complex to form.

Earlier and even ancient therapists suspected "malevolent spirits" coming up from the earth in certain places to cause cancer. How right they were! They called it "the geopathic factor" and recommended moving.

As the world's growing population squeezes its housing onto rocky lands, we get closer to the radioactivity. Tiny gas bubbles of radon work their way up through the cracks, attaching themselves to a dust particle for a tiny magic carpet. They sail into our homes and through them with the air currents, getting stuck here and there, and suddenly, without warning shooting off a bullet as if it were a mighty cannon. The bullet is an **alpha particle**; it is positively charged. Along its path it attracts negative charges, causing great disruptions in our body chemistry as it crisscrosses through our tissues. Each tunnel it digs in our organs could cut a chromosome in two, or dot its path with smaller gene mutations. The harm is easy to see through a microscope.

Polonium, uranium and radon give off similar alpha particles as they shoot their pathways through our bodies.

Cut chromosomes are evidence of an alpha emitting radioactive element. After shooting off an alpha "ray", the element is lighter and has an entirely different nature. In this way uranium turns into thorium, thorium turns into radium, radium turns into radon, radon turns into polonium, and polonium turns into lead. But not ordinary lead. This lead is radioactive, shooting a "**beta**" **particle**, which is an electron and very tiny compared to an alpha particle. It is negatively charged and can travel long distances. This again leaves a new element behind. This kind of radioactive "decay" is going on around us and in us as we inhale radon gas along with the oxygen and nitrogen of the air. The whole "family" of radon's "daughters" is called the **radon decay series**. Of course we inhale radon's "daughters" too, if we are living in a "radon house", where a large amount comes up from the earth.

Many radioactive elements, including uranium itself, give off gamma radiation. This is similar to x-rays. These have no particles but the electromagnetic rays can travel long distances, right through most solids. All this radioactivity, alpha, beta, and gamma, makes up a "background" we can measure with a Geiger counter. A lot of damage is done, but our cells have ways of healing all kinds of radiation damage. Even damage to our genes, called mutation, is regularly healed using special enzymes called DNA repair enzymes. Nevertheless, it would be a good idea to move away from uranium rocks and certainly not build our homes underground or with a below-ground level.

Lanthanide Elements

Nor did we have any idea, ever, that we are wading in lanthanide elements. Notice the row of 14 elements in the chemical table, page 37. They all belong in one little square where lanthanum (Ln) is located to make 15. After WWII there was a determination to "put them to use", and "get them into commerce". The study of health effects lagged far behind the commerce, so gadolinium and others were injected into people to make scans more visible. When health effects did show up, it was too late. The FDA and EPA, in fact, all governments protect commerce. True protection for society can only come from the people themselves. Thulium, ytterbium and yttrium were put into reverse osmosis membranes. Cerium expanded its use in fire-lighters to plastics because it was so reactive. While putting them to "use" we did not realize that we already had been knee deep in them from birth because they, too, came up from the earth. They, too, combine so eagerly with phosphates that they are found in the same rocks as uranium. Only one of the 15 lanthanides is radioactive, **promethium** (Pm). The Syncrometer® shows that at all times our air is full of Pm, our bodies are full of Pm and we constantly sweat, eliminate and excrete it. Does it do harm or good? Most elements do some of each. We should study and understand what to expect from them if we live on top of uranium rocks. Which of the 15 are most abundant will depend on what is present below, and the weather. Rain and snow seals over, temporarily, the rising lanthanide mixture as well as radioactivity mixture. When the earth dries again, they both burst upward again. Cold weather increases the flow upward; maybe new cracks develop to allow more travel.

Each radioactive element does its own kind of damage. Radon is inhaled and while it is in our bodies its family is produced, giving us radioactive lead, bismuth, and the others. Lead moves into our bones, as usual. Little is known about the attracting organs for the others. The polonium produced does not stay free because it quickly reacts and combines with other metals and our phosphates.

We sweat and excrete all the radioactive elements all the time, but many linger in us because they attach themselves to our bacteria. Our Salmonellas, E. coli, and others routinely have polonium, promethium, cerium and terbium attached to them.

As our WBCs attack these bacteria they are confronted with the radioactivity on them. Almost immediately the WBCs' vitamin C is consumed. The germanium and selenium are not depleted, but vitamin C is quickly depleted. Unless they get more vitamin C the WBCs, namely your entire immune system is stalled. It takes large amounts (grams, not milligrams) of vitamin C to keep radioactivity flowing out of the body. Laundry bleach and consequently the public water itself is treated with radioactivity inadvertently, through use of phosphate buffers and anti-scale treatments. We must increase our vitamin C consumption in rather large amounts. By constantly consuming our vitamin C and stalling our WBCs we are left with lowered immune power. The radioactivity in us is constantly producing mutations; those that emit alpha rays can cause whole chromosomes to break, called "aberrations", besides the smaller gene mutations.

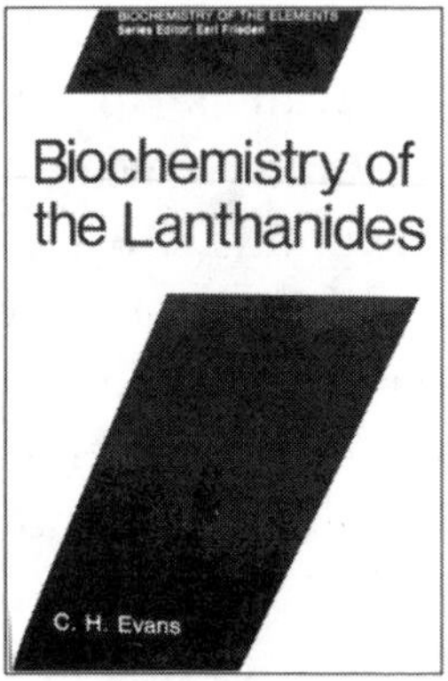

ISBN-0-306-43176-9

Fig. 86 Lanthanides disrupt DNA timing for transcription and replication

Lanthanide damage is seen on a grand scale in their reactions with our energy supply…our phosphates, especially our ATP, ADP, and AMP. Older people and sick people have almost no free ATP or ADP or AMP to get the body's work done. It is all attached to the lanthanides. Fatigue is felt. The lanthanides are so much more abundant than calcium that they crowd out the calcium, specifically. Problems with bone density, blood clotting, muscle action, that have been attributed to insufficient calcium, vitamin D, or sunshine are a toxicity effect of lanthanides according to the Syncrometer®. We must supplement these.

Terbium, especially, competes with our calcium. Different locations and different times and weather greatly affects our terbium intake and calcium levels. Terbium gives you tiny blood blisters and bruises by sticking to your thrombin*. Finding ways to keep terbium, cerium and other lanthanides at low levels in our homes would surely prevent a great deal of low-calcium caused disease and be helpful in recovering from cancer, as well as providing us with much more energy.

Bromine and fluorine are newcomers as toxins. Both belong to the group called halogens, along with chlorine and iodine. Bromine is added to our drinking water to help disinfect it. Fluorine is added to reduce tooth cavities. The possible harm done by the protection is far greater than the original problem.

The Syncrometer® finds that bromine and fluorine attract polonium! Instead of allowing it to pass through us as quickly as possible, it is accumulated in the spleen in large deposits. We now each have a reservoir of polonium in our spleens in the form of polonium-bromine and polonium-fluorosilicylate. These levels are especially high in the gold-related diseases (HIV, SV40, Prions, AIDS). We must find ways to reduce them. Find unbrominated and unfluoridated food and water.

---

* Testers, search for thrombin and thrombin combined with (touching) terbium.

Banish Sickness Again

We had learned that feeling sick is not due to the cancer itself. It is due to a half dozen well known bacteria and viruses. But they could not be identified or killed the usual way (with culturing and antibiotics). They were given advantages by carrying radioactivity. But we had found their vulnerability...they still need their metals to make their enzymes! It will be a simple matter to cut off their metal supplies and get relief from sweats, fever, coughs, bloating, organ failures, deep pain, and plain sickness. It can be done in less than a week. Here are their daily requirements.

Pathogens' Daily Requirements Table

Items in "*italic*" need further confirmation.

Pathogen	Requires
Adenovirus 16	copper (trigger is linoleic oil, *quercitin*)
Adenovirus 36 (obesity)	copper, chromium
Adenovirus, respiratory	copper, chromium, *cobalt*
Aspergillus (fungus)	cobalt, chromium, nickel
Avian Flu	gold, vanadium
Bacillus cereus	copper, cobalt, aluminum
Borrelia (Lyme's)	copper, *radon*
Chaetomium (fungus)	strontium, gold
Clostridium	nickel, *cobalt*
Cytomegalovirus (CMV)	strontium
Dirofilaria	chromium
E. coli	vanadium, molybdenum, manganese, chromium, nickel, copper
Epstein Barre Virus (EBV)	aluminum, gold, chromium, vanadium, *house dust*
Flu (Influenza A & B)	vanadium, see also Avian Flu
Herpes I & II	lead
HIV	gold (attached to core), strontium (attached to reverse transcriptase)
JUN	strontium (trigger is palmitic oil)
Measles	(trigger is linolenic; source is Ascaris)
Mumps	manganese, copper, zinc; source is Ascaris
Mycobacterium avium/cellulare	strontium, vanadium

Pathogen	**Requires**
Mycobacterium phlei (causes Schizophrenia and Multiple Sclerosis)	chromium, vanadium, gold, *house dust;* source is dog saliva
Mycobacterium tuberculosis	strontium
Mycoplasma	strontium
Mycoplasma arthriditis	vanadium; source is Bacillus cereus
Norcardia (Parkinson's)	titanium, *tantalum*
Papilloma (common warts virus)	(trigger is ASA); source is Echinoporyphium recurvatum
Penicillium (fungus)	copper
Plasmodium falciparum (malaria)	copper, ruthenium, selenium
Pneumocystis carinii (coccidia)	strontium
Potato Ring Rot	gold, source is Macracanthorhyncus
Prions	gold, ruthenium, source is free hypothalamus cells
Pseudomonas aeruginosa	strontium, gold
Salmonella enteriditis	gold, ruthenium, molybdenum, rubidium
Salmonella typhimurium	gold, ruthenium, molybdenum, rubidium
Salmonella paratyphi	gold, ruthenium, molybdenum, rubidium
Shigella (both types)	Strontium, gold, nickel
Staphylococcus aureus	chromium, gold, nickel
Streptococcus G	chromium, vanadium, nickel
Streptococcus pneumoniae	chromium, strontium, copper, gold, nickel
Streptococcus pyogenes	cobalt
SV40	chromium, strontium, gold
Warts	see Papilloma
Yeast (bread and alcohol variety)	chromium, nickel, cobalt, gold

Fig. 87 Our pathogens' daily requirements

If you have been sent to Hospice and can hardly endure living, a loved one can still rescue you. You may have all the symptoms mentioned in *Sickness Be Gone* (page 249). But you can banish them all in this simple way.

Hermits' Program

Go to live on a property that never had municipal water. There should be well water—unchlorinated, for all purposes. Test it for Total Chlorine with the most sensitive test paper (.05 mg/L or ppm). Drink only this.

Plant a garden. Tend it every day if the sun is shining.

Extract all artificial teeth and trim the gums as well as cleaning each socket. Harden any dentures after testing for radioactivity or do without. Start mouthwashes promptly with EDTA after each dental visit for 2 hours a day. Start as you slide out of the chair.

Cut off your dyed hair; use no more.

Bring a small chest freezer.

Lie flat till pain disappears without pain killer (10 days). Sleep upstairs in a well ventilated room or test the dust for radon.

For soap, use borax only. Use alcohol and white safe detergent for first shampoos, laundries and cleaning (see *Sources*).

Then start the program.

Early success could bring you new hope and soon a goodbye forever to Hospice. They did their best. They are to be commended on carrying on without hope. But your life beckons as you see you can succeed.

Summary — Chapter 13

1. The immune system is a vast network of guardian cells, called white blood cells. They have special powers, like traveling wherever they wish, mobilizing other white blood cells to help them, going to conferences at different lymph nodes, and listening to the beat of a different drummer that understands our lives much better than we do...perhaps including electric and magnetic fields.

2. In cancer patients many of these white blood cells cannot see, hear or taste; some cannot fight, some cannot travel nor capture trespassers, our invaders. They are disabled. Others are clogged. They had to eat so much motor oil, wheel bearing grease, dyes, and heavy metals, they cannot disgorge it all for want of enough organic selenite, vitamin C, and germanium.

3. The WBC cargos are south pole materials stalled on the way to the urine for dumping.

4. Iridium seems to have physiological importance. It appears to be linked to nickel removal as well as iron reduction. Although iridium is plentiful in rainwater, and can be drunk there, it is not advisable to take iridium chemicals as supplements. Only Nature, as in rainwater and certain herbs, could be trusted.

5. Metals can be divided into natural and unnatural varieties. Natural metals are those used by living things.

6. If NSF bleached water can be found quickly, the chance of recovery is excellent. Otherwise, no matter how good a cure or a clinical remission it is, it will soon fail again. Moving away from your "cancer-house" is by far the best advice, landing in a water zone that delivers NSF chlorinated water and in a house that never had filters or softeners attached to the plumbing.

7. Metals and minerals are one and the same element, but in different form. When they are used in an enzyme or by a living being they are in organic or mineral form. They are sensitive to strong oxidizers, or high heat cooking, losing their structure, so the element gets oxidized to metal again. Metal forms are toxic to organic forms.

9. We can destroy all our invading bacteria and some viruses by taking away the metals they need to survive. We do not need antibiotics to rid ourselves of them. Starving bacteria and viruses is faster than using medicines or herbs although they should not be condemned. A long recipe of homeographic antibiotics and herbs can kill many pathogens in 24 to 48 hours.

WANTED DEAD—OR DEADER

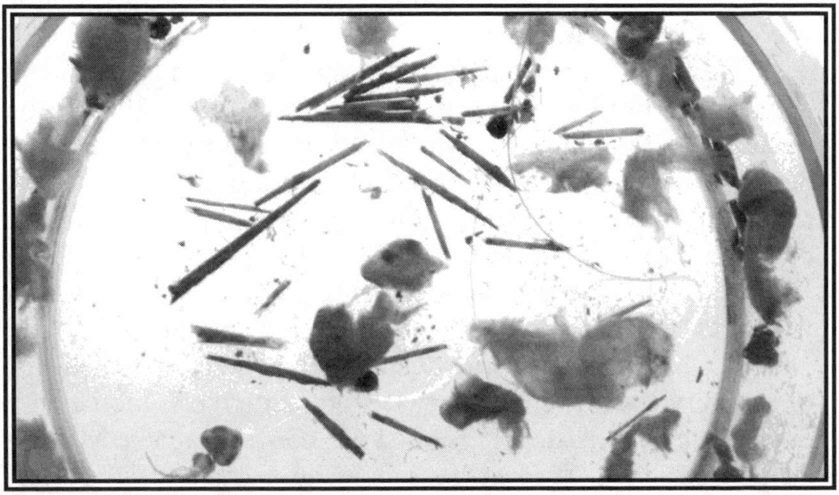

Spear-like E. recurvatum is a fluke, often 1 inch long. Other flukes and tapeworm segments make up the remaining "parasite soup" gathered during a liver cleanse diarrhea.

WARNING: DO NOT EXPERIMENT ON YOURSELF to remove tapeworm. The recipes were not complete at time of publishing.

CHAPTER 14

MAGNETIC HEALING

The commonest metal of all, plain iron, displays magnetic forces the most obviously. Yet, scientists have hardly begun to study its role in our bodies. It may be the most important actor in our metabolism and also the most important disruptor of metabolism in cancer and many diseases. In illness it has become the victim of other metals.

As a mineral, iron is essential. It is in your hemoglobin, for instance. But after it is oxidized to the ferric form, or to ferrite, Fe_2O_3, it is quite harmful in the wrong places. I believe this is partly because it is so easily magnetized. Any little bit of metallic iron can become strongly magnetized, even if it seems not to be magnetic, like a tack or paper clip. Take the cans on your food shelf for example. They are easily magnetized because they contain iron.

Even the tiniest pin would not stick to a can of food, though, because the can's magnetism is not strong enough. Still, you may be surprised to detect the force yourself with a small compass. Choose a can of food that has sat on the shelf a long time (weeks) with the same end up. Measure it at the top—your compass might find it is actually north pole. Measure it at the bottom, it will be south pole. You may find two places north, side by side, or a north and south pole on the sides, across the can. For every north pole there is a south pole somewhere. Numerous poles are possible, even side by side and upside down. Nearly anything is possible with iron, a situation that the body could never allow for its iron and survive.

The earth's magnetic field magnetized the tin can and does this rather quickly. You can turn the can upside down and a few days later find the poles are reversing! The same thing could happen to iron deposits in you if they were allowed to develop. Your body is not shielded from earth's magnetic field; in fact your body depends on it. Small deposits that are free to turn would behave like compasses. The earth's magnetic field, about ½ gauss in USA, is actually very powerful.

The total amount of iron in the body is quite small (about the size of a pea); probably for this reason…it must be so carefully protected! Some varieties of iron are obviously magnetic. Others are not. Simple oxidation or reduction, done in a second by your body, can make it non-magnetic or switch its poles, a drastic change. Iron supplies almost half our enzymes and all the hemoglobin in our red blood cells and myoglobin in our muscles. The cytochrome enzymes in every cell and P450 detoxifying enzymes are iron-enzymes. Even the very enzyme that makes DNA from RNA, called **ribonucleotide reductase**, contains iron. Maybe this is the critical iron atom that senses the magnetic field. Its traveling electron has an extra long path to take as it shuttles back and forth to make DNA, long enough to be the sensor, perhaps. Such iron could not be allowed to change its form uncontrolled. Perhaps this is why we have evolved such a good salvaging method for used-up iron. After red blood cells die and abandon their iron or when your enzymes need replacement and abandon theirs, it is quickly salvaged. Special white blood cells shuttle it all into a little ball of protein called ferritin (also see page 310). Inside the ball, it forms a tiny clump of thousands of molecules. Perhaps it can't be magnetized inside this cage. Perhaps the cage is a magnetic shield. The Syncrometer® finds the iron going into this cage to be south polarized but no magnetic field or polarization can be detected from ferritin afterwards. It also finds iridium molecules, the oxidized kind, inside ferritin. Are they sheltered together? Is the iridium reducing the iron back to usable form? Read more about ferritin on the Internet.

When iron is deposited outside of this little living cage it becomes magnetized into a strong south pole. A north pole may be presumed to be present somewhere, but has never been found by Syncrometer®.

The same thing could happen inside your body as happens inside the tin can. The food near the north part of the can will be north polarized. And the food just inside the south part will become south polarized. You cannot see this with a compass or even a magnetometer, but a Syncrometer® finds it easily. It is an effect of the north or south pole force nearby. The molecules have turned in one direction under the influence of the north pole and the other direction under the influence of the south pole. The Syncrometer® distinguishes them. They coincide with the letters d- and l- given to sugars and proteins.

l-molecules of amino acids have north polarization; d-molecules of these same amino acids have south polarization. Sugar molecules seem to have the opposite rule but are much less studied. A mixture of d- and l-, such as in citric acid made in a laboratory has no polarization.

The water surrounding a deposit of iron is given the same magnetic property as the deposit. I called such water north polarized or south polarized earlier (see page 242).

The Syncrometer® finds that an organ with iron deposits becomes south polarized when it should be north polarized. The white blood cells there do the same. When the iron is safely inside ferritin, it does not polarize the region around it, the organ stays north polarized when it should, daytime.

Certain organs are naturally south polarized by day, the whole brain, spinal cord and nerves, for example. The eggs inside the ovary and sperm inside the testis are also south by day.

Organs that are south polarized are capable of experiencing a powerful growing force, as if the ribonucleotide reductase enzyme had been turned on explosively. In the body, growing yeast can turn this enzyme on. We must stop its intrusion in your growth regulation. When a manufactured magnet is held within inches of the skin (back of neck) the north side turns off DNA, the south side turns on DNA. The south pole opens all the doorways into the cells, called channels, allowing them to feed constantly. These cells are treated like queen bees or sumo wrestlers.

When Nature is in control, the small molecule called stem cell factor arrives at these locations (south), presumably to stimulate the stem cells into growth and to feed them with all the essential minerals at the same time.

The true Nature of the growing force streaming from south pole magnets through water and living matter to produce south polarization is still not clear. Is it simply the opening of all feeding conductance channels? Is it the simultaneous turning on of DNA-manufacture? Is it the arrival of stem cell factor? Is it the bending of light to the right? A study of this force may reveal a fascinating story of how non-chemical life forces are transmitted and maintained.

The body will excrete the iron that was abandoned by cells and didn't get salvaged promptly, even using the nighttime to do this. It evidently is urgent to the body. But if there is an overwhelming amount of south pole iron it can get stuck in the kidneys on its way out. Then the kidneys become south polarized. This is the critical damage done to a cancer patient. All cancer patients have disabled kidneys even when nothing appears to be wrong with them.

It could be fixed, though, by removing nickel, including radioactive nickel. Your job will be to unload all the metal you can, most importantly, nickel, uranium and polonium. When this is done your cancer will turn around, bringing back your health and energy. This is the project undertaken in this book.

You now have a map that shows you the scientific path we will take to reach the goal. The goal is a scan or x-ray with the tumor missing, the illness gone, and the toxicity diseases gone. It is a more demanding goal than we had in the advanced cancer book or the *Prevention* book. We were satisfied then with the tumor missing. Notice how many patients were completely surprised even by this. Yet, it should come as no surprise now because it is rational and can be monitored with a Syncrometer®. The various apoptotic steps fall in place, the digestive enzymes appear at the tumor site, and the white blood cells can be seen eating the leftover tumor cells.

You are now ready to start the *2-Week Program*, knowing why you are doing everything. And why it has to succeed.

Syncrometer® testers can follow the *Tester's Guide* on page 437, to help avoid mistakes and speed up the cure.

WANTED DEAD—OR DEADER

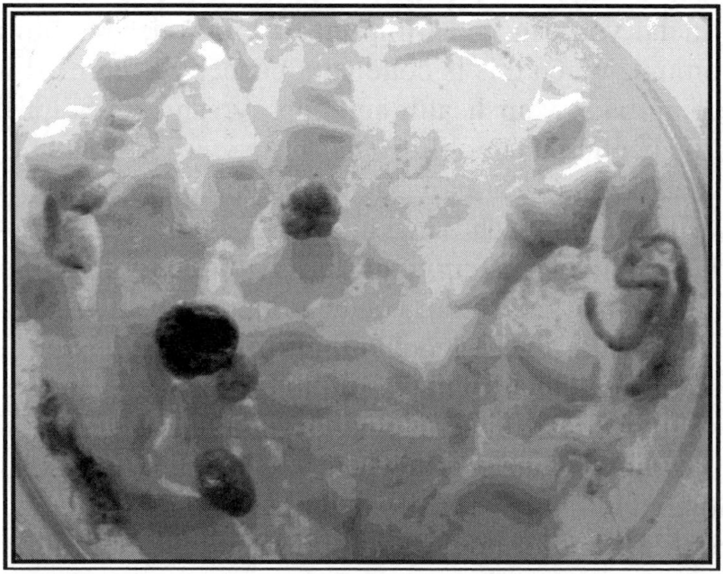

Taenia pisiformis tapeworm lies in a heap (lower center), like porridge, grey to tan colored. The scolex (head) was there, hopefully, since the bile duct remained *Negative* for this tape up to 2 weeks later. Starting the morning with 2 doses of Epsom salts, 2 hours apart, nothing more, and waiting 2 hours more before eating, produced this dog-tape.

***WARNING: DO NOT EXPERIMENT ON YOURSELF** to remove tapeworm. The recipes were not complete at time of publishing.*

CHAPTER 15

2-WEEK CANCER-CURING PROGRAM

Most Important

What took 3 weeks in the past now only takes 2 weeks. There are fewer supplements to take. And success is closer to 100% than ever before. It is because each tumor can now be tracked to its Po source.

We have known a very startling fact since 1999. All cancer patients, with any kind of cancer, are drinking the same kind of water, everywhere in the world. It is quite different from the water that healthy people are drinking.

It seems unthinkable that half the USA population is drinking water that is contaminated with polonium. It is responsible for all our cancer cases as well as other serious diseases and genetic diseases. Even novice Syncrometer® testers can find these toxic substances. Commercial labs do not find them because they are not on the list of required tests.

All water (about 99%) in the USA is disinfected with chlorine gas so that is not the problem. Only half of society gets cancer.

Bleaches are a second kind of chlorination given to all water. But cancer patients have water with bleach in it from the supermarket, called chlorox. It should have had food-grade bleach in it with NSF (National Sanitation Foundation) rating.

My top priority for every cancer patient in 1999 was to immediately switch their water to the variety without chlorox. The results were even better than expected. Those that managed to make the switch <u>all</u> got well at home to give the shockingly good success rate of about 95% for the cancer cure.

Now, the results are even better, reaching 100%. Only the new oscillator technology could make this possible by discovering the hidden polonium, as well as chlorox disinfectant, in our tooth fillings, food, as well as water.

Your most important change will be the same, to flee from anything that brings you Po, namely chlorox-treated water, food, or dental supplies.

The chlorox variety of bleach in water does not all come from the water department. It also comes from filters, softeners and previously contaminated pipes.

The most common source of the chlorox bleach variety is **filters**. All kinds of filters (about 95%), no matter how highly they are rated and advertised have themselves been disinfected with chlorox bleach, not NSF rated bleach. Any water passing through them will pick up the cancer-causer, not filter it out. Filters, even as small as a single refrigerator filter, all contaminate the rest of the house water pipes with chlorox, namely, polonium. All water occasionally refluxes and passes through pipes not intended for it. A single pass with chlorox-treated water would permanently contaminate it. That is because this bleach has sticky wheel bearing grease and motor oil in it. It is not required to have extra clean handling during its production. They are only traces to be sure, but traces of chlorox are very significant because they bring ultra traces of polonium. The ingredients of chlorox bleach can be dug up by heavy machinery without attention paid to dripping wheel bearing grease and motor oil. This sticks to pipes in a single pass and can't be washed out without about 100 gallons of piping hot water.

Filters had brought in the chlorox in about half the cancer cases. About ¼ of the cancer cases had a water softener attached. Even after disconnecting it or disconnecting the filters the pipes kept their contamination with chlorox. The city itself was using chlorox in the remaining quarter of cases.

You can clean your pipes by removing filters and softeners and replacing the pipes and water heater.

In spite of the many toxic chemicals in chlorox bleach (see page 62), I do not know of a single test that a commercial laboratory can do, to tell you what kind of bleach your water has. Nowhere can you test for the commonest of pollutants, malonic acid, isopropyl alcohol, azo dyes, PCBs, benzene, or asbestos in amounts that are realistic. This shows a glaring deficiency in our agencies' understanding of what is toxic and needs to be tested. Without an understanding of toxicities, our agencies cannot make useful water regulations. We must do something about that. It reminds us of a time when we entered a doctor's office feeling sick and feverish and the first thing you were told to do was to step on the scales and have your height measured. We were astonished at the instruction to pursue an irrelevant task. Skipping tests for added cyanides and radioactivity in drinking water while mandating a test for turbidity and taste seems to reverse the priorities. Yet, no concerned private consumer has the opportunity to check into their own water quality because commercial labs for these tests do not exist. The privately owned labs are at universities that would not allow private citizen use. We must do something about that, too. Citizens pay for the universities!

Wheel bearing grease and motor oil can be easily found by Syncrometer®, but not by a lab. Labs do exist that test samples for oil companies to keep them in compliance with the regulations but they cannot test for trace amounts. The public needs to engage their own lab analyst and equipment to feel secure about their water supply, especially as water gets scarcer and communities begin using recycled water. We must be much more wary about uranium and polonium in our water. Such a debacle as this 100-year cancer epidemic should never happen again. Not only our government, but our health must be "by the people".

Does this mean that the NSF grade bleach and water is good for us? NOT AT ALL. It, too, has cyanide added to protect the pipes. Only, it is ferricyanide, not ferrocyanide. Ferricyanide poisons us all, too. It merely does not give us cancer. It gives us our serious diseases and uranium caused genetic diseases!

For this reason it is best to install a hot-backwash filter that cleans itself so it cannot fail to remove iron cyanides of either variety before they reach you. Even such a backwash filter needs to be specially prewashed and tested for all the toxins that need to be removed from the charcoal itself before use.

Other Solutions

Another solution is to rent or lease a large, new, uncolored HDPE plastic tank on wheels, holding about 300 to 600 gallons. Purchase NSF chlorinated water from a source you have had tested by a Syncrometer® tester. Test for ruthenium and thulium, as well as oils like linoleic and linolenic. These come from contact with plant charcoal filters and reverse osmosis filters. Do not buy filtered water. Engage 2 or 3 testers so that differences in sampling and other details can be ruled out. Connect the tank to your plumbing at home wherever the force of gravity will be enough to supply the water pressure you need. Fill this stationery tank regularly with a duplicate tank that is kept on a pick up truck, covered and in the shade. Purchase a water-lubricated pump (see *Sources*) to transfer the water to the stationery tank. Test the pump first in a bucket of clean water by sampling the outflow and testing for toxins besides chlorox bleach. Keep extra pumps, tanks, and hoses to a minimum and test your water again as it arrives in the kitchen at the cold faucet.

The house water pipes and water heater should be changed at the same time since the new good water will not clean them. You may test your water heater by sampling the water from the bottom of the heater at the spigot. If it is not contaminated you do not need to replace it, but simply hot wash the pipes with 3 tankfuls of the hottest water possible. Attach a garden hose to the spigot and run it into both hot and cold pipes to the kitchen and bathroom. Do not use flexible hose for your drinking water, not even washing machine hose. Arrange for PVC pipes, even for temporary use. Rubber and soft plastic clog kidneys. Then attach the hot backwash filter.

Yet another solution is to rent an RV and connect it to an RV park water line after you have tested their water. The cost will be low since you are not driving anywhere. Pipe the water in through a new flexible hose to your plumbing system, bypassing your pipes. Keep it as short as possible. Buy a new storage tank and water heater (not electric) for the RV. Attach the hot backwash filter that removes iron cyanides and polonium where it will also remove the plastic and rubber from this hose. A week later send a sample of cold kitchen tap water to a Syncrometer® tester. Test for chlorox bleach, NSF bleach, polonium, lead, copper, Teflon tape (used in plumbing), methylene blue, ruthenium, and coconut oil. They should all test *Negative*.

Second Most Important

...are your teeth. When the radioactive element, polonium, is built into your teeth in the form of a solid, there is no solution besides removal. Plastics and plasticizer can be hardened so you can prevent seepage of metals, dyes, malonic acid and even cerium from them.

But when the contaminant is polonium, or uranium which breaks down into polonium, all of it capable of piercing bones and tissue in every direction, hardening does not help. Consider yourself very fortunate if you can even identify your radioactive teeth so they can be picked accurately for removal.

When dental supplies have been "disinfected" with chlorox bleach instead of NSF grade, you will, of course, acquire the polonium that way. And when porcelain is used to make your teeth "sparkle", this will bring spent uranium. All uranium is radioactive, spent or not. It stimulates growth while polonium stimulates malignancy. The Syncrometer® found that half the amalgam in use has uranium contamination!

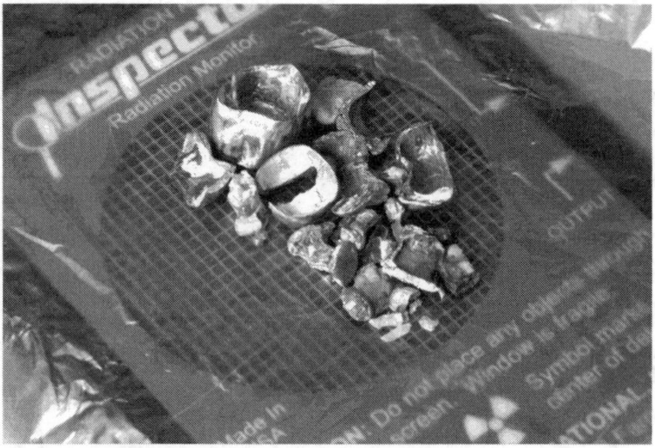

These caps, crowns, and other bits of artificial dental materials had radioactivity of 79.0 counts per minute (for 50 minutes). The background radiation was 46.7 CPM. No corrections of any kind were made. This is very significant.

Fig. 88 Dental supplies on a Geiger counter

Evidently, the toxicity of dental supplies has had no attention. Our commercial radiochemistry labs are excellent but are not used to protect people from toxic radioactive dental supplies. There are no regulations. The public should be encouraged to use these labs to test dental supplies, food and water.

Third Most Important

...is cleaning your house. After the kitchen faucet water has been changed to NSF grade bleach as its disinfectant, you can easily clean the kitchen and furnishings with a chlorox-free strong detergent, together with chlorox-free cleaning mixtures (see *Sources*). Wherever you place your foot or rest your arm, it must be free of chlorox contamination. Send carpet and furniture wipes to a Syncrometer® tester when you think you are done. You can see it would be safer and faster to move to a house that never got contaminated.

Sources to suspect are telephone, contact lenses, eye lubricant, scissors, eyeglasses, wristwatch, toothbrush, comb, brush, bedding, slippers, shoes, shaver and supplies, all the dishes, pots, bracelets, wig, dyed hair, clothing, floor, carpet.

As soon as the water and house are cleaned up you can start to remove each cancerous tumor from your body.

Perspective On The Program

We can wonder at so many other people who are drinking the same water but do not have cancer. This is like saying, Why doesn't my neighbor get a wet carpet when it rains, like I do? Actually, <u>nobody</u> knows which other people will get cancer even though it can be predicted that half this nation (USA) will get cancer. Perhaps everyone who consumes this water for more than 7 years (this is the average time a family lives in 1 house) is targeted. Only a Syncrometer® test can find the very early cases.

Now that we know exactly what the cancer-complex is made of and how it forms, we do not need to be panicked or in constant fear of it. We can create our own security. We will be able to see some easy chemistry we can do to take the complex apart, to cure the cancer, and then prevent it from ever coming back.

After taking the complex apart we can wash out the pieces of the complex and test ourselves to see if it is truly gone. All OPT should be gone, too. We can work on all the parts of the complex at the same time to speed up progress.

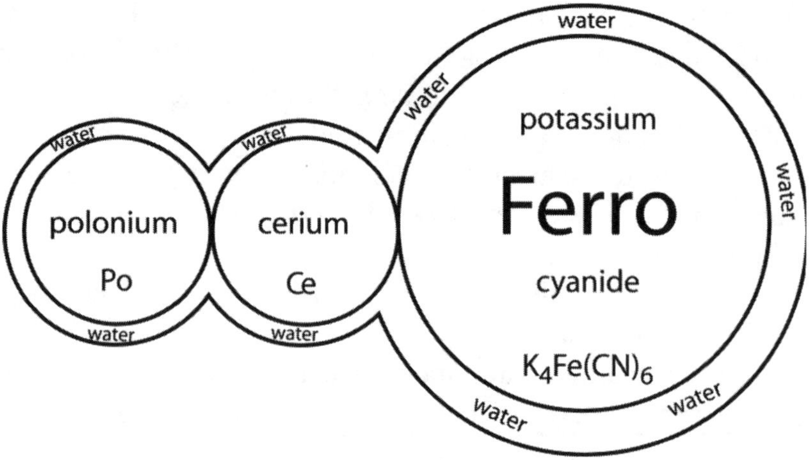

Fig. 89 The basic cancer-complex

The first 3 parts of the cancer-complex are basic. It can already produce OPT as a mutation when it attaches itself to your DNA. It comes to you from the chlorox bleach. It will attach itself to your DNA or an alkylating agent or bacteria or F. buski. Any of these combinations will all produce OPT and other cancer related substances. The small and the large complexes are landing in your genes at precisely the place where they can fit snugly (making coordinate bonds). There they cause mutations that produce substances like HCG or HGH, for instance. These are Human Chorionic Gonadotropin and Human Growth Hormone. Our immediate goal is to remove these cancer-complexes from your DNA.

> We only need to loosen the parts from each other to stop the complex from working and the OPT from forming.

Fortunately for us, when the cancer-complex is removed from your genes, the cancer is **gone**. We did not expect this. We have been taught, and believed, that "once a cancer is started the causes are no longer relevant; it can continue on its own". That may be true, but each cancer still has to be "in production" from its cancer-complex. The OPT and other cancer mutations must be ongoing to preserve the cancer. If we can access each one of its 5 or 6 parts, body-wide, with our simple chemistry, we will have a body-wide cure.

Cerium is the heart of this complex. It can attach to 4 things at the same time (only shown with 2 on the diagram) and choose many things to combine with. It reacts with isopropyl alcohol and malonic acid, besides attaching to bacteria, viruses and the tumor nucleus. Fortunately, cerium makes ionic bonds—weak and watery. We could weaken them further; maybe even break them apart, with just more water! We could flood the complex with water. Then sweat it outward. Water could loosen the "ferro" connection on one side and the polonium connection on the other side. These are all easy bonds to break.

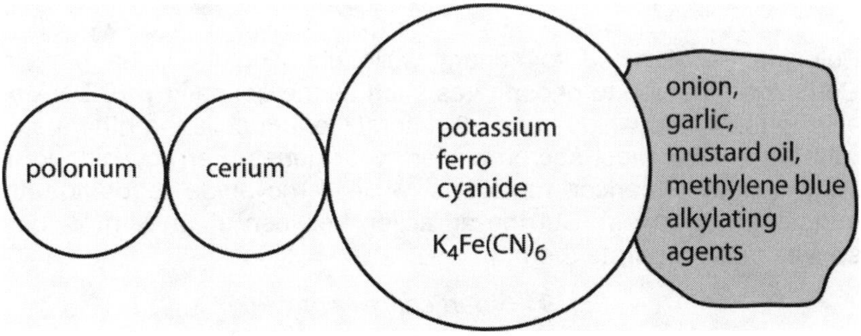

Fig. 90 4-part cancer-complex

We could oxidize the ferrocyanide with any suitable oxidizer like a **quinone** to change its form to ferri. This will at the same time kill malaria stages and bring an immediate sense of well being.

We could complex the alkylating agents with MSM (methyl sulfonyl methane), a supplement, to make them unavailable for making more cancer-complexes.

As the complex breaks apart and gets pulled off your DNA one of the first mutations stops. Instantly, the enzyme Rhodanese is made again. Then both iron cyanides can be detoxified into **thiocyanate** again and no free cyanide is made to poison metabolism. All the various iron enzymes and compounds get back to work and life becomes normal. We could then remove the scattered pieces of the complex so they can't find each other anymore, and will get swept out by sweating and water exchange.

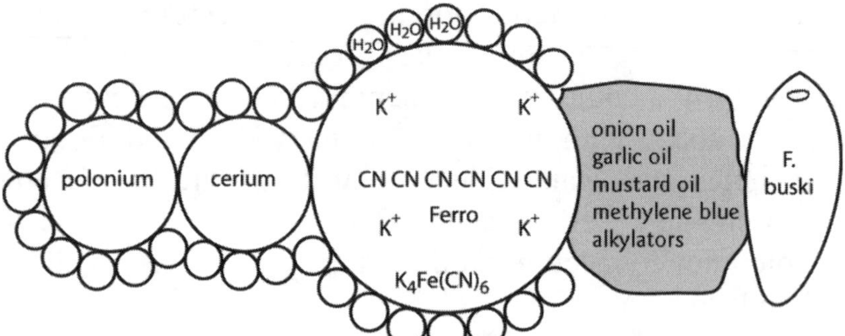

Polonium is attracted to cerium while shooting its alpha particles. Cerium is attracted to phosphates such as the genes in your DNA and also to the iron cyanides and alkylators. Cerium pulls the others along with it into your most sacred places, your genes. Ferrocyanide in this troop leads to cancer mutations while ferricyanide leads to other mutations (diseases). But the attraction between all of them is loose, so water can separate them.

Fig. 91 5-part cancer-complex, drawn from Syncrometer® data

Fortunately, the alkylating agents that attach to F. buski do not attach to the ferricyanide, they only attach to ferrocyanide and vice versa. The alkylating agents that combine with other parasites do not combine with ferrocyanide, only to ferricyanide. So only chlorox bleach, which brings ferrocyanide, not another variety, can cause cancer. The NSF bleaches act in a similar way, to make mutagen-complexes that give us our other major diseases.

It will not take long to break loose the complex from the DNA in each tumor, taking only 2 to 3 days.

Each ingredient of the complex had been constantly supplied. The supply line for each part is easily broken by water currents we can create. But the supply lines can also repair themselves if there is an ongoing source. The supply line for polonium tends to repair itself again and again when it comes from a tooth filling. This tooth filling, being stationary, can easily find a nearby medullated (insulated) nerve. These nerves can cross the body to a distant buski parasite's DNA and replenish the Po there. This raises many fascinating questions, but they must wait for more research. It is easy to see that a broken polonium connection forms again, within a day, if the polonium-tooth was cleaned, or repaired or replaced, but not moved away. Sometimes a new connection is made right beside the old one if the old one has already healed from some treatment given. The pace is extremely swift (all in days). This is fortunate, since we have many more cancerous lesions than our x-rays and scans ever showed. The Syncrometer® finds them by searching for the marker, OPT, and the increased growth rate, namely excess **thymidine** and DNA, rather than the clinical markers. Thymidine is always made just before DNA is made and reflects directly on the growth rate.

You cannot search every organ by name or even every slice of tissue in a set of microscope slides for leftover small malignancies. This is too laborious. But you can find even the smallest one after you absorb sweat from that location. By wiping the skin and keeping all the "body wipes" for testing, you can find any leftover chlorox bleach or polonium or OPT or excess DNA or other cancer mutation. X-rays and other scans routinely miss them. If the body wipes are numbered (see torso chart) you can see where the OPT came from, such as pancreas or stomach, and test it daily. As more and more malignancies disappear, finding the remaining ones gets easier. Finally they are all gone. But only if all the polonium connections stay broken.

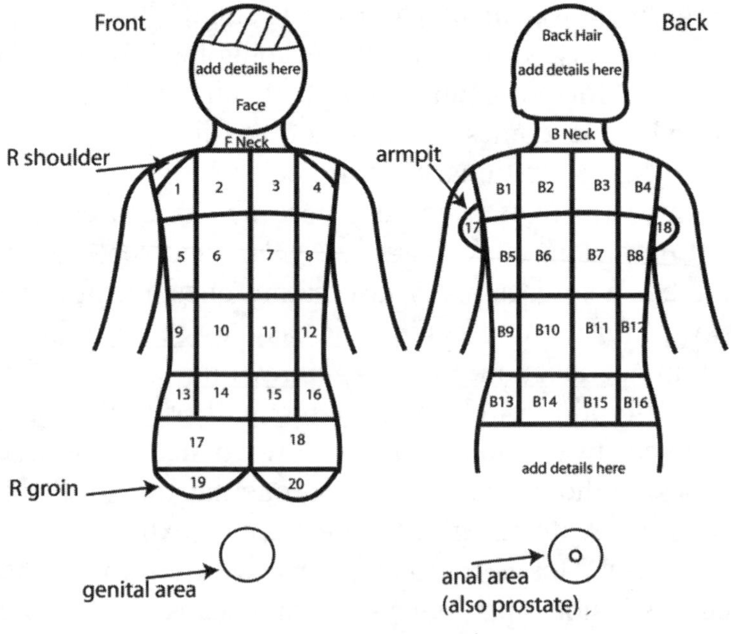

A skin wipe over one area can be tested repeatedly to see the progress made there. Mark your skin in imaginary squares and number them. Make body wipes every 2 days to follow progress with removal of cancer-complexes.

Fig. 92 Syncrometer® "x-ray"

If your dentist or you could use magnifying glasses and an electronic dental probe you would find dozens of grey specks all over your inside cheeks, but especially along both jawbones. These could have chlorox and polonium, besides mercury and uranium. If your dentist could snip away the entire gum surface and its margin, as well as remaining bits of "papilla" you might see instant shrinkage (1 day) of some tumors and disappearance of pain here.

He or she could cut away any tattoos, using magnifying lenses (see *The Tooth Truth* by Dr. Jerome). Trimming the gums at new extraction sites clears away a large amount of mercury, other metal and radioactivity that would otherwise be left behind to give you metastases and ongoing disease. Doing this at the time of extraction is best.

It is not possible to identify the radioactive elements except with a Syncrometer® or by sending samples to a radiochemistry lab. But if a tumor shrinks or a pain disappears you know you are on the right track.

Polonium, uranium and chlorox bits can all be locked into old extraction sites that were not properly cleaned using Dr. Hal Huggins' principles. Small bits that drop off the brittle fillings of teeth that are now being extracted fall easily into the cavity being made. Now, 10 or 20 years later, it can still be done as a belated cavity cleaning, called "*Socket Therapy*". Belated cleaning can still rid the mouth of about half of its trapped polonium and uranium. Left over will be those tooth fillings with hard imbedded chlorox and polonium that are now linked to your remaining malignant sites. The polonium locations can be the dental canals, the dental gum margin, the pointed "papilla" gum between teeth, or the gum surface itself. Removing these has been pioneered and developed by Dr. O. Solorio of Mexico. The dental canal (sulcus) can be cleared with prolonged (2 to 3 days) mouthwashes and gargles using common chelators (see page 353) by yourself.

As soon as you remove these sources of polonium and uranium, by any means, the connected tumors begin to shrink (less than 24 hours). If you do not extract a polonium-containing tooth, but choose to **drill and replace** instead, there will be polonium-drillings throughout the mouth and even through the entire body, having lodged there. Metastases proliferate immediately from these because new pathways will be made.

Be patient with your past dental history. The dental profession will always prefer repair. My best suggestion is to move from dentist to dentist, after you have already identified your own radioactive teeth, until extraction and *Socket Therapy* are completed. See *The Advanced Dental Program Step-By-Step*, page 413.

Chromium-containing dental debris and fillings are responsible for the most excruciating pains, with or without a cancer, and deserve the same dedicated search by yourself. Then find a dentist willing to extract the culprit teeth and remove selected gum tissues. Chromium causes bacterial invasion by Streptococcus pneumoniae as well as terminal yeast invasion of your body. Rising clinical markers, CEA and AFP, points at spreading Yeast and informs you of the chromium problem…namely, residual amalgam.

Cobalt is especially damaging too, because it invites abscess bacteria, Streptococcus pyogenes. These migrate to the spine, hip bones, and brain. Be patient with yourself, again. Chances are quite good that you could find all the cobalt locations and abscess areas yourself with a dental probe and could find an alternative dentist to remove them.

Whatever shrinkage you can see in some tumors is still not enough if you want to cure your cancer and thereby save your life. Any tiny bit of uranium or polonium will be relentless and claim you. You must hurry and you must be thorough.

It seems unwise to try to shrink the last remaining tumors by radiation or chemotherapy, or by cutting them away unless they are immediately life threatening. These procedures do nothing to remove the trapped radiation. Tumors are sure to grow again in another place.

> Each radioactive tooth has a "medullated" nerve leading away from it that is jammed with polonium, cerium, iron cyanide, and uranium.

Fortunately, the nerve clears itself when the radioactive tooth is removed.

Needless to say, if a tumor that had begun to shrink starts to grow again, another bit of polonium or uranium has found the nerve pathway to it.

It seems wiser to stay near the dentist who is willing to help you with this life-salvaging agenda. The dental work is not very invasive and may not even require anesthesia for parts of it. But it requires patience and persistence and your own Syncrometer® skills. Meanwhile, be sure to do your part conscientiously, keeping the dental canal clean with at least 4 hours of EDTA swishing daily. Your reward will be finally walking away from the dental office without any malignancies and with tumors shrinking, pains all gone, and your future ahead of you again.

Meanwhile you can, while working at your dental clean up, proceed with the rest of the program. If you are seeing a clinical doctor at the same time as doing this curing program, which is encouraged, try to get the cooperation of your doctor in:

a) **not** using isopropyl alcohol on your skin; bring an unopened high strength ethyl (drinking) alcohol instead

b) **not** giving contrast injections with your scans because they fill the body with lanthanide metals and dyes, which create effusions; request ultrasound or MRI's in spite of less detailed views

c) **not** doing a bone scan or whole body scan without evidence of bone or further disease; getting radiated till the whole skeleton or body glows is too invasive just to satisfy your or the doctor's curiosity

d) **not** using plastic IV bags; to avoid the PVC, the diallyl phthalates and other plastic derivatives. Use glass (see *Sources*)

e) **not** doing a new biopsy when chemo is a dubious choice anyway and when a history of cancer makes malignancy the most probable description; avoid this new trauma and the possible spread of cancer cells to gain insurance coverage

f) **requesting** allergy testing so you can minimize PGE2 formation The RAST food test is most helpful. If you have corn allergy, request saline instead of dextrose in your IV as far as possible

g) **recommending** alternative therapy to you when hope for survival fades, or as an adjunct; if your doctor could not do this, go elsewhere

There are about 50 things to do in this program. The speed is up to you. Going too fast is likely to give you unnecessary detox-illness. Do not confuse detox-illness with cancer-illness. Find a helper to get you through detox-illness faster and help you prevent it.

Items you will need to purchase are underlined.

Try to reach the Black Walnut parasite program by the sixth day. This gives you a significant kidney cleaning before you do intensive detoxification and parasite-killing. The advanced patient usually has 4 or 5 parasite varieties systemically attacking them! You can go slower and still succeed. Remember the priorities: water, teeth, house, food. Never use an untested supplement, no matter how highly rated it is. Always give a dental appointment the first choice. Each item is discussed further at the end of the program, page 394. Use the *Tester's Guide* on page 437 if you have a Syncrometer® tester to help you. You may test yourself. Test at least 3 times a week, at body wipes and paper bedding, to know your status. Be patient with your own mistakes.

THE PROGRAM

The program has 2 parts: the projects and the supplements. Between these is a reminder of our goal and how we are getting there. Please be sure that the water coming into your kitchen sink does not have the cancer-complex before starting. *Carrying in "good" water cannot work. Only removing filters and cleaning the pipes can work.*

The Projects

These are the projects to get started on as soon as possible. Mark each one as you complete it. Do not leave any out. It is better to do part of a project than nothing. Add them at the end if you missed any. Even if you feel all "done" and well after 1 week, add all the projects and program parts even if it takes you months to complete them.

Project #1 - If you must stay at home to cure yourself.

It is a huge handicap to be forced to stay in your "cancer-house". It is like trying to take a shower while standing in a mud puddle. You must also have help if you are too sick to cope with the house clean up or personal clean up. Don't try to go on without changing the water or cleaning the house. But if you are offered another home, that never had a filter or softener attached, take the opportunity to recover there. It will be easier to stop the cosmetic habit away from home, too. It will be easier to be away from pets, the needs of children, tobacco smoke, the refrigerator and critical neighbors who all mean well.

But if stuck in your own home begin by tearing down every filter, water treating device, distiller, softener, no matter how small, or how far away from the kitchen. Don't overlook those devices that include a small filter. All water mixes with all other water in the house, even the refrigerator dispenser. Do not use refrigerator water or ice even if you remove the filter.

F again (very hot). Use a garden hose attached to the bottom drain faucet of the water heater to lead hot water wherever you need it. Never use flexible hose to pipe your drinking water.

If you are not allowed to remove or add anything to your plumbing, install a parallel PVC pipe. It is easily removed. Then retest for chlorox. After this you may attach the whole house hot-backwash filter. Its backwash feature automatically cleans the filter for you. But it must also have the prewashed activated carbon of the coconut shell variety (see *Sources*) not containing **methylene blue dye**. It must be found free of **ruthenium** seeping out of the charcoal as well as many plant oils seeping from the coconut shells. These oils will prevent it from filtering out motor oil or wheel bearing grease. Only the coconut shell variety can be washed free of it all—do not buy the "animal-black" variety nor coal-derived kind of carbon filter, which cannot do this.

Set the backwash cycle to 5 or 6 days for a small family. Later test your cold kitchen water on day #5, just before the backflushing begins; test for chlorine getting through to your kitchen faucet. If it is, iron cyanides are getting through, too. Set the cycle shorter.

Purchase a bottle of "**Total Chlorine**" strips (see *Sources*) to do your own testing. Finally, test for NSF bleach, ferrocyanide, ferricyanide, methylene blue and

PVC solvent, copper and lead to be secure. There should be none.

> Your newly filtered water should not run through copper pipes because it will dissolve a lot of copper and toxic lead from the pipes, much more than unfiltered water would. Use only PVC piping from the filter to the water heater and from the filter to the kitchen and from the water heater to the kitchen. Changing it all is by far the best. Cities are changing the rules restricting PVC, check yours again.

If your water heater is contaminated with chlorox bleach, you must buy a new one.

<u>The new water heater should not be electric</u>. The latest ones have very soft metal electrodes. They are arranged to stick right into the hot water you will use. There is no separation of electrodes from the drinking water. You would be getting very toxic trace metals like tungsten, chromium, vanadium, palladium, nickel, etc. …about 40 of them. Buy a glass lined <u>gas</u> water heater. The water is much cleaner. This is opposite of the situation in the past.

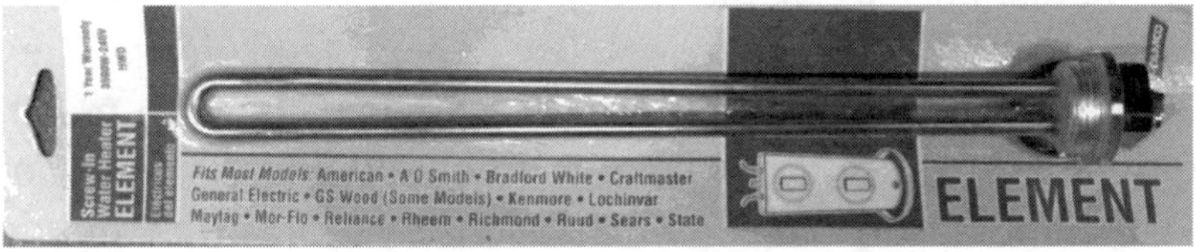

Fig. 93 Water heater electrode

It would be much wiser to leave your cancer-house forever, or at least immediately, until your family has made all the changes for you. When done, you should send a paper wipe from each carpet and floor, plus kitchen counter, shelves, dishes, bedding and clothing to the tester to search for chlorox. Be as thorough as if you were cleaning up poison ivy.

Be sure to purchase chlorox-free detergents, cleaners, and household bleach for all kinds of household uses. Do not save the toxic ones for your animals, nor store them or give them away. Throw them out. Get powdered detergents for laundry and heavy-duty cleaning at first. Borax is not strong enough to remove chlorox or motor oil and wheel bearing grease; nor are liquid varieties. See *Sources* for all these. These are not ideal cleaning agents, but they do not bring polonium, uranium, or ferrocyanide or alkylating agents. Don't risk others. After your home is clean again, you may return to borax, citric acid, vinegar and baking soda for all purposes.

Project #2 – Find well water for drinking and cooking.

NSF food grade bleach in your drinking water allows you to take your malignancies out, clean your house, and get your immunity back. But it is not good enough to shrink large or numerous tumors nor to get your health back. This is because it is also radioactive and has cyanide and methylene blue dye. It merely does not have polonium or ferrocyanide. All chlorinated water contains radioactivity easily found by Syncrometer®. It is added as an incidental part of the phosphate buffers or anti-scaling chemicals or anti-corrosives used to protect pipes. They keep the water from "eating" your pipes if they are metal. Obviously you will not be able to completely shrink your last tumors due to this radioactivity. But by finding unchlorinated water to drink and cook with you could still reach this goal. **In the meantime, drink and cook with the hot-backwash filtered water**.

> Our food needs to be safe from anti-corrosion and anti-scaling chemicals, radioactivity, isopropyl alcohol, methylene blue dye, azo dyes, malonic acid, cyanides, asbestos and automotive oil and grease.

Search for an unchlorinated well by using a bottle of "**Total-Chlorine**" test strips to see if the water has received any chlorination. If it has not you will be avoiding all added radioactivity. It will be easy to disinfect any well water with an ozonator. Do not install a commercial ozonator, though, because it will have a filter attached. (You could remove it.) Five minutes of ozonation in a HDPE gallon of water kills bacteria, viruses, and parasite eggs. The ozone would be good for you, too. Do not use 5 gallon or other large size bottles to carry or store your water. Blue ones diffuse lots of cobalt (it causes fatigue). Clear glass diffuses thallium and gold. Use HDPE 1- or 2½-gal. used bottles. Store water in a cool place, keeping a gallon refrigerated. Repeat chlorine-testing next day and several more times. On this hangs your life! Do not accept any person's reassurance. Even a Syncrometer® tester cannot test accurately if they are full of the same substance they are testing! Using a paper test strip is better, provided the sensitivity is at least 0.05 mg/L (50 ppb).

If you dig a well, be careful not to use paper or cloth strainers; they are disinfected with chlorox. The stainless steel variety is fine. If you use a pressure tank for storage, be sure to remove all filters first or you will contaminate your water yourself. For well cleaning and "shocking" provide your well digger and maintenance person with the correct food grade bottle of bleach, such as Desert Star, Target brand, Sani-Clor, Water Guard. Take theirs in trade. There is also **calcium hypochlorite**, meant for wells, and never contaminated. Find this and others at a pool and spa shop.

You now have the safest, best-tasting, and most nutritious water on this planet. Or so it seems, whenever there are really no options. Nearly all bottled water has radon because each bottle was capped so quickly by the capping machinery there was no chance, not even 3 seconds, to let the radon gas escape first. The accumulated radioactive "daughters", lead, thorium, or bismuth in the bottle can be shocking. When I uncapped any bottle, a damp paper held above it trapped escaping radon instantly. It was already gone from the bottle in 3 seconds!

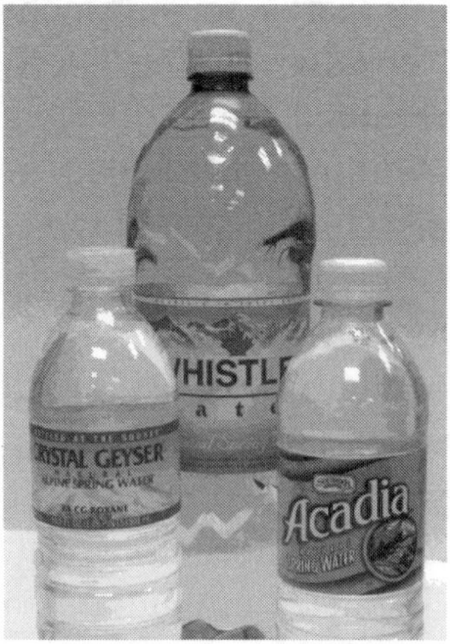

Fig. 94 Kosher bottled water has no radon or "daughters"

But the marketplace for bottled waters has been changing. There are now (as this book went to print) several unchlorinated, radiation-free bottled varieties (see photo). Use bottled water only in emergency because the plastic sheds plasticizer, etc. and a disinfectant is required.

Rainwater may be better than well water in many ways, but is quite inconvenient to strain without carbon-filtering. Carbon filtering would defeat the very purpose of drinking it. Make your own collecting system and cheesecloth filter.

If you are dependent on someone else's choice of well water, do not drink it. Many advanced cancer patients who had cured themselves already, chose a well they were "absolutely positive" had never been chlorinated. But they chose wrongly. The Health Department had anticipated them and installed regular chlorination based on chlorox bleach. Choose rainwater for certainty.

Spring water, is of course, excellent when it comes out of the earth or rocks. Radon has time to escape and it tastes delicious. The hazard is chlorination. A number of unchlorinated springs have been found in Europe (see page 642) to the great delight of European patients. In fact, most of Switzerland delivers unchlorinated public water, as refreshing as it is health-promoting. Only the hotels, rentals, business offices, public laundries, buildings and restaurants have poisoned their waters to preserve their water pipes and boilers. (Another solution could have been to change all metal pipes to PVC or HDPE.) With this warning you could choose this progressive country for your recuperation.

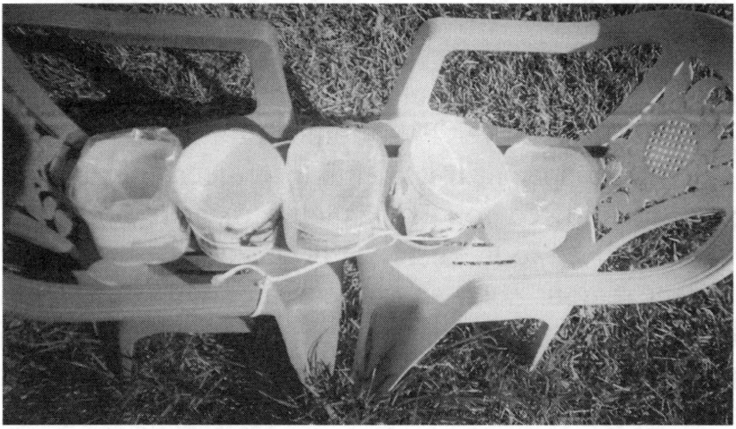

Catching rain in large clear zippered bags that line buckets or baskets is an efficient way to collect and store it. Bungee cords hold it all in place between two plastic chairs.

Fig. 95 Rainwater collecting system

You might think that you could carry "good" water to your kitchen while avoiding your kitchen water, showers, and laundry. All such patients became fatalities although they had cured themselves earlier. The reason is that you cannot just reduce your contact with chlorox, but still wash your hands, wear clothing, walk on floors that give it to you again. You absorb it instantly through hands, feet and from clothing as if it were poison ivy.

Your family should not be blamed for differing from your or my beliefs. Although religion is not involved, philosophy of living is very much involved. We, too, must live up to our beliefs: that life is worth fighting for, that we must not yield to authority when there is no hope there, that we should explore new avenues before giving up, that we should trust in our common sense before trading it for expert advice based on hopelessness. We all know that miracles happen—that very improbable things happen constantly. The paths leading through our biosphere are full of surprises for all of us.

Remember to be kind to those who differ; they still want the best for you, but your life's decisions are best made by yourself, in fact they are your birthright.

You can even get well in a motel if the management told you they have PVC pipes, no filters or water softeners, no special treatments to protect their boilers or pipes, and allowed you to see their furnace room.

Hopefully, food lists will become available for different regions soon so you can go shopping and know which brands have no chlorination in your area. This would protect you from chlorox, and hopefully you would find the old fashioned disinfectants, steam and Lugol's iodine. Which foods have the common allergens that give you inflammation and which foods test *Negative* for all radioactivity, detectable by the Syncrometer®, have the next priority. Such information would serve the cancer patient best, and any other sick person, too. The most important labeling on a processed food is not calories, nutrients, and portion size, but safety.

Project #3 – Getting ready to cook.

Buy new time saving kitchen devices; they have been getting better in the past decade. All metal has been getting harder, to its great credit. But BE CAREFUL. All plastic has been getting softer, so that very toxic metal now seeps from the plastic, enamel, ceramic, Teflon and glass kitchenware. Only the newer stainless steel does not seep (but still needs testing). The 18/10 stamp on the bottom of pans helps to identify it, but not with certainty. Glass and Teflon seep **thallium** (rat poison) in large amounts! If your shins hurt, send food samples or rubbings of your cookware to a Syncrometer® tester. Ceramic and enamel ware seep so much you can often see the dye left behind! The only safe plastic that does not need testing is HDPE; everything else must be tested. Cutting your dishes out of opaque water jugs (the 1-gallon size) will keep you safe. Buy a conductivity indicator to help you (see *Sources*), though it is not perfect.

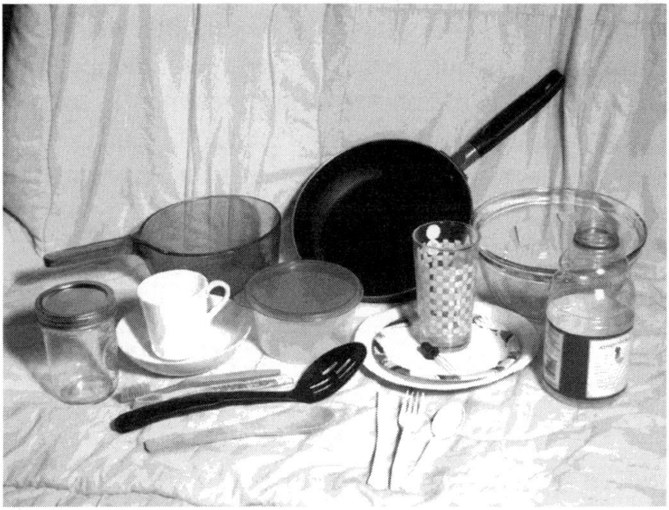

Glassware, canning jars, Teflon, toothbrushes, paper plates, plastic ware, and "good" china seep heavy metals, malonic acid and thallium! Ceramic and enamelware also seep.

Fig. 96 Kitchenware that seeps

- Buy several stainless steel saucepans without glass or gold trim on the lids.
- Find 2 or 3 hotplates to cook on if your stove at home uses gas. Fossil fuels, like gas, have **vanadium**; it benefits E. coli, your major bacterium.
- Find a Farmers' Market and small ethnic food stores, health food stores and natural food stores and the kosher and ethnic sections of supermarkets. Their food must still be tested, but is much safer.

• Purchase a small chest freezer to sterilize your food (see *Sources*). Also get a freezer

- F should be quick and easy).

E. coli is extremely hardy. Find the temperature control and learn which places must not be obstructed to keep it coldest. Defrost it regularly or attach an automatic timer (see *Sources*).

• Buy an ozonator. It is to sanitize your food and make ozonated water. Test the water for nickel with the diffuser removed and for thallium and dyes with the diffuser returned. See *Project #14*, page 373. To be safer, remove the diffuser.

• Make a rubbing of the blades in a blender or grinder in a utility store at a clerk's invitation. Use a slightly damp piece of paper towel, rubbing quite hard. Bring several dampened towels, each in its own zippered bag for testing different items. Buy only the ones without chromium, nickel, vanadium, or cobalt on the paper. Test other appliances and cutlery the same way.

• Purchase a bread maker without an aluminum or Teflon coating. Test it in the store by taking a rubbing of the inside basket and stirring blade. Test the sample for thallium and gold. Throw away the bread around the blade.

Finding Food

Most of the problems in the past with food, making you believe you were allergic to it, were actually due to bacteria and bits of metal and disinfectant. If your food is tested for heavy metals you can avoid pain reactions, yeast growth and much more. If your food is sterilized by ozonation, or freezing, your whole appreciation of food could change. Even sauerkraut and scones can taste good when your tummy stays flat and nothing can be felt or heard inside. Sterilize the flour, salt, sugar, canned food, packages, in fact, everything. Sterilize the rice, baking soda, corn starch, drops of vitamin D or A or IP6 and all prescription medicine. Finally, sterilize the kitchen sponge, and any cloth towels. Make up your mind you shall not pick up Salmonella or E. coli again! Check the freezer temperature daily till you are familiar with the freezer. Prove your determination by not putting your fingers to your mouth unless disinfected.

True allergies must be respected; do not be coaxed to "try a bit" when you know it is suspect. Your cancer-specific allergy is most important, even if it bars carrots or something healthful.

Get enough food tested in your area so you have the staples. Find Syncrometer® testers and give each one assurance in writing, that no lawsuits will ever be initiated, that you understand this is not a government test, that it is manual, not automated, and mostly a "labor of love" at present. As a tester, use a handwritten and signed disclaimer, at the very least. Appreciate each others' intent. This is a new science.

Purchase inexpensive stainless steel cutlery that is not likely to be plated with silver or nickel. Soak them together in a big plastic zippered bag. If the soak water is *Positive* for metal, track it down and eliminate the item.

Obey the new food rules. Do not eat any foods that include the 3 cancer-allergens. They are chlorogenic acid, phloridzin, and gallic acid. Find which foods these are on the *Food Table*, page 97. Do not eat foods from the ONION-GARLIC-MUSTARD families nor beans (except black beans) or lentils. They will supply the alkylating agents for the cancer-complex and feed F. buski larvae. Finding ethnic and kosher foods will be a great help. Search for unchlorinated items. Finding a cheerful cook will be the greatest help so that laughter and optimism surround you.

Find the allergen that belongs to your kind of cancer in the *Cancer Location Table* page 292. Do not eat this food even though it seems healthful to you. If it has a strange name, find the foods that have it in the *Food Table*.

Use the mail order catalogs where good food has already been found (see *Sources*). Kosher food, Amish and Asian foods are superior to USA food but must still be tested item by item.

Project #4 – Request these blood tests.

- CBC and Differential
- Blood chemistry (called SMAC) of about 24 items
- A cancer "marker" test, but only if your oncologist used one; we will use orthophosphotyrosine, HCG, CEA, AFP and PSA (if there is prostate cancer).
- Blood clotting tests
- Serum iron
- Urinalysis

Ask for a copy of your blood test results. Analyze the results yourself using the chapter on *How To Read Your Blood Test Results*. Decide if you have an emergency or very nearly do. Skip to the *Emergency* chapter, page 455, without waiting for anything else, if you sense you do.

Other tests are seldom necessary and create needless cost. Cancer patients regularly have too low cholesterol. It makes no sense to measure amounts and varieties. In fact, our clinic always <u>accepts</u> advanced cancer patients with the higher cholesterol level because they will be the easiest to cure. The test results will give you a starting point to compare with new tests to be done after the *2-Week Program*. Use *Blood Test Results* on page 481 to understand your test results and to know what to do about each one.

Project #5 – Stop using <u>all</u> commercial cosmetics, over the counter drugs, and jewelry.

Body products such as soap and shampoo, as well as herbs, teas or supplements cannot be used unless they are tested by Syncrometer® for chlorox bleach, malonic acid, dyes, isopropyl alcohol, PCBs, and benzene. This applies to prescription drugs, too. A single bad one taken daily will hurt you. It will supply the polonium or cerium or iron cyanide to replenish your cancer-complex. Find unpolluted, uncolored, prescription drug varieties before going off your own. Your pharmacist can often help you in 1 day. Stop using metal jewelry, including rings; harden all plastic items in a sonicator (20 min.) or in steaming (not boiling) hot water for ½ hour. Get kitchen towels, toilet paper, plastic zippered bags and facial tissues tested.

Project #6 – Cut a place setting from HDPE water bottles.

The amount of metal coming from small plastic items like spoons, glasses, contact lenses and toothpicks can keep you in constant pain and your cancer markers high. Eat, cook, and store food only in containers tested for heavy metal seeping. Test them yourself with a conductivity indicator (see *Sources*). If you are in pain, test for chromium. Choose stainless steel and HDPE for all needs. Use your water jugs to cut place settings.

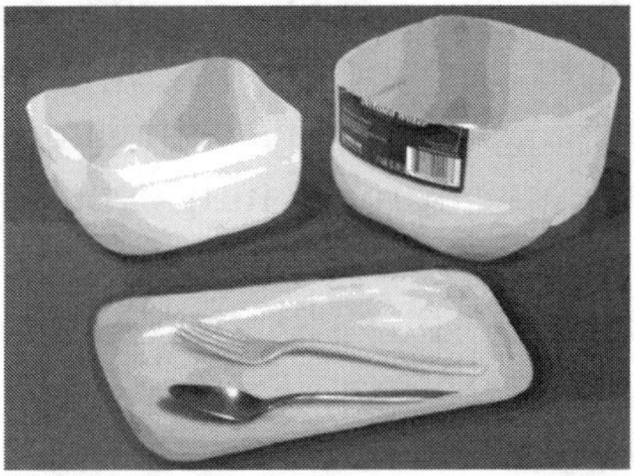

Fig. 97 Temporary place setting

Project #7 – Stop brushing teeth.

Throw away your current brush; it cannot be washed clean. Buy the straight, narrow handled ones, not motor driven; they can be hardened quickly (see *Sources*). Cut floss from a shopping bag that has been tested free of chlorox (see Sources). Cut strips ¼" X 4". Wash under hot water tap and set to dry. After flossing, rub teeth gently with finger wrapped in a strip of paper towel, dampened and dipped in toothpowder. Make toothpowder in a zippered plastic bag from: 10 level tsp. baking soda plus 10 drops oregano oil. Each of these must be frozen to -20° F for 24 hrs. to sterilize. Squish until mixed. Use it once a day. Do not buy any "homemade" variety. Do not use any that you did not make yourself. The manufacturers, including "homemade" ones are certainly not Syncrometer® testers! nor will they disinfect for you. Many advanced patients stumbled on this project and became statistics! Don't take risks. Brush a second time with hydrogen peroxide ("peroxy") only.

Project #8 – Stop wearing rubberized or Teflon clothing.

All elastic and rubber sheds huge amounts of cerium, the second element besides polonium we are trying to get out of our bodies. Teflon sheds thallium and gold—soon to make your shins ache and bring obesity. Until you have a new wardrobe, turn over your waistband several times. Buy mostly silk, it avoids chlorination of all kinds. Wear leather or plastic shoes. Never go barefoot in your shoes—it is too toxic. Stop wearing rubber shoes. Don't go barefoot indoors until the carpets and tile have been cleaned with safe powdered detergent. A wipe with paper towel should show no chlorox. Laundry detergent and dishwasher detergent are often colored blue. This is methylene blue and a cobalt compound. Methylene blue is an alkylating agent that facilitates attachments to your DNA. Buy non blue and non green detergents. Cobalt is a heavy metal, especially toxic to the heart, bringing fatigue.

Project #9 – Stop regular shampoo.

Mix ½ cup non-chlorox laundry detergent powder with enough water to be used for shampoo. All other varieties are not strong enough to remove the chlorox, cancer-complex, wheel bearing grease, and motor oil from your hair and scalp. Choose safe varieties (see *Sources*). It will take 4 shampoos, one after the other, to get it out of your hair. Dry between shampoos using safe paper towels only. On the 2nd day rub hair lightly all over with a paper towel to get a sample for testing. Test for chlorox and OPT. If OPT persists, make a "body wipe" sample of your scalp to test for brain cancer. Metastases come from your hair, teeth, clothing, pillow, places where the cancer-complex still exists.

After the chlorox and OPT are gone, shampoo once a day with any liquid detergent of a safe kind (see *Sources*). If you are advanced use only borax and citric acid. Mix 1 Tbsp. borax with 2 cups very hot water. Mix 2 tsp. citric acid in 1 cup water to condition your hair. Leave in hair 1 minute.

Project #10 – Make appointment to change glasses frames to plastic, even if there appears to be plastic coating on the temples. Do not delay this. The nickel in them will delay return of immunity.

All metal except hinges should be covered with plastic but not bulging. Do not buy gold-hinged or gold-framed glasses. Avoid gold, it invites Salmonella and any of the new diseases (see *Pathogens' Requirements* page 328). Harden the plastic immediately in a saucepan. Cover them with water and bring to steaming temperature. **Do not actually boil or you could warp them.** Turn off heat when bubbles start to burst, cover and let stand for ½ hour. Do not use them till you have tested them. If you can't do this, harden them 2 more times. (To test, cover with new water and let stand 2 hours, then send sample of this "soak water" for testing.) Wrapping the hinges or temples with tape does not work. Plastic items can also be hardened in a sonicator, or small jewelry cleaner (see *Sources*) for 15 minutes. Immerse item in water while keeping it dry in a plastic bag.

Project #11 – Prepare for *Dental Aftercare* (read page 422)

Buy water pick, blender, stainless steel strainer. Practice with water pick. Test blender blades for seeping metal by making a rubbing of them. Buy safe painkiller to get through the first night in comfort (see *Sources*). Buy or make *Dental Bleach* in a HDPE dispenser bottle (see *Recipes*).

Project #12 – Get panoramic x-ray of teeth and jaws.

Ask your dentist for a referral to the best radiology lab he or she knows of. Request 2 copies, one for the dentist and one for yourself.

Find a dentist or surgeon willing to work with you interactively where you supply Syncrometer® based information and they are flexible enough to do what is needed for you, individually, instead of their usual "protocol". After they see some of your malignancies disappear by their treatment in the first few days, they may be more interested.

Ask your dentist to list and evaluate each tooth, from #1 - #32, such as: "missing", "metal crown", "broken at gum line". He or she will need your panoramic to do this. Ask your dentist to make impressions with chlorox-free supplies. This means sending them to a Syncrometer® tester or finding a list of tested ones on the Internet. Hopefully, such lists will become available soon. Be prepared to supply one yourself or take responsibility for the testing (see *Sources*).

The dental goals are:

- to remove radioactivity from your mouth
- to remove abscess bacteria and Clostridium from your mouth
- to remove metal from your mouth

The chief steps to be taken are in this order:

1. Remove all gold.
2. Remove all root canals. Clean the socket left below using special burs (drills) that can shear the rubber and plastic off the bone all the way to the bottom. You may need 3 sizes. Clean the sockets of <u>old</u> root canals, removed in the past. Reach your former dentist to check which teeth had them.
3. Remove all caps, bridges, inlays, crowns, and veneers, cement, or porcelain coating. Do this without drilling into them. This removes about half the radioactivity in your mouth. They are all easily replaced with non-radioactive materials. Extraction is not needed if old dental material can be completely removed. Teeth need testing before replacement.
4. Identify and extract radioactive amalgam teeth, leaving the non-radioactive remainder to replace. This will be about half of all amalgam-teeth.
5. Identify and extract radioactive composite teeth, leaving the non-radioactive remainder to replace. This will be about ½ of composite-teeth.
6. Identify old or new sockets containing crumbs of uranium or polonium. Drill clean. This will throw radioactive particles into your mouth with great force. These will give

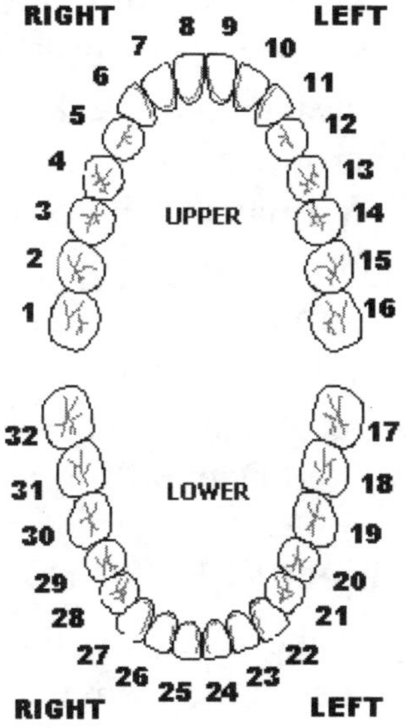

Fig. 98 Tooth number chart

you metastases in a month or so unless removed immediately from your mouth. Plug sockets with earplugs till ready to suture.

7. Clear the mouth of dental debris constantly from the time of leaving the dental chair all the way home, using a water bottle and a plastic bag with paper towels in it to spit into. Continue at home, for ½ hour periods using EDTA mouthwashes done very gently not to disturb the clotting process.
8. Do dental power wash using citric acid on all gums.
9. Surgically remove a 4 mm wide strip of gum, including gum margin that rests against the tooth, and the papilla. The depth is about 2 mm - 3 mm. Include all tooth locations from #1 to #32 whether teeth are missing or present.

Start each morning with EDTA mouthwash and 4 more hours later each day for 3 days. Thirty hours after the last dental work you may assess the results with a Syncrometer®.

A final test by Syncrometer® or dental probe should find no connections (resonance) between any teeth and the cancerous lesions. In other words, every cancer patient should be able to walk out of the dental office free of cancer when done. But there is more to do. See the Step-By-Step Dental Program, page 413.

Project #13 – Purchase tooth zappicator and L-1 zapper.

Make a saliva sample for chlorox testing as soon as you get home from the dentist. Later, when it is tested you can judge whether chlorox-containing supplies were used on you. Make a new saliva sample each day upon arising so you can see if it has dissipated. If it doesn't leave in a few days, the implication is that it was used for the dental work and has already been built into the new structure, accidentally. Or, that the extractions and cleanings are not complete. Have all dental radioactivity removed as soon as possible. To guard against accidental recontamination, it is best to leave teeth "open" until they have been tested for remaining radioactivity or mercury. Zappicate any new repairs as soon as they are completed (same day or next day), to avoid seeping to your tumors. This appears to harden the plastic while removing nearby toxins. You should be on kidney cleaning drops for heavy metals and dyes during this time, or on the kidney cleanse. The zappicator is powered by its own 1000 hertz zapper (called L-1) with only one wire attached. If 2 wires are attached, give it to any electronics person to fix, along with the diagram, page 532.

Project #14 – Purchase ozonator, the kind without rubber or black plastic tubing (see *Sources*). Remove diffuser at end of tube; it introduces more hazard than there could be benefits.

The kidneys easily "clog" with soft plastic or rubber. Both release cerium. Cerium attracts polonium and more polonium-cerium-duplex is formed. Start drinking 2 cups ozonated water a day, but only after testing the finished water for cerium, azo dyes (from a colored diffuser stone), nickel (from hot fan blades), thallium (from the diffuser), common plastics (from the tubing), and finally your WBCs themselves to see if they are busy removing the water. If your water is being removed by your WBCs it is toxic, do not drink it. Search for a better ozonator. Meanwhile, use "peroxy" drops in your water, only a few drops per glass. This supplies your cyanide-poisoned tissue with oxygen and is very beneficial even though it does not truly correct all the poisoning action. It is only First Aid. Avoiding all cyanide in water is necessary to stay well.

Ozone is chemically very active. It can easily oxidize rubber or soft plastic. Even the tiny diffuser at the end that is making the bubbles can be attacked so it sheds large amounts of plastic and dyes. It would be better to remove it. It would be better not to use ozone than drink a daily dose of plastic, rubber and dye.

Project #15 – Purchase zapper plus zap plate.

Buy rechargeable batteries, charger and voltmeter. Use instructions and zapping schedule on page 173.

Project #16 – Place food, supplements, and herbs in deep freezer for 24 hrs at -20° F or colder to disinfect. Learn about other methods of suitable disinfection.

Being 1 degree too warm or 1 hour short does matter. Do not miss disinfecting a single item, such as baking soda, salt, your freshly bought fruit and vegetables and each supplement, or you will get very ill soon again. Do this at home till your health has returned completely (1 year). Test the first few batches by Syncrometer® to be sure there is no Salmonella or E. coli surviving. Mark all frozen items so you cannot get them mixed up. The best or next best methods of disinfection are ozonation and sonication. Ultraviolet rays are an upcoming method. Use the most suitable method for different foods.

Project #17 – Get ready for your first day of curing.

- Buy 6 apricots and wash the pits, but do not crack them nor refrigerate, nor freeze. Read the instructions and get ready for your first apricot suppository tonight (see recipe, page 590). They do not need to be tested. Chlorox does not penetrate the pit.
- Buy a plastic drop cloth from a paint store to cover the whole bed, pillow and sheets (no need to change). You will only need one (see *Sources*). Cover furniture, too, like chairs.
- Buy 10 or 15 paper drop cloths so you can put a new one on top of the plastic sheet each day. After getting into fresh night wear and going to bed, wrap the other half of the paper

sheet around you to raise your temperature and soak up any perspiration. Be sure your head and arms are touching paper, not bed sheets or pillow case. Paper is more absorptive.

- Buy a supply of paper towels and toilet paper, previously tested for chlorox bleach. Remove all cloth towels. Spread a strip of paper cut from the paper sheet to put on the tile or carpet if they have not already been cleaned. Do not walk barefoot on the floor unless it has been cleaned and tested. Buy tested paper goods only.
- If you are very advanced, also wrap paper towel around body parts with internal cancers, like breast, neck, armpit, groin. Tape it securely with masking tape so it acts like a blotter for sweat on the skin. Do not tape your skin nor use other tape. They commonly contain chlorox. Then get into night wear and into your paper bed.
- Read the *Laundry Recipe* (page 611). Wash everything as soon as possible using the strongest dry detergent you can find that does not have chlorox nor blue or green color. This could be methylene blue, another alkylating agent! Don't wear anything twice.
- Purchase powdered and liquid varieties of safe detergents and cleaners as well as safe household bleach (see *Sources*).
- Buy the supplements and extra items you will need and sterilize them, whether in bottles, boxes, or other packaging. Sterilize by deep freezing, sonicating, ozonating, or Lugol's.

Things You Need (packages or bottles)

SUPPLEMENTS		
3-Selenite (selenium)	1-Birch bark (bulk or capsules)	1-Vitamin B2 capsules
1-Hydrangea root capsules	1-Baking soda (sodium bicarbonate)	1-Hydrochloric acid (HCl) 5%
2-Rose Hips capsules	1-Reishi capsules	1-Magnesium oxide
2-MSM capsules	1-Stevia (herbal sweetener)	1-Potassium gluconate
1-Burdock root capsules	1-Vitamin D_3 (with PE dropper bottle)	2-IP6 (with PE dropper bottle)
1-Uva Ursi	1-Oscillococcinum	3-Turmeric

capsules	package	capsules
1-Ginger capsules	1-Pantothenic acid	3-Fennel capsules
1-Eucalyptus capsules	1-Ornithine 2-Vitamin C capsules	1-Pepsin capsules
1-Boneset capsules	1-Wormwood combination	1-Digestive enzymes
1-Citric acid (bulk) 1-Rutin	1-Cloves (capsules) 1-Hesperidin	2-Pancreatin-Lipase
1-Citric acid capsules	6-Green Black Walnut tincture (Extra Strength) 1-oz. bottles	1-Oregano oil (with PE dropper bottle)
1-Bromelain (not for malaria)	1-EDTA 1-pomegranate peel or seed capsule	1- liquid vitamin A (with PE dropper bottle)

MISCELLANEOUS	
2-Melatonin, 3 mg., Benadorm (Mexican pharmacy)	½ oz. amber PE bottles with flat lid
Sodium chloride (pure salt)	Tea ball, stainless steel
Borax bottle and refill Dental Bleach	Hydrangea-Marshmallow-Gravel Root (kidney herbs)
1-pint water bottle, HDPE	Lexan Cutlery
½ oz. amber PE bottles with dropper, nozzle, cap	Plastic Bags, 6"x6", zippered, no color, no fragrance
Nuts in shell, mixed, tested	6-Marathon paper towels, or tested brand
Nutcracker or heavy hammer	1-Bread Maker (tested for thallium and gold at walls and paddle)
Raw beets	Enema bottles (Fleet) 2 adult size
Epsom Salts	Decaris (from doctor) levamisole, 50 mg.
Blender	Water pick (Target stores, others)
Thyroid (prescription, 1 grain, from doctor, tested)	1-Colgate-Palmolive white detergent powder, tested
Lugol's iodine for disinfection (2% iodine in USA, or 5% homemade)	Flour, Mexico (El Rosal) with no bromine, fluorine, gold
Stainless steel saucepan, 18/10	Eggs, Mexico (unbleached)
1-plastic drop cloth 14-paper drop cloths	Rice (tested for thallium, bromine, chlorox)
1 set measuring spoons	Honey (Mex) tested for chlorox, gold
Hot plate	Pomegranate, fresh (tested for chlorox)

You are now set for the big adventure that will set you free of illness, pain, and cancer. You can see that you need a helper to get everything organized, at least at first.

THE GOAL – A Reminder

The main goal of this cancer cure is to stop making OPT and to remove it all from your body. As soon as the cancer-complex is broken up, the mutations including OPT stop. Your WBCs can eat the cancer-complex parts and spill them into the bladder, but the WBCs and bladder must be ready for this. Also the individual pieces of the complex must not find each other again. Fortunately, they are so water soluble we can draw them out through the skin just by sweating and showering. Amazingly, the cancer-complex behaves like a "mutation-machine" and must constantly be fed. Even more amazing is that every malignancy stops within 12 hours after its polonium feed-line is stopped or F. buski is killed. Perhaps malignancy is just another mutation we have not yet identified. We were all taught that "once a mutation, always a mutation", but it is not so. That is why we only need to pursue 1 goal: to break up the cancer-complex. Other goals are minor, like killing bacteria, stopping toxicity and relieving symptoms but we will achieve these, too.

When we look carefully at the drawing of the cancer-complex (see page 349), we see it is surrounded by water. In fact, the polonium, cerium, and ferrocyanide are very wet molecules, barely holding together. With a little more water they would float apart without any pulling force needed. How fortunate! If we drink more water, wash ourselves more, sweat more and urinate more, we will have flooded the complex. We can next find the pieces in our perspiration and in the urine where they had stopped arriving previously. We can even draw them out through the skin with paper.

This is how we reach that goal:

THE CURE

On DAY 1: Place a plastic sheet over entire bed and pillow to avoid contact with contaminated bedding. Wherever the skin touches chlorox, it will absorb it and the cancer-complex with it! That is how cancers are replenished. Next, place a paper sheet, like a painter's drop cloth over the plastic sheet; fold it over to wrap yourself in it. It will absorb sweat and prevent contact with top sheet. You may wear fresh nightwear. Launder clothing and bedding next day. Do not wear or use clothing twice. Do not use any cloth towels. Use paper towels only and throw away immediately. Chlorox with its polonium is on them and it behaves very much like poison ivy. If you touch it with even one fingertip it is on you. It does not "go away". If you next touch your finger to your face you will transmit it to your face. Next morning roll the paper sheet into a "fire log", taping it tightly, and replacing it in its original package to be tested. The caregiver should do this so the cancer patient has no contact with it. Use masking tape only or the "fire log" will test *Positive* for chlorox.

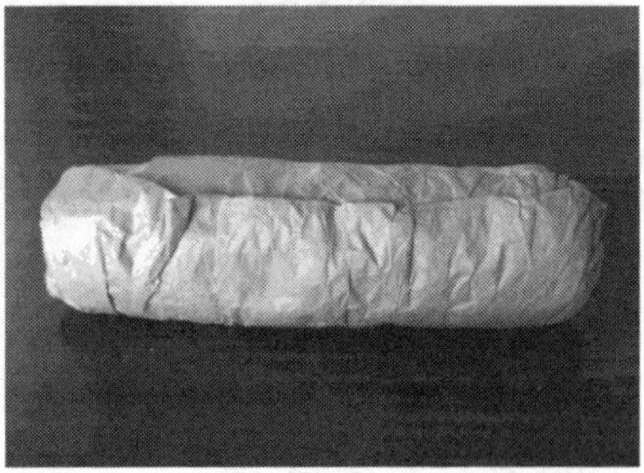

Fig. 99 "Fire log" paper bedding

Take 3 hot showers daily to make you sweat. This is the "slow system". If you could take 5 or 6 showers a day, avoiding chills, it would be much faster. Use a handful of paper for a washcloth. Dip it in powdered safe detergent for armpits, groin, and the skin over tumors. Do not rub, but wash briskly and keep hot water striking the tumor areas during showers. Do this every day. Go to sleep with dry paper towels wrapped around the tumor areas to help draw the perspiration from them. It only takes days.

Make a set of skin wipes after each 6 showers or 2 days. These are to be tested for leftover OPT or chlorox. Use the torso diagram on page 350. Use a paper towel folded 4 times and slightly dampened to wipe your skin in the morning when rising (not after shower). When all the wipes are free of bleach and OPT you may stop. Continue making wipes at suspicious locations.

It will take 36 hot showers and 4 shampoos to be free of all the accessible cancer-complexes…those easily reached. The shampoos should be one after another, using safe dry laundry detergent, and drying hair with paper towels each time. Send a hair wipe next day. If it still has chlorox, repeat 4 shampoos. If it still has OPT, consider cutting it short (to ½ inch). If it tests Positive for chromium, or lead, stop dying the hair till a non toxic variety is found (see Sources). You may have missed clearing the brain, skull, eyes, nose, face, salivary glands if these did not get enough paper contact. If face wipes still have chlorox or OPT, make a greater effort. Wrap your face, scalp and back of head in 2 layers of paper towel for the night. Do not put tape on your skin. Next day, stuff the paper in a plastic bag for testing. And you may have accidentally eaten and drunk chlorox which resupplies the complex. Then they will appear in the saliva. Do not take risks. It is mainly polonium in tooth fillings, root canals, caps and bridges that will still find its way to your leftover cancers to replenish them. Getting dental work done with supplies that contain chlorox is a common mistake. It is better to delay dental work till the supplies are tested than to put a fresh polonium source into your teeth. But when all the radioactive teeth are gone, the cancer is gone too, coming closer to a guaranteed cancer cure than any previous method. Aim to be free of cancer in 12 days instead of 2 weeks. Many have succeeded.

Use the apricot suppository before bedtime, following the instructions given on page 590.

On DAY 2: Do laundry using the special recipe (page 611) to be sure all chlorox comes out in one wash. Shop for all the supplements listed or underlined. Start taking the WBC supplements as soon as they are sterilized. They should be marked if frozen properly. The most fail-safe way to sterilize anything is to freeze it for 24 hours at -20° F or colder. There are several other ways, but more difficult to do. A single unsterilized item will hurt you. Write the time on the items as you place them in the freezer. Use a thermometer. Put an automatic timer on the electric cord for defrosting. Set it for 1 defrost per week.

Continue to remove chlorox with dry detergent and alcohol from your surroundings and products so you do not contact it. Wash slippers, sandals, eyeglasses, watch, comb, brush, toothpicks, doorknobs, toilet seat, carpet, counter, drinking straw, cutlery, contact lenses. Dry all items washed, using paper towels and throw away. Make a wipe of each article later for testing.

Cook the protective herbs and teas (see page 405) or take the capsules after sterilizing them. Start the kidney cleaning drops. The *Kidney Cleanse* is second best. **Do not refrigerate or freeze homeographic drops nor apricot pits** (they will lose their activity). As soon as you get your supplies, sterilize them. Just a few bacteria, far less than you could find by culturing them will easily grow in you! These few will pick up radioactivity in your body and wear it like a shield to protect themselves from your white blood cells. Soon you are sicker than ever. Healthy people will not even notice them, being able to eat unsterilized food with relish, cooked or raw.

Start with the WBC supplements, the first 3 sets of kidney drops, and all the protective supplements and teas. If you do not have the drops yet, start the *Kidney Cleanse* recipe exactly as given in the book without shortcuts or substitutions (see page 592). Use the apricot suppository recipe again as on the first night. After 3 nights in a row you can expect one malignancy to be gone. Then take 1 or 2 days off, if needed. Add 3 more nights for each tumor you have. In general, there will be 2 or 3 times as many tumors as your oncologist found by scanning, so you have a bigger task than you expected. But your success can be certain.

On DAY 3: Make your first set of body wipes using the torso chart to guide you, page 350. Most of all, be sure to wipe over every painful spot, lump, or problem area, numbering it or labeling it for testing. This is so you can tell what is happening inside, and what needs to be done next. You should be on all the protective herbs and supplements now. Do not wait for everything to be together. An easy way to keep track of them is to line them all up along the edge of the kitchen counter. The dose is mostly a few capsules 5 times daily. Going from bottle to bottle at this low dose is not so overwhelming. Those that are taken 4 times or 3 times get pushed out of line and marked on the cap. It is a full time job. You should find a helper who can help you get all your chores done. You are the doctor, the hospital, the nurses and the patient rolled into one. Keep notes. Unfortunately, you can't get reimbursed by any insurance company for wasted premiums. But life itself is a fine reimbursement.

Start Your Protective Herbs And Teas

Short Herb Set

- Eucalyptus, 2 cups tea a day or 1 capsule, 3 times a day
- Boneset, 2 cups tea a day or 1 capsule, 3 times a day
- Epazote, 2 cups tea a day or 1 capsule, 3 times a day
- Birch Bark, 1 cup tea a day or 1 capsule, 2 times a day

- Burdock, 2 cups tea a day or 1 capsule, 3 times a day
- Reishi mushroom, 1 capsule, 3 times a day
- Turmeric, 6 capsules, 3 times daily as tea or capsule
- Fennel, 6 capsules, 3 times daily as tea or capsule

This **short herb set** can cure and protect you from most bacteria that cancer patients get. You can feel decidedly better from just this set. There are several spices that you can add to make the teas more tasty (any mentioned in *Recipes*). Do not use sugar or syrup since they feed bacteria too easily. You may use Stevia or inositol, disinfected, besides spices as sweetener.

If you know which bacteria you have you can pursue them individually, too, with faster results (see page 252).

The following are the most important bacteria and how to protect or cure yourself from them.

Protection From Salmonella:

Salmonella bacteria are the consequence of killing parasites(!) and of eating unsterilized food. Nobody escapes them if they are succeeding! You must constantly kill them to keep up with their arrival throughout the program.

• Lugol's iodine solution, 6 drops in about ½ cup water, 4 times daily, best after meals and bedtime. If you have a diluted form of Lugol's (2%), use 10 drops instead.

• short herb set

• The individual recipe on page 253 is for stubborn cases of Salmonella.

Salmonella appears after killing Fasciolopsis buski parasites.

Protection From E. coli:

This is the cancer patient's worst enemy. Every patient has it upon arrival.

- 6 capsules turmeric, 4 times daily
- 6 capsules fennel, 4 times daily

Take them at any time. Do not separate them or reduce the dose. You may mix them in a little "cocktail" that you make from fruit or vegetable juice. This dose can eliminate E. coli in 2 days and you can be in much less pain after that. It will then stay away if all your food, supplements, and hands are kept sterilized. Do not lick your fingers or other objects unless dipped in alcohol or *Lugol's* solution first. This includes stamps, envelopes, book pages, the telephone and newspaper. Consider your mouth off limits. You do not "catch E. coli" from kissing, singing, talking, laughing, or even sex. You do catch it from your fingers, your toothbrush, sucking on a pencil or pen, kissing a pet, unsterilized supplements, going into or coming out of a washroom. Wash your hands. Turn the doorknob with a piece of paper. E. coli appears after killing Macracanthorhyncus.

Protection From Clostridium:

These appear after killing Fasciolopsis buski parasites.

- Take 10 drops oregano oil in an empty capsule once a day at first, more later. CAUTION: Oregano oil is very fierce; even ½ drop cannot be tolerated by the mouth, but does not affect the stomach. After 3 days of killing F. buski with apricot suppositories, you will be growing many more Clostridium bacteria and should increase oregano oil to 3 times a day for 3 days.

Protection From Flu Virus:

Take 1 tube of Oscillococcinum at bedtime whether you feel sick or not. It is a homeopathic treatment. Follow the label instructions. It needs disinfection. Also take the short herb set in tea form or in capsules.

Protection From Avian Or Bird Flu:

These have acquired the ability to use gold as a mineral, as have certain other modern pathogens.

- Remove gold from your teeth
- Remove gold jewelry including glasses and rings
- Stop eating supermarket breads because they all contain gold.
- Trim all the gums where teeth once were and where teeth still are. Gold diffuses and spreads broadly.
- Do EDTA mouthwashes, they remove more gold.

Avian flu does not respond to the homeopathic treatment, but does respond to the herbs. The chief danger is supplying still more gold to prions, which make you dizzy and disoriented. For such symptoms stop the program until all gold is removed. Some flours do not have gold; use a carefully chosen bread maker to supply yourself with gold-free baked goods.

Take all the short herb set in tea or capsule form.

Protection From Adenovirus: (the common cold)

- Take each of the protective herbs in the short herb set, 1 capsule or ½ cup tea, 3 times daily.

Protection From Prions: (disorientation and dizziness)

- Remove all gold from teeth and jewelry. Prions require gold and can be starved this way.
- Stop eating USA bread because it all contains gold. Always take this seriously. Go back to the high dose of *take-out* drops

for heavy metals, to remove gold more completely from the kidneys and lymph.

- Take Birch bark, 2 cups tea daily or 1 capsule, 3 times daily. Reduce dosage again when recovered.
- Take Reishi, 1 capsule, 4 times daily. Reduce dose when better.
- Trim all the gums where teeth once were and where teeth still are to remove every trace of gold (see page 371).
- Make and take gold-out-of-the kidney set and lymph. Gold can be added to nickel first so both come out together.

Using the *Protective Herb* list in the short herb set will prevent and help cure many other infections too. Do not neglect them because you "feel so well" or "are willing to suffer". Your hidden infections delay your recovery. They are some of the most useful herbs for all circumstances.

If you make teas or take capsules of them, they should be frozen first. Cooking does not sterilize them but does produce fewer bacteria. Making teas gives you much more "water" to drink than taking capsules. This will help you get the amount necessary to wash the cancer-complex out of your body. You should make no less than 2½ qts./liters of urine in 24 hours but not more than 4 while you are washing out the cancer-complex.

Feed Your White Blood Cells

- Selenium (sodium selenite) 3 capsules, 5 times a day
- Hydrangea root powder (organic germanium), 2 capsules, 5 times a day
- Rose Hips (organic vitamin C) 3 capsules, 5 times a day
- Rutin and Hesperidin in the form of currants contain the organic part of vitamin C. Do not heat them or get them wet. Eat straight, after freezing, 1 tsp. X 3.
- One Tbsp. of peanut butter keeps your WBC supplied with both germanium and selenium for a day. Eat 1-2 Tbsp. daily to be able to stop these supplements for a day.

First Aid

When your body can no longer detoxify the iron cyanides that you are drinking it will start filling up with real "free" cyanide. All cancer patients arrive in this condition. One of the first mutations made by the cancer-complex is absence of the enzyme Rhodanese. This enzyme normally detoxifies organic cyanides, those that are part of our food. Without Rhodanese they will form free cyanide, the kind that kills. You need more oxygen at once, besides stopping the iron cyanide that is present in all chlorinated water. You already stopped drinking chlorinated water on **Day 1**.

- Drink ½ cup ozonated unchlorinated water (see *Sources*), 3 times daily for 1 week at least. If you use chlorinated water you will be giving yourself more cyanide. Ordinary filters do not remove the iron cyanides. If ozonated water is not available or has not been tested use hydrogen peroxide.
- Take hydrogen peroxide, 17%, called PEROXY, 1 drop in a glass of water, 2 drops in the next glass and so on till slight discomfort is felt in the stomach. Stay at this "tolerance dose" 3 times daily. Continue till there is no free cyanide (sodium or potassium cyanide) in your saliva, at least 1 week.

Alkalinize

- Take ¼ tsp. baking soda dissolved in water morning and night to help kidneys excrete the allergenic chemicals. Phenolic food allergens are quite acid and can stall the kidneys. These were forming your tumor nucleus before switching to the new diet. The baking soda must be free of benzene and sterilized.

Start Protective Supplements

- IP6, 20 drops, 5 times a day (transfer to plastic dropper bottle before using). Use no rubber or glass dropper, nor an untested pipette. This removes polonium. Be sure to sterilize.

Reduce to 2 times a day after 5 days. Take before or between meals.

- Oregano oil (transfer to plastic dropper bottle before using and sterilize). CAUTION: Do not touch lip or mouth with even a drop of it. Take 10 drops once a day (put in empty capsule). This kills Clostridium bacteria. Stop after 2 weeks or if stomach has pain. If depressed or crying or uric acid is low on the blood test take it 3 times a day.
- Ginger root, 2 capsules, 3 times a day for 5 days. This removes methyl malonate from kidneys to unblock them.
- Uva ursi, 2 capsules, 3 times a day for 5 days. This also removes the malonate block from kidneys.
- MSM, 3 capsules, 5 times a day. This pulls the buski-ONION-GARLIC-MUSTARD chemicals away from the cancer-complex. Sterilize. Reduce to 2 capsules 5 times a day after 2 weeks.
- Quinone drops, a set of 5; these transform the ferro to the ferricyanide compound. After this the ONION-GARLIC-MUSTARD compounds cannot keep themselves attached to the rest of the cancer-complex. Do not refrigerate or freeze.
- Fresh pomegranate seeds or dried peel, ½ tsp., 5 times a day. This prevents detox-symptoms. Test for chlorox; wash in Lugol's water and refrigerate, then cut fruit in quarters. (Pomegranate peel capsules are second best.) Dump contents of fruit in Proctor Silex blender or other brand with non-seeping blades. Blend 4 seconds at a time till the seeds are drinkable. They supply organic vitamin C.
- Citric acid, 1 or 2 capsules, 5 times a day to supply the mitochondria with raw materials to help make energy.
- Vitamin C, 1000 mg., 5 times a day, plus organic varieties, to detoxify radioactivity.

Start Kidney Cleaning Drops

Start the first day with the pyruvic aldehyde set followed by the kidney and lymph set. Take them as if they were homeopathically made, behind the bottom front teeth under the tongue. Hold the bottle about 6 inches (15 cm) higher than your nose so you can see and count the drops. Do not swallow for 1 full minute. Then swallow to clear your mouth for the next bottle. Keep a kitchen timer so no less than 1 minute passes between bottles; more is fine. The order of bottles does not matter. Do not touch your mouth with a bottle. If you do, wipe nozzle immediately with paper towel. Use a mirror or get help till you manage it accurately. Count the drops, do not squirt. You may go directly from one set to the next or to any other bottle.

It would be good to copy all your bottles when you receive them, in case you run short or something happens to one. Learn to copy, and have your first 3 copies checked by a tester. Use rainwater only, not treated in any way, nor filtered, and in contact only with HDPE. Collect it yourself (see page 246). Hot-backwash filtered water is second best.

All dosages for drops are 6 drops. But the number of times a day can change. On the first 2 days, take them 6 times each day. It will be convenient to take supplements on even number hours and drops on odd number hours or the other way around. If you fall behind your schedule, simply catch up by taking them closer together. Do not skip. Do not take supplements or drops after 8 p.m. or sundown not to burden the kidneys.

You can take drops very close together if needed. Pain or sleep sets can be taken 10 minutes apart.

Notice, again, that this is a full-time job; you will certainly need a helper to get any other chores done.

After the first 2 days, reduce the drop-taking from 6 times to 3 times daily, for all sets. Continue at this rate for the entire program. Then stop. Do not copy your own drops to continue because you may have gotten bacteria in them. Copy only new bottles or order 2 sets. Bacteria will be magnified by copying.

Start any new set at the 6 times daily rate. After 2 days reduce it, too, to 3 times daily. You are now taking 3 sets, all three times a day and finishing by sundown. Don't have food in your mouth or talk with drops in your mouth.

After 2 more days, start the 4th set of drops at 6 times daily. Continue all the earlier sets at the 3 times rate. After 2 more days start the 5th set while going down to 3 times daily for the earlier set.

Finally, you are on 7 sets, all 3 times a day. When they are gone switch to the *Kidney Cleanse* to help them excrete (see page 592).

Start the gold-out-of-kidneys and lymph set. Combine gold with nickel first so you can take both out together. Remember to make a copy of Au and Ni beforehand, not to destroy your only masters. Place them side by side, touching each other and place the blank at either end. Then throw away these "combined" masters (see page 207). Starting this take-out set last gives you time to remove gold from your mouth first. Gold causes dizziness, difficulty breathing, swallowing, Alzheimer's disease, new rare diseases and fatigue.

As soon as you are caught up with the drops, ozonated water, WBC supplements, teas, and protective supplements and have done the first 5 days of this program, you may do your first regular *Parasite-Killing Program*. Not sooner! Actually, your body has already started on its own! If you are not fully protected, with your WBCs fed and the kidneys ready to excrete, you could feel worse than when you started. This is called detoxification syndrome. You may also lose some time getting well and remotivated, but your cancer-curing will not be set back. Catch up before going on.

Of course you were killing parasites with the apricot suppositories. But if you can manage to keep up with everything so far, you are ready for the Black Walnut Hull method too.

If you can't keep up stay on this first part as much as you can. You will still succeed if you watch your priorities (no chlorox-water in your home, no chlorox food or contaminated clothing, no chlorox-contaminated dental fillings and no porcelain fillings nor root canals, or uranium-containing amalgam in your teeth and gums).

Start Regular Parasite-Killing Program

- 9 wormwood capsules
- 9 clove capsules
- 1 tsp. up to a whole 1 oz. bottle of green Black Walnut Hull tincture Extra Strength. Store this in your freezer.

(Always test a new herb first by trying 1 capsule or ¼ tsp. liquid. Although reactions are very rare, be cautious)

The following are optional additions to the Green Black Walnut tincture to improve taste:

- 1 tsp. up to 1 Tbsp. fresh pomegranate (see recipe page 387).
- 1-2 Tbsp. extra heavy whipping cream tested for chlorox (see *Sources*) and previously sterilized with 5 drops *Lugol's* (or 10 drops 2%) per ½ cup. This prevents nausea.
- 1-2 Tbsp. maple syrup (see *Sources)* tested for chlorox and gallic acid and sterilized.

Freeze the tincture beforehand. It will not solidify and it stays green longer. Freeze the capsules to disinfect. But the cream and syrups can be disinfected by standing them opened in a shopping bag and putting the ozonator hose in the bag beside them for 10 minutes (see page 548).

Now you will be killing many more parasites and you can expect the side-effects called "Detoxification symptoms". Fortunately, you are ready for them with all the protections in place. If you do get sick, try to see the humor in getting sick from getting well. But be more vigilant after this. While sick force yourself to eat regardless of appetite; you should not lose weight. If you miss half your meals for one day, have each food blended for you the next day, so you can drink it without tasting or chewing. Add spices and digestive enzymes. Also expect to see all your symptoms get worse for 2 days. If you have diarrhea, use the opportunity to find your parasites (see page 181).

Do not try to "weather" the Flu and Salmonella symptoms. They could get worse and worse to the prion stage. Then you feel dizzy and disoriented. Do not try to outlast a prion attack either. Sip birch bark tea all day long made as a tasty beverage. Take hydrazine sulfate drops to keep yourself eating even without appetite. And take melatonin and ornithine to help sleep. Disinfect these also. As soon as you are better and can handle the program again you may add the remaining supplements.

Remaining Supplements

- Take a thyroid pill in the morning, starting with ½ grain, then switching to 1 grain in a few days. Be alert to possible reactions, even though they were tested and sterilized. If you do react, find a different brand. This is not a synthetic variety. Sonicate to destroy any prions. Elderly patients should stay with ½ grain to avoid stress on heart.

5 Minutes Before Meals Or Earlier

- 3 times a day, take 1 capsule magnesium oxide and 2 capsules vitamin B_2. We will leave out the iron of older programs because it can reduce the ferricyanide to cancer-causing ferrocyanide in the cancer-complex. If you take magnesium too close to food you will get indigestion. If you are constipated take 2 magnesium capsules instead of one.
- 2 capsules Decaris (levamisole, 50 mg.)

If all these upset your appetite, move them to an earlier time, like 20 min. before meals. If you can't take 2 supplements but could take 1, do that. They help greatly to stimulate the stomach to make pepsin. The levamisole kills Strongyloides, Ascaris, and the filaria parasites, dog heartworm and Onchocerca. It also removes ferritin coating on WBCs. Sterilize all pills. Pepsin kills prions.

With Each Meal (Sterilize each item)

- 15 drops HCl (hydrochloric acid), 5%, stirred into your food and beverage with plastic cutlery. If you don't mix it, it could eat your tooth enamel. You may put them in a capsule.
- 1 capsule potassium gluconate, tested for radioactivity besides chlorox. Add it to a salt-loving food.
- 1 drop vitamin D_3, 5 times daily, totaling about 2,000 units. More is better. It can destroy the cancer-complex.
- Betaine hydrochloride. Start when dental work starts. Take 3 capsules, 3 times daily for 3 days. Then reduce to 1 X 1.

After Meals (Sterilize each item)

- 3 capsules pepsin
- 1 capsule multiple digestive enzymes
- 2 capsules pancreatin-lipase
- 1 bromelain (not if malaria is present)
- 6 drops *Lugol's* iodine or 10 drops diluted *Lugol's* in water (do not combine with anything)

The enzymes can also be taken with meals or just before. Lugol's can be taken whenever the stomach feels bloated, gassy or hurts.

Between Meals (Sterilize each item)

- 1-3 multiple digestive enzymes, 5 times daily. They can digest unusual things like yeast and chitin.
- 2 drops vitamin A, 5000 units each, 3 times daily (not the dry form).

- 15-pancreatin-lipase, 2 times daily. (You may combine these with your dose of turmeric or fennel in a beverage IF drunk promptly.)

All of these varieties of enzymes remove the undigested food as well as dead parasites that litter the tumor zone.

Bedtime

Do not take B-vitamins or drops nor zap at bedtime. The kidneys will be stressed and sleep can be disturbed. It often helps sleep to take 2 capsules of rose hips or 1 vitamin C, 2 capsules of pancreatin-lipase, 1 capsule of milk thistle seed and 6 to 10 drops *Lugol's* iodine in a bit of water at bedtime. Take Lugol's first so it can't oxidize the supplements. Give it a 3-minute head start.

If you have gurgling and gas, take 6 fennel and 6 turmeric near bedtime and repeat at bedtime. These two doses help you get through the night without waking. It is caused by unsterilized supplements and food.

If your insomnia is severe, take 9 to 12 ornithine capsules plus 2 or 3 melatonin, each 3 mg. The cause is always bacteria, the same kind you are trying to kill by daytime. Kill them before going to bed and then take the insomnia treatment right at bedtime.

Cutting Down

After 2 weeks on the full program, cut all dosages in half. It does not have to be precise. This will help you find and stop anything that you have become allergic to or that may have bacteria or other contamination. Stop these as soon as you notice them. You may skip every other day instead of reducing the dose.

After the 3rd week, at half dosage, cut it in half again, so you are on about ¼ of the starting dosages.

Your Accomplishments

You have learned to sterilize your food, simplify your life, and hopefully how to zap yourself in several ways. If you have salvaged yourself from Hospice or other dire predictions, please form a Self-Health-Survivors' Group so others could benefit from your experience.

If you learned to use a Syncrometer® please apply for a diploma* to the International Syncrometer® Educational Science Center (ISC). You are the first generation of self-health testers, although many before you have succeeded in their own way.

Tips For The Program Projects

***Help* #1.** Flee first, fix later. Don't wait for anything if you have a cancer diagnosis. Flee to a friend or relative that has no filters attached to the water system anywhere, nor softener. This already raises your chance of success to 50% (from zero). Unfortunately, there is no test or lab that can tell you which kind of bleach is used in your city water. *The search is on for a test that tells the difference between ferrocyanide and ferricyanide in trace amounts in water.*

As soon as you have found a Syncrometer® tester, test the kitchen cold water and move again if it has chlorox bleach. Test other waters immediately, too. (Hot water tests have many more errors than cold water, don't request these.) Attach the hot water backwash filter for security.

***Help* #2.** All active wells are required to be disinfected by the Health Dept. Do not guess, even if the well is isolated and looks unused. Purchase test strips called

* Apply to International Syncrometer® Educational Science Center (ISC), please use our fax 011 52 664 683 4454 in Mexico if possible. Thank you. Send name, date, and 12 small items (not fruit), enclosed marked *Pos* or *Neg* for chlorox bleach or polonium.

"TOTAL-CHLORINE". If the well seems unchlorinated, send a sample to a Syncrometer® tester to check by testing for chlorination of any sort (hypochlorite test).

***Help* #3.** After you have done your own testing, send samples to a Syncrometer® tester to check on your results. Sets of pans or cutlery cannot be assumed to be the same in quality; test each item separately. Ask questions at the Farmer's Market; do not assume the produce is home grown. Open the plastic wrap on all produce as soon as you get it home to let out the accumulated radon. Be sure to use chlorox-free paper towels and plastic bags for testing.

***Help* #4.** Even if you have an emergency and must take the advised treatment, try to analyze it by Syncrometer® so you can begin the healing process at the same time.

***Help* #5.** Prescription drugs should not be stopped until the exact replacements have been found without chlorox bleach. When hardening your plastic watch or glasses you could warp them if the water gets too hot. Don't leave the stove while heating them. Stop heating them before they boil. Place them in zippered bags first.

***Help* #6.** Many more HDPE containers are available on the Internet. Sanitize them in the dishwasher.

***Help* #7.** The baking soda must be frozen to sterilize it first, as well as the toothbrush, floss, and oregano oil. Salmonella and E. coli are everywhere.

***Help* #8.** Although you may be living in a good water zone, your dishes, furnishings, bedding, and carpets could be washed in chlorox-containing cleaners if you chose these or are in a hotel. New clothing probably has chlorox residue; launder it first with special recipe (see page 611). Silk is ideal, having no chlorination.

***Help* #9.** Do not use alcohol on your hair or scalp. It could cause hair loss. Powdered detergent is strong enough. Don't miss any small scalp area or bit of face. The excessive fragrance and other chemicals must be endured since nothing else strong enough for this task exists.

***Help* #10.** Miracles can be done in many optometrist or ophthalmologist offices. Your glasses can be "copied" into a different lens and frame by many. Your prescription can be looked up and put into new glasses with an all plastic frame. Glasses' temples are a big source of cerium (plastic) for cancer of the eye, optic nerve or brain. Sonicators in the form of jewelry cleaners are easily obtained to harden glasses. Items must be held below the water level to be effective. Place in zippered plastic bags first. Sonicate for 20 minutes.

***Help* #11.** Find a medium quality water pick; practice seating the basin carefully and snugly. Harden the plastic basin first by pouring steaming hot water into it and covering it for 30 min. Run hot tap water through the hose. Practice adjusting the settings for your mouth sensitivity. You may add pure salt or a few drops of *Lugol's* iodine to a tankful to keep it sterile in use. Buy it now to avoid a single day's delay.

***Help* #12.** Ask the dentist a few weeks before your appointment for a set of supplies to be used for you, even the anesthetics, sealer, adhesive, gauze, sutures, and other "minor" items, besides the main ingredients. Nothing needs to be out of its container for testing. Explain your chlorox sensitivity briefly. Offer a full deposit on them to cover cost in case they are lost, since you need to send them to a Syncrometer® tester.

The dentist can often see a dark rim around a plastic filling where leftover amalgam remains. You may need to call your earlier dentist to find out which teeth had work done and what it was, or supply name and access numbers to your new dentist who needs to know. Your dentist may be able to use a current measuring meter to find out which teeth still have metal. A Syncrometer® tester could search for mercury, gold, nickel, copper, chromium, etc. Teeth that have been drilled out twice may be borderline in survival and not a candidate for their third filling.

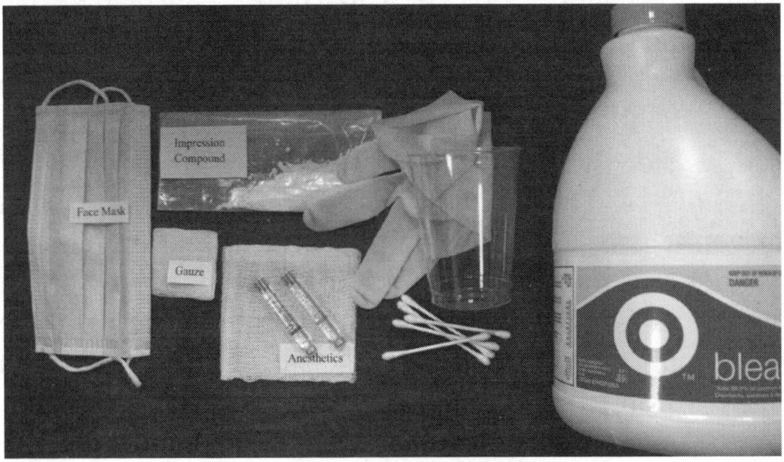

Fig. 100 Test all Dental Supplies

If you prefer certainty of survival to keeping your original teeth, you should choose extraction of all filled teeth. Any accidentally leftover polonium or uranium whether in a tooth or behind the gums or stuck in your gums will give you a new malignancy, called a metastasis. Polonium that is just a chip or crumb or dust in an old socket is just as dangerous.

While teeth are "open", keep food away from them. Floss and brush and water pick them after each meal. Sterilize the brush by dropping into *Lugol's* water for 20 min. Frequent use of *Dental Bleach* becomes too much chlorine for you. Dilute it further by squirting 1 or 2 squirts into a small cup of water. Only use *Dental Bleach* this often during dental work.

***Help* #13.** Do not zappicate metal. Be sure to store the tooth zappicator in a zippered plastic bag at all times, but not air tight. Do not place it on the TV or zappicator food box; it has a very small and easily overwhelmed magnet inside. Test your tooth zappicator with a compass before use to make sure it has not switched to south pole. Dropping it could switch its polarity. Do not put it in your mouth uncovered. Put it in a plastic bag, head first, and tape around the handle to use it.

The L-1 zapper refers to LOW frequency, 1000 hertz. There should only be one wire connection to it, the *Positive* side. It will function like an antenna.

***Help* #14.** The ozonator has a very important job to do for you—give you FIRST AID treatment for your chronic cyanide poisoning. Acute poisoning comes from sodium cyanide or potassium cyanide because this reacts directly with your iron-enzymes. Chronic poisoning comes from the two iron cyanides in our 2 kinds of bleach added to water. We all thought and were reassured that the iron cyanides "had rather low toxicity".

We also thought that added cerium hydroxide, to lower arsenic levels, would be of low toxicity. Now the Syncrometer® finds both chemicals to have huge toxic effects by joining the cancer-complex.

***Help* #15.** There are many zappers in the market place. How can you know which work and which do not? While the device is under warranty, you should do 2 things: 1) Take it to an electronics shop and ask the technician there if he/she could put it on the oscilloscope to see the output. A picture of the expected output is on page 525. Also ask the technician if there is any "spiking" and if there is ¼ volt *Positive* offset. Return spiking or no offset or part *Negative* units.

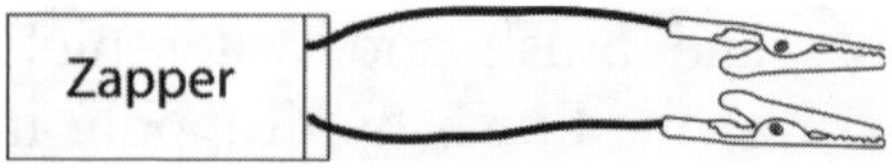

The next test you can do yourself. Arrange the zapper with the leads attached, but nothing attached to the electrodes. Place a plastic bag under them for some insulation. Next, fill a ½-ounce plastic or glass bottle with water up to the neck. Close it with its lid. The water should be room temperature. Place the bottle across the metal electrodes so the ends lie on the 2 electrodes. Keep it all in horizontal position lying flat. The body of the bottle should be just a bit above the table, not touching anything, as shown. Turn on the zapper for about 5 minutes. Turn it off again. Label the bottle "output of Test-zapper 5 minutes". Test it for magnetic polarization. It should be north, and only north. If the zapper fails this test, it is not up to the quality standard expected. Do not be surprised if any of the tests fail. Hopefully, the vendor will take it for its trade-in value and set it right before selling it again. Vendors are often not in control of their electronics technicians who may feel they know best. Often one product is superbly made while others fall short. The market place will get better from expecting high standards. It benefits us all to have the best quality devices.

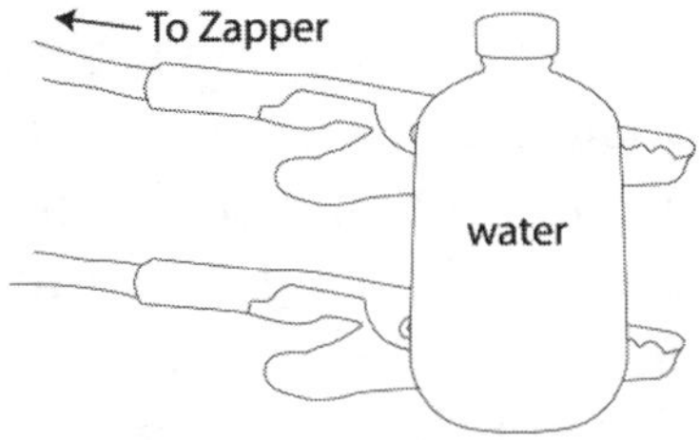

To test the polarization of the bottle you just made you will need to send it to a Syncrometer® tester who will match it to a north or south testing bottle. These can be easily made (see page 333). CAUTION: If these bottles are shipped by air, or frozen, or passed through a security check point they will not give accurate results. The tester must remedy this first (see page 200).

***Help* #16.** Nothing is absolutely sterile in the market place, not cooked food or canned food, not prescription pills or intravenous solutions, not vitamin capsules nor products unopened straight from the manufacturer. It is even very difficult to achieve in a bacteriologists' clean-room! All cancer patients have systemic infections that are untreated and untreatable with clinical methods. To get well you must stop eating these ever-present bacteria. The easiest way is to freeze everything to -20° F for 24 hours. With such a helpful boost, your 2 chronic infections, Salmonella and E. coli, will yield to your recovering immune system in 2 or 3 days! You will feel the difference in your well being. A single supplement will hurt you if you neglect this.

***Help* #17.** You will not be able to see the sweat on your skin in the morning, but it is there and will be picked up by the paper you use. When this is tested for the different parts of the cancer-complex, you can see how much progress has been made in breaking it up and washing away the parts into your urine and sweat. This way the only new cancers that can be made must come from polonium sources like teeth and from touching the cancer-complex to your skin, like your ear against a contaminated pillow or your arm on the arm rest of contaminated furniture. Cover everything with thin plastic or wash it clean. Remember, alpha radiation, the most harmful kind, coming from polonium, uranium and radon, cannot pass through even a thin plastic sheet. But once inside you it wreaks havoc. Paper towels and toilet paper are very important, too. Use them to wrap around the body part that does not get good contact with the paper sheet at night. Aim to get all chlorox out by the 3rd day, half the OPT out by then and only the dental work incomplete by the 12th day.

THE PROGRAM AT A GLANCE

PROJECTS
Switch to unchlorinated well water for drinking and cooking.
Switch diet & avoid personal antigen (page 292). Stop chlorine, bromine, fluorine, cyanide, motor oil, alkylating agents and polonium in your water.
Blood Test
Make toothpowder from 10 tsp. baking soda plus 10 drops oregano oil in plastic bag. Do not purchase already mixed.
Stop brushing teeth with current brush. Throw away. Cut floss from shopping bags tested for chlorox. Cut ¼ x 4" strips. After flossing rub teeth gently with finger wrapped in damp paper towel and dipped in tooth powder. Later, buy straight, narrow brush. Harden. Test before using by soaking in water ½ hour. Test soak water for dyes, DAP, PVC, urethane, chlorox.
Stop pills till tested and replace with tested brands. Keep only essential ones till replaced.
Stop wearing jewelry, cosmetics, hair accessories, plastic items until tested for chlorox. Harden and test new ones.
Stop wearing rubber & elastic clothing, including Spandex & Lycra. Turn waistband till new ones are found.
Cut dishes from water bottles. Save plastic bowls and cutlery to reuse. Do not use other cutlery, dishes, cookware.
Stop regular shampoo. Mix ½ cup dry laundry detergent with enough tap water for shampoo. Do not get in eyes. Dry with paper towels. Shampoo 4 times. Later use borax and citric acid (page 606). Send hair wipe to test.
Make eye appointment to change eyeglass frames to all plastic rims. Harden new glasses. Make soak water. Test.
Get Panoramic of teeth and jaw (2 copies). Give 1 to dentist for tooth evaluation. Remove gold first, then root canals. Then test amalgams for radioactivity. Replace non-radioactive amalgam with composite after testing each one for residual mercury. Repeat for composite. Do Huggins cavity cleaning, Jerome tattoo search, Solorio gum-trimming and non-radioactive restoration.
Get water pick (Target or Wal-Mart), stainless steel strainer, and read *Dental Aftercare* (page 422).
Get Tooth Zappicator plus L-1 zapper. Zappicate new plastic teeth as soon as possible.
Get ozonator with non-black tubing. Test for nickel and chlorox. Start whole body ozonation.

Get zapper plus zap plate, rechargeable batteries, charger, and voltmeter. Use zapping schedule in book (page 173).
Get food zappicator; treat all food (in bowls) for 10 minutes.
Place all food, herbs and supplements in chest freezer for 24 hrs. at -20° F. to disinfect. Do not miss a single one or you could get very ill. Continue at home with a new freezer, thermometer and timer for automatic defrosting. Disinfect food with ozonator or by sonicating if more suitable.
Send home water and dust samples for testing by Syncrometer®. Send 3 frozen samples for testing disinfection.
Start apricot seed suppository for first 3 nights. Then take 1 night off and repeat till cured (see instructions page 590).
Start WBC supplements, teas and protective sets as soon as frozen. Do not freeze or refrigerate drops or seeds.
Start each morning with several EDTA-mouthwashes (see page 420).

On Day 1 – Place plastic sheet over entire bed and pillow to avoid contact with contaminated bedding. Place paper sheet over plastic sheet and fold over to wrap yourself in it to absorb sweat and have no contact with top sheet. You may wear fresh night clothing. Launder clothing and bedding next day. Do not wear anything twice. Do not use any cloth towels. Use tested paper towels only and throw away immediately. It contains the cancer-complex, as transmissible as poison ivy.

Take 3 hot showers daily to make you sweat. Use a handful of paper for a washcloth. Dip in powdered safe detergent for armpits, groin and skin over tumors. Do not rub. Go to sleep with paper towels wrapped around tumor locations and held with masking tape. Send a set of skin wipes after each 6 showers (2 days). Use a paper towel folded 4 times and dampened with well water to make wipes in the morning when rising (not after shower). When the wipes are free of OPT you may stop. Continue wipes over tumors or painful spots.

On Day 2 – Do laundry daily (see instruction sheet page 611). Every 2 days roll paper bedding into a fire log shape, using masking tape to keep it tight for testing. Place in plastic bag with nothing else in the bag to prevent cross-contamination.

WHITE BLOOD CELL SUPPLEMENTS	Start 1st day with these & continue Freeze everything at -20° F for 24hrs	DATE	DATE	DATE	DATE	DATE
Selenite (Selenium)	3 capsules 5 times a day					
Hydrangea Root (organic germanium)	2 capsules 5 times a day					
Rose Hips capsules (organic vitamin C)	2 capsules 5 times a day					
IP6 (transfer to ½ oz. plastic dropper bottle before using)	20 drops 5 times a day in glass of water; reduce to 2 times after 5 days					
Oregano oil (transfer to plastic dropper bottle) CAUTION	10 drops once a day on empty stomach (put in capsule)					
Ginger Root	2 capsules 3 times a day for 5 days					
Uva Ursi	2 capsules 3 times a day for 5 days					
Vitamin D3 (tested for lead)	1 drop 5 times a day					
Vitamin C, 1000 mg., plus frozen Sun Maid currants, eaten straight, 1 tsp. 3 X daily for organic vitamin C (hesperidin) Sun Maid or Kosher only	2 capsules 5 times a day					

DROPS TO CLEAN KIDNEYS AND LYMPH	DATE	DATE	DATE	DATE	DATE
Pyruvic Aldehyde set (also hematoxylin, R & L hypothalamus, rhodanese)					
Kidney set & lymph					
Quinones drop set					
Heavy metal out-of-kidneys & lymph set					
Dyes out-of-kidneys & lymph set					
Wheel bearing grease out-of-kidneys & lymph set					
Plastic and rubber out-of-kidneys & lymph set					
Gold and nickel out-of-kidneys & lymph set					

PROTECTIVE SUPPLEMENTS	
Lugol's Iodine	6 drops (10 if 2%) in 1/3 glass water 4 times daily, NOT IF ALLERGIC
Oscillococcinum	1 tube at bedtime
Hydrazine Sulfate (for appetite)	6 drops 6 times daily for 2 days, then 3 times daily for 2 days
MSM (methyl sulfonyl methane)	2 capsules 5 times a day
1 fresh pomegranate, tested	Peel and grind all seeds till smooth (1/2 tsp. 5 times a day)
Ozonated (5 min.) well water	½ glass 3 times daily (ozonator tubing should not be black)
Pantothenate	1 capsule 5 times a day
1/4 tsp sodium bicarbonate (baking soda) in 1/2 glass water upon rising and bedtime (must freeze)	
3 capsules Betaine Hydrochloride 3 times daily for 3 days when you start dental work. Take with food.	

PROTECTIVE HERBS & TEAS (Add ¼ tsp. Stevia herb sweetener to improve taste)	**DATE**	**DATE**	**DATE**	**DATE**	**DATE**
1 cup Eucalyptus tea or 1 capsule 3 X a day					
1 cup Boneset tea daily or 1 capsule 3 X a day					
1 cup Epazote tea daily or 1 capsule 3 X a day					
1 cup Birch Bark tea daily or 1 capsule 2 X a day					
1 cup Burdock tea or 1 capsule 3 X a day					
½ tsp. Reishi mushroom, raw, daily or 1 capsule 3 X a day					
2 capsules Turmeric 3 X a day not with meals					
10 drops Fennel 2 X a day not with meals (put in capsule)					

**2 cups of each tea is much more powerful, as quoted on page 381. Add them to food for blending. You may also add spices.*

You MUST be caught up to here before going on…

PARASITE PROGRAM for 3 days in a row, same days as apricot treatment	**DATE**	**DATE**	**DATE**	**DATE**	**DATE**
Black Walnut Tincture (Extra Strength) 1 tsp to whole 1 oz . bottle					
9 capsules Wormwood combination					
9 capsules Cloves					
ZAPPING SCHEDULE (follow schedule page 173)	**DATE**	**DATE**	**DATE**	**DATE**	**DATE**
1 X Regular zap daily					
1 X Vascular set daily					
1 X Plate-zap of organ with tumor daily					
1 X Plate-zap of tumor daily					

OTHER SUPPLEMENTS (all items, even prescription pills must be frozen first)	**DATE**	**DATE**	**DATE**	**DATE**	**DATE**

MORNING					
1 Thyroid, 1 grain (from doctor). Test for chlorox bleach and freeze.					
1 EDTA, 2 times daily on empty stomach (in addition to EDTA mouthwash)					
5 or 10 MIN. BEFORE MEALS – 3 times daily					
2 capsules Vitamin B2					
1 capsule Magnesium, 5 minutes or more before meals to avoid indigestion					
1 capsule citric acid					
1 capsule Vitamin B6, 250 mg.					
2 capsules Decaris to kill "roundworm" parasites					
WITH MEALS					
15 drops HCl (hydrochloric acid 5%) mixed in food or beverage					
1 capsule Potassium gluconate, mixed in salt-loving food					
1 capsule Cascara Sagrada if constipated, or other treatment (page 586).					
AFTER MEALS (or during)					
3 capsules Pepsin (freeze first)					
1 capsule Multiple digestive enzymes (freeze first)					
2 capsules Pancreatin-Lipase (freeze first)					
1 capsule Bromelain (freeze first) NOT with malaria					
BETWEEN MEALS					
15 capsules Pancreatin-Lipase, plus 1 to 3 multiple digestive enzymes					
2 drops vitamin A x 3, daily					
BEDTIME (Do not take B vitamins, drops, nor zap at bedtime)					
9 to 12 capsules Ornithine plus 2 to 3 capsules Melatonin 3 mg. (for insomnia)					

CHAPTER 16

ADVANCED ALTERNATIVE DENTISTRY

We thought the worst part of amalgam fillings was the mercury. But now there is a much worse toxin that we had never guessed. Only a Geiger Mueller tube could find it. It is radiation coming from polonium, the same polonium as makes the cancer-complex. It has immediate urgency. A malignant tumor will always grow again if polonium can be supplied by your teeth. The Syncrometer® finds polonium right beside any uranium, in fact, touching it, in any radioactive tooth filling as well as in a tumor. It has actually made a path to your tumor! This makes cancer a part-dental disease!

The biggest new challenge for dentists is to remove the polonium and uranium from the patients' mouth.

The polonium came from the uranium. Uranium is allowed by government regulation* in amalgam. Every kind of uranium is radioactive, even if it has been depleted of one variety. There are several varieties, usually mixed. They produce **α**, **β** and γ radiations. The **α** and **β** radiations make the larger mutations. The gamma radiation makes the most distant and mostly gene mutations. These radiations make tissues grow, just what cancer does. It is common to downplay the importance of uranium radiations. This is like downplaying the significance of a serial killer in a big city because he's only one man in half a million.

---

* Radioactive Compounds In Dental Materials? by Ulf Bengtsson, 2000 http://www.gbg.bonet.se/bwf/art/radio.doc

Every malignancy is receiving polonium, and the polonium finds its partners, cerium and ferrocyanide quite easily in your body. Although cancer is started by polonium, cerium and ferrocyanide in the water, these ingredients must be constantly replenished to maintain it. Replenishing the cancer-complex can be from any source and depends no doubt on its "turnover rate". Polonium and cerium do not come from your own natural teeth! They come from the artificial parts glued or fastened to them. If they could be somehow removed without making any radioactive dust or tiny particles to get away into your body, you could leave the dental office, cancer free. All malignancies could be made benign in less than 1 to 2 weeks of dental repair. We can reach this goal by means of this advanced dental procedure.

By removing the polonium and uranium stuck fast in your teeth you can destroy all your malignancies. Cancers are not independent. They depend on a stationary polonium supply and a constant supply of living energy called "reducing equivalents" from the parasite. Stopping either one is just as effective.

> The most important mission to our species could be to stop the spread of uranium and polonium from dental supplies, from chlorox household bleach, from our drinking water and products made with it.

There are more dental supplies with polonium than just amalgam.

We are going into an age of radioactivity that we did not choose or foresee. It was something the early geneticists feared, something that the "peaceniks" and "flower children" feared, as well as unpopular religious groups and a few scientists. At that time we left the dilemmas in the hands of "green" people and "activists". Where can we turn now? Could it be the dentists?

It is important to own a Geiger Mueller counter (see *Sources*). Test a sample of fertilizer before you buy it. Test water softener salt before you buy it. Test your teeth with a **black light** to see if they glow in the dark. If they do, replace them.

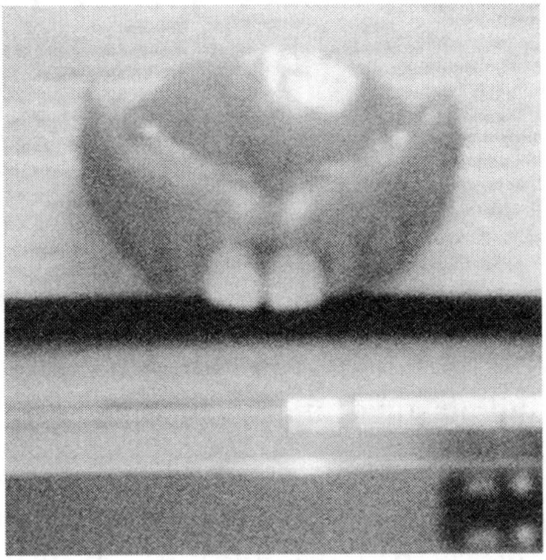

After exchanging all his other glowing teeth, the owner found his asthma improving, but couldn't bear to part with these last 2 "headlights". But he took the plunge and found he could go camping, hike trails and sleep (walk) upstairs again.

Fig. 101 Glowing teeth, the ultimate toxin

To replace them, test the new supplies for chlorox bleach and for NSF bleaches with a Syncrometer®. They should have <u>no</u> bleach because all chlorination with bleach brings radioactivity. Find bleach-free supplies, where iodine was used to disinfect instead.

It is very fortunate that some corporations still use steam or Lugol's iodine to disinfect.

Don't choose dental supplies that are porcelain, or "veneer" or "cement" nor, of course, containing chlorox.

Test all the supplies used in any procedure for alpha (α), beta (β), and gamma (γ) radiation. This much can be done by Syncrometer®. The anesthetics, adhesives, as well as composites are easily tested.

The danger is that tiny bits of polonium and uranium in the chlorox disinfectant will be hardened along with the polymer as it cures, never to be removed by the body's immune forces.

The purpose of dental work in earlier books was to destroy Clostridium bacteria and to remove metals.

Now the purpose includes these, but even more urgent is:

- to remove Po and U from your mouth
- to remove chlorox and other hardened bleach from your mouth
- to remove cerium from your mouth. This is in the rubber of root canals and plastic of many composites.

Once the composites with these metals and bleaches is solidified the radioactivity cannot be removed by your WBCs, nor by brushing teeth or with mouthwashes. They are permanent. They will make permanent connections to your tumors, even as far away as the groin or ankle. Now you have a polonium- or uranium-tooth.

The Polonium-Tooth

There are 3 ways a tooth can become a Po-tooth: one is from a plastic filling that had chlorox bleach as its disinfectant; another is from an amalgam filling that also had uranium; a third way is from any dental device with uranium or chlorox contamination, such as a crown, bridge, inlay, retainer or denture.

Amalgam fillings had uranium contamination in about half of the samples I tested 10 years ago! It had already been legal for some time. It was devastating news. We all know what uranium does…it breaks into 2 parts, both radioactive. It makes Po out of itself, in a process called radioactive decay. Devastating because the government allows such a dangerous element to be placed in teeth to make them sparkle! …or visible when x-rayed! Such frivolous purposes show that our government agents have no idea of the real hazard to our society. The fact that it is "spent" uranium makes no difference. The fact that U has a long half-life makes no difference. The high energy radiation of U means it will reach our most sacred organs where reproduction for the next generation occurs, besides the more local ones.

In a society where the incidence of genetic disease and birth defects is sky rocketing it makes no sense to put any mutagen in the body, particularly teeth, since they become a permanent fixture.

At the very least, the rate of birth defects for parents with uranium in their mouths should be compared with parents without uranium. The parents of a neighborhood could do this independently, hiring only a project manager for guidance.

Now it is important to remove all uranium and polonium from the teeth as quickly as possible.

Preparing The Dental Office

Most important is to have radiation-free water and supplies in the office. Send a cold water sample to a Syncrometer® tester to search for chlorox bleach, polonium, and uranium.

- Locate the office in a "good water zone" where only NSF-rated bleach was used to disinfect it. This will not be radiation-free, but you can make it so.

  Radiation-free water does not come from city water in the USA, although it does in Switzerland.

- To become radiation-free, attach the hot-backwash filter to the main water intake.
- Replace all cleaning agents with chlorox-free varieties. Throw away the present ones.

- Test all dental supplies for chlorox bleach. Acquire chlorox-free varieties.
- Send 1 or 2 staff-persons to a Syncrometer® teacher for a 2-day course, to do your own testing.

It is not difficult to achieve perfect success with a Syncrometer® tester near you. Success is turning out patient after patient without radioactivity in their teeth and free of all cancers (and pain!) at their next doctor visit regardless how advanced they were.

What Is It Worth?

Some Mexican prices in 2007 are: tooth extraction using *Dental Bleach* and socket plug protection plus Huggins socket cleaning about $100.00 per tooth; Socket Therapy (socket cleaning at old missing tooth site or old Root Canal site $100.00 per tooth; non metallic, non radioactive crown (Targis) $300.00; temporary acrylic crown $100.00; tattoo search is included in regular initial examination, altogether, $50.00. Gum trimming per set of 8 teeth (margin of gum, gum, tip of papilla) $250.00; extra denture hardening, 20 minutes in sonicator $10.00; non radioactive partial or full denture $300.00, upper or lower, chlorox free, pink or clear, post-hardened by sonicating, temporary or final product. Ask about all these details before making your appointment. Share the news of your satisfaction and health benefits later when you see them.

Syncrometer® tester's charges for testing dental products: $30.00 per hour (about 15 sample products).

Syncrometer® tester's charges for testing teeth and finding mouth status: $20.00 per hour.

For Geiger Mueller tube counting of dental supplies or related products, with background and product readings for 50 minutes: $30.00 per hour (2 hour minimum).

The Advanced Dental Program—Step-By-Step

1. Obtain a panoramic x-ray of teeth and jaws in duplicate, one for the patient, one for yourself.
2. Remind the patient to stop taking vitamin C for 12 to 24 hours before your appointment. This will minimize the amount of painkiller needed.
3. Take your own painkiller at home. This is to reduce the pain of the pain shots. You may also use baby-teething liquid to be applied by yourself (see *Sources*). All this reduces pain by about one-half.
4. Describe each tooth to make discussions of them quick and easy for both yourself and the patient. It is called the **Tooth Evaluation**. Provide tooth map with numbering system (see page 371).
5. Supply *Dental Bleach* (.05% sodium hypochlorite, NSF-rated) to each patient as they are seated in the dental chair. Label the cup "DISINFECTANT! DO NOT SWALLOW". Rinse, and spit out. Provide a "dental bag" (a plastic bag with paper towels inside to absorb then put inside a brown paper bag to be discreet) to empty your mouth for the trip home later.
6. First remove all gold. Mental confusion, depression, dizziness, indecisiveness and apathy frequently accompany the terminal stage of any disease. It is due to prion formation. To stop this immediately and even reverse it in the advanced patient, remove gold from the mouth first. Gold supplies prions with their essential metal. Removing it corrects breathing and swallowing problems and the risk of coma with their disease later. Be patient till all gold is removed before proceeding with dental work. It should also be removed from jewelry and food as well as from the gum tissues. Gum trimming will be described later.
7. Second, remove and replace all prostheses (caps, crowns, bridges, dentures) that can be removed **without drilling**. They can be expected to contain about one half of the total radioactivity in the mouth. It is easily replaced with non-

radioactive supplies. Drilling into them scatters the radioactivity, multiplying the rate of metastases many fold. Be patient till all are pried off or cut off, but not sawed, filed, or drilled in the process. Native tooth substance can be drilled, filed or sawed since it never has radioactivity and can not spread it. A Syncrometer® tester cannot find individual radioactive teeth until the high background from prostheses is removed. If one tooth is so decayed it is not a candidate for crown replacement, there is no need to remove the crown.

8. Leave these teeth "open" till tester finds each one free of gold, uranium, polonium, mercury and chlorox bleach. Then repair with materials tested free of radioactivity. If they are filled prematurely, they may need to be removed again. Keep them disinfected with *Dental Bleach*.

9. Extract all root canals and clean the sockets below with bur type drills selected to shear the rubber off the cavity wall and reach down to the bottom. The tester should find no cerium present later.

10. Clean old root canal sockets, called *Socket Therapy*, with similar techniques. Identify old root canal sockets by searching for adhering cerium (rubber, plastic), chlorox, uranium, polonium. Ask the patient or former dentist where old root canals were.

Advise the patient to make a liquid diet or blend each food, similar to baby food, to avoid weight loss till teeth are functional again. Keep open teeth disinfected with *Dental Bleach* 4 times daily. Use it undiluted for infections. Dilute in half or even one fourth for sensitive patients.

11. Next, find radioactive amalgam teeth. To do this the gum canal (sulcus) must first be cleared of radioactivity to avoid confusion. Start the patient on mouthwashes with chelators to flush out chips and crumbs of radioactive teeth already removed (see instructions page 419). This could take 2 days of non-stop mouthwashes. Be prepared to see symptoms change as the location of Po chips changes during the mouthwashing. They will then find new landing spots and reach different tumors and organs through the tooth nerves.

12. The tester should check the dental canal at several missing tooth locations to see if it is clear. When clear of uranium and polonium ask tester to find uranium and polonium at tooth locations*.

13. Extract amalgam-containing teeth that have polonium or uranium. Clean each socket with the Huggins technique, namely burs that shear away the tiny ligaments that had attached the tooth to the jawbone. If left inside, a chronic bone infection can result to prevent solid bone from replacing it. This cleaning also fetches out any radioactive crumbs that accidentally fell into the cavities. Future metastases are caused by these crumbs. After washing and suctioning vigorously plug the socket to prevent further entries into it (see *Sources*).

14. Next trim away the gum for 3 to 4 mm, and the gum margin for 2 mm along the whole length of the tooth space. It is saturated with mercury, chromium, copper and other metals besides the radioactive elements. Trim away the whole papilla. Leave the plug in place till ready to suture.

15. After 30 hours test the new sockets, made during recent extractions, for mercury, polonium, uranium. There should be none. If still contaminated, test canal and gingival tissue (gums) for left over bits. Then test the socket (bone). Arrange the socket test with tooth number first, then the bone slide, followed by chlorox or uranium or polonium.

16. If no more radioactivity is found in remaining amalgam-teeth and the patient requests replacement, drill out the amalgam for replacement. Use the Solorio designed dam with wax strip around the tooth under the dam as well as a wax collar on top of the dam. This is to reduce the number of drillings that escape below the dam. They slide into the canal

---

* Testers, place generic tooth on Right plate. Add mercury, then uranium. If it resonates with patient's saliva or body wipe remove generic tooth and replace with tooth #1, 2, 3 and so forth, to 32. Include missing teeth in search. Repeat each *Positive* find by approaching it from the higher number downward instead of upwards as you did before. This reduces the local stimulating voltage and false *Positives*.

To find if the radioactive particle is in the tooth socket, place the bone slide (compact bone) between the numbered tooth and the Hg, or other, test bottle.

as well as getting caught by salivary glands and other soft tissues of the mouth.

17. Wait 30 hours from dental surgery before testing to get valid test results. If the patient had chronic pain also test for chromium. If the patient had leukemia, also test for copper. If the patient had nervous system disease also check for thallium (Tl is the constant companion of Hg). Leave teeth open till tested for residual metals.

18. When all amalgam or other metal has been removed replace with chlorox-free composite or a paste variety to suit the need of the patient.

19. Advise patient to rinse once with *Dental Bleach* while leaving the dental chair and then resume gentle water-mouthwashes on trip home. Do not miss the first critical half-hour when radioactivity is still loose in the mouth. Continue mouthwashes till the canal is clear again. This can, again, take 2 days, non-stop.

20. Next, old composite fillings can be tested for radioactivity. If the composite fillings were placed on old amalgam sites arrange the test* with the Hg next to the tooth number followed by plastic (Ce).

21. Extract radioactive composite-teeth. Since composite is brittle and much radioactive dust is created, use a Solorio dam as before. The extraction procedure itself produces dozens of fairly large crumbs that easily fall into the cavity being created. Clean cavity using Huggins method with several burs. Wash and suction intensively. Then plug the socket with earplugs, suitably cut (see *Sources*). Trim away the gum surface, margin,

* Testers, place saliva sample or lesion wipe on Left plate. Place generic tooth on Right plate followed by mercury, then chlorox or uranium, then polonium. Replace generic tooth with each tooth in turn, from #1 to #32. At missing tooth sites, immediately search for its precise location. Make a space between tooth number and the mercury test bottle. Insert the 3 gums, the canal, the bone slide, the medullated nerve slide, the cerium test bottle, one at a time. When repeating the test, move from number to number in opposite direction. This will dissipate the extra voltage that has built up with speed of testing and reveal any error.

For composite teeth that were not placed on old amalgam, omit the mercury in the arrangement.

and papilla with Solorio technique. Use undiluted *Dental Bleach* as disinfectant. Follow with gentle water mouthwashes immediately to avoid return of uranium or other particles through settling. At home switch to gentle EDTA mouthwashes, non-stop. Healing is substantial in 2 days.

22. The patient must clear the canal again to prevent radioactive dust and crumbs from settling. Mouthwashes with EDTA alone are sufficient if done for 2 to 3 days throughout the day. If not perfectly cleared each left over particle will start its own metastasis later.

All old and new extraction sites need Solorio gum-trimming to remove chromium in pain diseases, mercury and thallium in brain disorders, uranium in abscess diseases, and polonium in cancer.

23. Repair tooth cavities (caries) with paste varieties (phosphates) for sensitive patients and composite for others, chlorox-free.

24. Ask tester to search for left over abscess bacteria, Streptococcus pyogenes in all 4 jawbone quadrants and at suspicious teeth. Clean such areas with pressurized water and *straight Dental Bleach* (.2% bleach). Note: If periodontal or other cleaning is done before all radioactive teeth are removed, it spreads the uranium and polonium to other teeth and all soft tissues of the mouth.

25. Replace crowns and other prosthetic materials with non-radioactive replacements. For final testing, make soak water and test by Syncrometer®. The Geiger counter cannot test liquids or wet materials. Test for α, β and γ radiations.

26. Repair infected or broken teeth.

27. If you, the patient, still have pain, anywhere, make a body wipe at these locations and test for OPT, chromium, chlorox, and Strep. pyogenes. *Positive* results mean there is still Po for the cancer, chromium and chlorox for the pain and S. pyogenes for the abscesses.

28. Continue EDTA mouthwashes 4 hours a day or more, followed at bedtime with application of calcium supplement powder sprinkled on toothbrush to alkalize and protect teeth.

To Find Abscesses

Uranium seems to attract abscess bacteria, Streptococcus pyogenes. They require cobalt which is found where your tooth-uranium is found, in fillings. Each bacterium gets its tiny shield of U. Gradually, the abscess bacteria invade a small part of the tooth and then the jawbone itself. Finally, they try to enter the brain at the base of the skull. The uranium sticks tightly to the abscess bacteria, but is attracted to the brain, possibly because of its high phosphate content. The invasion of the brain is completely silent. There is no fever or swelling to alarm you. They pass quietly through the same hole as is used by the spine, passing upward into the medulla and then turning downward to the bottom of the spine.

From the bottom of the spine the uranium-cloaked pyogenes can travel back to the top of the brain with the cerebrospinal fluid. It can also travel sideways to the hip bones to start abscesses there. As long as the bacteria have room to travel they do not cause pressure and pain. But when they are blocked by an organ the pressure buildup can cause excruciating pain.

Back in the brain they might turn into a cyst or be held in check by the WBCs. The amazing fact is that the brain can be infected by bacteria and the victim feels no symptoms at all.

If you have attacks of excruciating pain in your body, suspect an abscess, and treat with antibiotic of the penicillin family first. If there is some reduction, it supports the abscess theory, since Streptococci are killed by it. This should lead you to your teeth for dental inspection first. A tooth abscess may give no symptoms as it spawns body abscesses.

Wherever uranium goes, our main neurotransmitters stop being produced. Epinephrine levels drop first, leaving that organ in poverty—the organ can accomplish much less now. Soon acetyl choline is missing, too. Now the organ goes into failure.

Mouth Chelation

EDTA, IP6, and citric acid taken as supplements and one after another as mouthwashes can remove the uranium by pulling it off the brain phosphates or kidney phosphates for excretion. This could also explain why chelation therapy is so useful for cancer patients.

There is no way to identify polonium- or uranium-contaminated amalgam and tissues except with a Syncrometer® or radiation detector. But a rubbing, made on any tooth, can give you the answer, quickly.

A sliver of emery board, 1 inch long and 1/8" wide, rubbed vigorously on the mercury filling may be enough for the Syncrometer® tester if each sliver is put in its own zippered bag. Label the tooth using a drawing (see page 371). No water should be added, but the rubbed surface should be faced downward on the test plate in the plastic bag. The tester should search for tooth number first to be sure the rubbing is from the correct tooth. Then search for Po, U, and chlorox. You could also test for lead, which can give frequent attacks of Herpes Virus I and II. Cadmium could give you high blood pressure or vitiligo. Chromium could give you pain or yeast growth. Use this opportunity to understand your health problems.

Mouthwashes

The IP6 Mouthwash And Gargle

- 10 to 20 drops IP6 in ½ cup of warm water.
- Take small mouthfuls, keeping each one about 4 minutes before spitting out.
- When gargling, tilt your head from side to side to let the water in deeper. Do not swallow this.

The EDTA Mouthwash And Gargle

- Empty 1 capsule, 500 mg., on top of a half-cup of water.
- Swish mouth and gargle for about 4 minutes before spitting out. Use small mouthfuls. Do not swallow this.

The Citric Acid Mouthwash And Gargle

- ½ to 1 capsule (¼ tsp.) citric acid in a cup of water.
- Swish mouth and gargle for 3 to 4 minutes before spitting out. Do not swallow this.

Each of these supplements must be frozen for disinfection as usual. Before bedtime brush your teeth with a calcium supplement capsule to restore calcium and alkalinity to them for the night. Use about ¼ capsule sprinkled on toothbrush. IP6 and citric acid are the most corrosive for the remaining teeth. If you have sensitive teeth or develop sensitivity, use only the EDTA but increase the time used for mouthwashing.

If you have neurological disease or malignant melanoma do not try to save amalgam-filled teeth even if not radioactive. For you, these should not be drilled either. Even mercury dust will worsen the symptoms. Extract them and replace with dentures. You can't expect to be much better, though, until you have removed the mercury from all the gums and dental canal besides old sockets. Do this by dental gum trimming and socket cleaning. At the same time, do gargling and mouthwashes. In malignant melanoma mercury is part of the "personal antigen" which includes phenylalanine, making you allergic to mercury as well as toxic from it. It contributes to PGE2 at each melanoma.

In between all these dental procedures, you, the patient, must avoid mouth infection most of all. You must not lose weight. And you should not suffer unnecessary pain or trauma. To accomplish all this, follow the *Dental*

Aftercare program (page 422). Focus on this during your dental work. Use a chlorox-free painkiller (see *Sources*). In addition, do mouthwashes throughout the day, beginning as soon as you leave the dental chair.

These will seem like near-miraculous procedures in their efficiency, absence of pain and low cost. Dentistry, at least Mexican dentistry, can be very rewarding.

Patient Responsibility

- Your responsibility is to keep the dental canal (sulcus) clear of polonium or uranium bits so the tester is not confused.
- Your other responsibility is to blend your food with so much liquid that you can drink it with a straw past the open tooth zone. This also prevents weight loss.
- Paint your fingertips with Lugol's drops to remind you not to put them in your mouth.

Congratulations to yourself and your successful dentist!

If you removed all polonium and uranium from your teeth, all malignancies will be gone, too, without continuing the curing program.

Tumors are forced to shrink. Even warts (papillomas), polyps, cysts, moles, "tags" and calluses will begin to shed without any effort on your part. Some skin blemishes and crusts will peel or rub off. They had been growing from the radioactive stimulation.

Parasites disappear in large numbers with little effort. Search after a liver cleanse when you are likely to see the most.

Give yourself excellent grades. You have saved your own life and shone a light on your path for others to follow.

Dental Aftercare

Extractions do not automatically clear up infections. And antibiotics cannot be relied on either. So a vigorous program is needed to clear up mouth infection even after the infected teeth are pulled. Clostridium bacteria are ready to eat all the tiny morsels of dying gum tissues. Strep pyogenes is ready to eat anything with cobalt or uranium in it, such as old amalgam mush. This *Dental Aftercare* program is successful in killing Clostridium and Strep pyogenes.

Copy the next few pages and carry them with you to the dental office. Your friend could review them while waiting.

You will need:

- a water pick
- hot water, towels
- pure salt (see Sources)
- *Dental Bleach*, NSF (see Sources)
- one or two stainless steel strainers for food preparation
- blender with non-seeping blades (see Sources)

Purchase these before your dental appointment. Practice using the water pick beforehand, too.

Also purchase chlorox-free painkillers to get you through the first night.

- In Mexico, purchase Dorixina forte (not regular). Freeze ahead of time. Take one hour before your appointment.
- In USA, purchase Tylenol Extra Strength, the quick acting kind. Take 2, 15 minutes before your appointment.

These pre-appointment painkillers are to reduce the pain of the anesthetic shots.

> Stop using vitamin C for 24 hours before appointment. It seems to counteract the anesthetic so much more is needed.

The immune power of your arterial blood is much greater than in your veins. How can you bring arterial blood into the jaw area to heal it faster after dental work? Simply by hot-packing it from the start!

Just before leaving the dentist's office, as soon as you are out of the chair, rinse with *Dental Bleach,* followed by gentle mouthwashes. Carry your own squirt bottle of each and a "dental bag". All the while you are traveling home, swish with water, using this bag to spit out discreetly.

The next 3 hours are the most critical. Uranium, polonium, chromium have all been set free like a swarm of wasps from their nest. When they land on your tonsils, salivary glands, or clefts in your cheeks who will get them out again? You must keep them moving constantly till they are outside your body. Your skillful dentist churned them up for you. But you have the job of getting them out of your body so they cannot start metastases. Keep the cotton plug in place for you to bite down on and reduce bleeding, even while swishing. Don't suction the water forcefully around your mouth.

> The first day of dental after care is critical. If you miss this, a massive spread of infection can occur because the mouth is always a "den of bacteria", and your own tooth infection is itself the source.

A few hours later apply a hot towel to the outside of your face where the dental work was done. Wring a washcloth out of the hottest water you can endure. Or fill a plastic bag halfway with hot water, zipping it shut securely and enclosing it in a second plastic bag. Do this for 20 minutes, 3 times a day and every time you feel pain for a few days. Then 2 times a day for a week—even when there is no pain.

Don't suck liquids through a straw till Day 2 when you need to pass food safely over your teeth. Don't allow your tongue to suck the wound site, and don't put fingers in your mouth. If this is an ingrained habit, paint your fingertips with Lugol's iodine.

As the anesthetic wears off there will be very little pain. But you could introduce bacteria yourself, by eating, or by putting fingers into your mouth. Consider your mouth a surgery site, off limits to everything! But the mouth cannot be bandaged and you must eat! To be successful, eat a big meal just before your dental appointment. Then drink nothing but water later on, the day of extractions. You may need a painkiller on the first night; choose a non-aspirin variety to minimize bleeding.

Bleeding should have reduced considerably by bedtime. The cotton plug put in your mouth by the dentist may be thrown away. If you need another one, make it yourself out of a tightly rolled paper towel the shape and size of a finger. Rinse it several times with pure water by squeezing it. Rinse your mouth with *Dental Bleach* once more before bed.

Dental Day Two

The next day (the day after your surgery) you need to be well fed, yet eat no solids, or liquids with particles in them. The particles easily lodge in your wound. Your choices are:

1. Soup broth, strained, with HCl drops added (see *Recipes* page 577).
2. Herb teas, sweetened, strained, with HCl drops added.
3. Fruit or vegetable juice, strained, with HCl drops added.
4. Puddings made of starch or flour, thinned with fruit juice to be drinkable, with HCl drops added.

5. Cream shakes made with heavy whipping cream (and other beverages), with HCl drops added.
6. Supplements that are in capsule or drop form.

Run foods through the finest strainer. All food should be ozonated or frozen or sonicated to sterilize it.

Drink through a straw to get the food past the tooth zone. Immediately after eating, rinse your mouth with a cup of warm water to which you have added ¼ tsp. pure salt. Then disinfect with *Dental Bleach*, using 2 or 3 strong squirts in ¼ cup water. So far our only cases of infection (2 per year) were patients who did not use their *Dental Bleach* due to misunderstanding. If pain increases instead of decreases on the second day use the *Dental Bleach* straight, with 1 or 2 squirts directly in mouth. Continue swishing and hot packing for one hour. Stop using sweetener. Devote the whole day to fighting this infection. If the pain subsides, the infection has been cleared. If not, you will need a more forceful stream of water. Begin using the water pick at its lowest speed setting. Water pick repeatedly until the pain clears. (It could take four hours!)

Hot pack the outside of your face just as on the first day. Even in the night, if pain strikes, hot pack it at once and rinse with straight *Dental Bleach*. If pain is subsiding on the second day, you are being successful. But the gums are <u>not</u> healed; you cannot take chances yet on eating solid food. Nearly all infections come from eating solid food on the second day.

Floss the remaining teeth with homemade floss, being extra gentle. For floss, cut strips of plastic shopping bags, ¼ inch by four inches. Rinse them with very hot water. Fish line floss and toothbrush are too harsh after dental work. Clean teeth by hand-rubbing, using paper towel wound around your finger and dampened, then dipped into oregano oil toothpowder (see *Program*).

Devote the whole day to spitting out the uranium and polonium particles that your dentist loosened and raised to the surface for you.

Also rinse your mouth with *Dental Bleach* 4 times during the day and bedtime.

When you can tolerate toothbrushing use peroxide (5 drops) on your brush once a day.

Dental Day Three

On the third day, you may drink blended solid food; do not try to chew solids with remaining teeth. Use a blender with blades that do not seep metal (see *Sources*).

Again, spend the whole day swishing your mouth. Particles that fall down may get into the gum spaces again and require redrilling. The first 3 days are critical. It may be your last chance to find and remove the radioactivity. This time add EDTA to the water, all the better to pick up metal dust that has returned to the canal.

Use your water pick now after each meal. It must be hardened first or you will get the seepage from it into your wounds and brain. Simply fill to the top with steaming hot water and let stand ½ hour. Repeat. Then fill the tank with hot tap water to which you have added a few drops of Lugol's iodine, or 1 tsp. colloidal silver, or pure salt. Set it at the gentlest level at first, squirting each site gently. Floss the front teeth and finger-rub them with oregano oil toothpowder and calcium powder at night.

No matter how carefully you eat, you will see food entering the gum spaces. Notice how difficult it is to squirt out any trapped food. Swishing is not sufficient! You need to water pick till all spaces are cleared; inspect each one. Continue hot packing. Continue disinfecting with *Dental Bleach*. If pain returns and all this has not succeeded in clearing it after 4 hours, you must hurry back to the dentist to search for the food particle. The wound will be opened and cleaned out for you.

Avoid Weight Loss

It is a handicap to your body's healing plan to lose weight. Blend all your solid foods, even meats, salads, desserts, adding an herb tea or broth. You may even regain lost weight this way and build up muscles again. Take more digestive enzymes with liquid food than solid food to help digestion.

Taking Out Stitches

Two days is all that a person with low immunity can wait when a dead object (stitches) is imbedded in the tissues; it will develop an infection of its own. Your stitches are being sterilized with the *Dental Bleach*. The dentist will grab the knot with the left hand, using forceps, pulling it up to make a space below the thread, and pushing scissors into the space to snip the thread. It is quite painless.

If you should get caught in Day 3 on a Sunday with an inflammation building, you could ask a friend to do it for you this way: Find a pharmacy that can sell you high quality small scissors and tweezers. Wash your hands in Lugol's water for a full minute or straight vodka. Your friend should do the same. Soak the instruments in a cup or zippered bag of the alcohol. Dry with a paper towel. Hold your mouth open toward a strong light. Use your freshly sterilized fingers to hold it open. Your friend can snip the free end of the suture knot again and again, without help of forceps. When the knot is reached, the loops will fall apart and can be pulled straight away. It is totally painless.

Dental Bleeding

A moderate amount of bleeding is normal, even days later. Bleeding caused by water picking is not too serious. But if you sense an emergency, apply ice cubes wrapped in a paper towel or washcloth. Bite down on them till bleeding stops. Continue ice packing for 4 hours. Check your pills for aspirin. Stop taking these. After bleeding has stopped for 2 hours return to hot packing. If ice packing does not stop the bleeding, go back to the dentist or emergency room. The usual cause is hidden infection.

If you have a very low platelet count or are on a large amount of "blood thinners", which promote bleeding you need special attention. Yet, oral surgery is a very skilled profession. Dental work is safe in the surgeon's hands. Platelets, or a transfusion, can be given just beforehand; blood thinners can be temporarily stopped. These same patients often state that they feel better, immediately after the dental extraction, than they can remember in months! It was the dental problem that was poisoning their platelets and their blood! It may be the last transfusion that will be needed, in spite of some unavoidable blood loss with dental extractions.

Be Vigilant the Next Week

Continue water picking and rinsing your mouth with *Dental Bleach* after each meal for a week. Continue EDTA swishes for 4 hours a day to avoid future metastases and more dental work. Floss and brush your front teeth once a day.

Clostridium can return even after a week of steady recovery. <u>If you detect an odor from your mouth</u>, at any time, it is Clostridium making a comeback. <u>Try bleaching, swishing, and water picking for half a day</u>, till odor is completely gone. Hurry back to the dentist if the odor persists. You cannot recover with a mouth infection.

If you got through the whole process without needing more than one nights' painkiller and without needing to return to the dentist for extra clean up, give yourself excellent grades. And if you got through, in any way, still give yourself very good grades!

It is common for dentists to recommend cold packing to reduce swelling after dental work. I recommend hot packing because I consider swelling less important than infection or pain. It is also common for dentists to rely on antibiotics to clear up infection. I find this is not sufficient. The whole *Dental Aftercare* program is needed.

MORE DENTAL HELP

Plastic Fillings

If a tooth with composite has never had an amalgam filling and does not contain chlorox, polonium or uranium, you could harden the plastic with the toothbrush zappicator (page 431) instead of replacing it. Next day a test of the saliva should show no plastic tooth materials*. If it does, repeat the zappication. If it still does, replace the filling with a "paste variety".

> Plastic fillings may now be saved by a technique for plastic hardening in the mouth. But risk is present since it is new and not yet widely used.

Such teeth can be kept clean by once daily brushing with oregano oil toothpowder and once daily peroxide brushing.

---

* Testers, search for azo dyes, acrylic acid, urethane, bisphenol A, cerium, DAP. DAP is most difficult to harden.

Only further research will reveal whether new plastic fillings can be so well hardened and kept so well fitting that no seeping occurs and no crevices develop.

Home Dentistry

Search your mouth yourself, every month, for a fresh cavity. It will be a small brown discoloration. Rub this spot twice daily, once with oregano oil toothpowder and once with calcium powder taken from ¼ capsule of a supplement powder (see *Sources*). Purchase a long-handled dental mirror (from automotive supply store) so your helper can see the backsides of your teeth.

There may be a time when dentistry can safely fill a small hole but it is not now. Research is progressing in other countries to bring healing methods to small tooth infections instead of new kinds of fillings. Search the Internet to keep pace with it. Remember that teeth are bones! Your diet should have calcium and vitamin D_3 in it. Ascaris parasites soften teeth and bones. Kill them regularly. Avoid sugar on your teeth and gums. Brush it out and alkalinize them with calcium powder before bedtime.

Each morning do a 5-minute mouthwash with plain water to wash the dental canal before drinking water.

Jerome Tattoo Removal

In the past, when amalgam was being put into your teeth or drilled out, tiny drillings and dust bits got away or flew away with great force into your mouth. It landed in your cheek folds, in neighboring gums, in exposed bone nearby and in the bottom of newly made sockets. Nobody will ever see these again, or so it was thought. (And guilt can never be laid.)

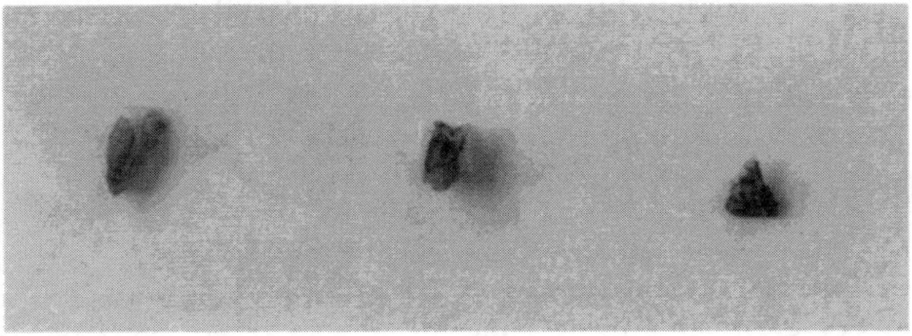

Bone and gum fragments black with mercury should be removed.

Fig. 102 Tattoos

The larger bits of amalgam, called tattoos, can be seen on the panoramic or digital x-ray. Your dentist has already spotted them no doubt. But smaller particles do not show up. You must ask the dentist whether he or she is equipped to search visually, with a **magnifier** and remove them all regardless how painstaking the job is. This and many more facts of dentistry are discussed by Frank Jerome, D.D.S. in his book, *Tooth Truth* (search the Internet). Each quadrant of your mouth needs a careful examination for mercury tattoos.

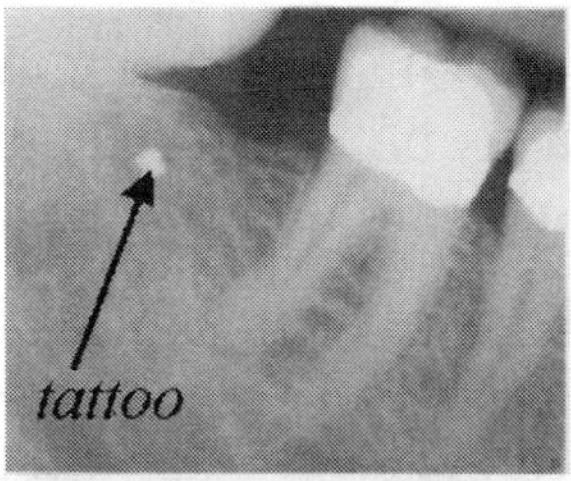

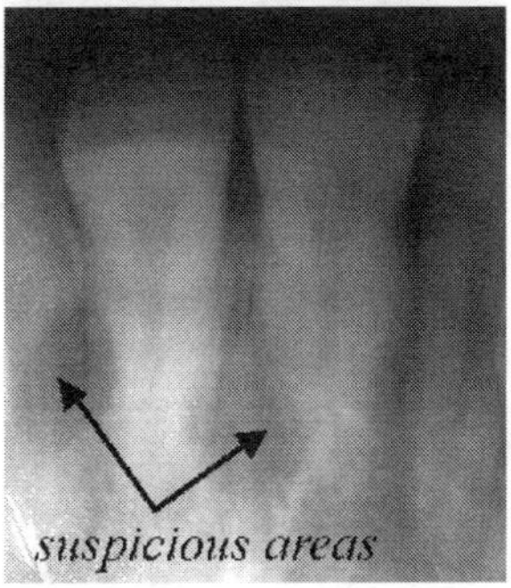

Fig. 103 Digital x-rays give superior view

Tooth Zappicator

A tooth zappicator is a small loudspeaker fastened to the end of a toothbrush. The speaker is attached to your food zappicator circuit, which produces a frequency of 1 kHz.

Cavitations are old unhealed holes in your jawbone.

Even when you are not able to search for them first, many hidden cavitations can be systematically cleared by zappicating along the whole ridge where teeth once were. Do it yourself to be sure it is thorough.

Repeat on inner and outer surfaces of the gums, making three treatments altogether. Don't miss the remaining teeth themselves.

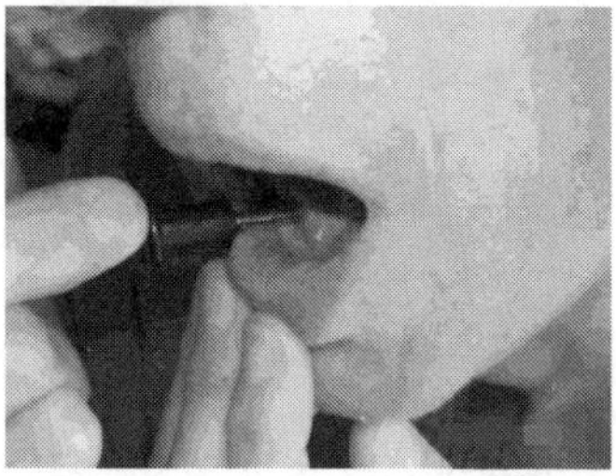

Find tattoos and cavitations in minutes.

Fig. 104 Dental Syncrometer® probe

The tooth zappicator can also be used to harden plastic. Press it against plastic teeth or teeth with plastic fillings to get this hardening action. For this purpose, treat for five minutes on top of each tooth location, then take a break for at least one-half hour. Drink water to help kidneys excrete. Repeat a second time on the inner surface of each tooth location. Take another break, and repeat a third (and last) time at the outer surfaces of the gums. The effect is permanent.

Using your Tooth Zappicator

1. Insert a 9-volt battery into the 1 kHz zapper carefully, to be sure polarity is correct.
2. Connect the *Positive* output of the zapper to the *Positive* terminal of the loudspeaker. Do not use any *Negative* connections. They should not have hanging wires either.
3. Tape the zapper to the tabletop to guard against slippage while in use. A loudspeaker that falls to the floor could change its polarity.
4. Protect the tooth zappicator by placing it in a plastic zippered bag, with the loudspeaker in a bottom corner. Wrap the bag around it, handle and all, snugly. Tape in place. Be sure to keep saliva out of the plastic bag and off the bare tooth zappicator.

5. Wipe with ordinary ethanol or any alcoholic beverage or Lugol's water before first use. Do not get liquid inside.
6. Turn the zapper on. Place loudspeaker firmly on jawbone ridge for three (or five) minutes.
7. Start at the extreme end of one jawbone and work toward the other, skipping nothing. When you come to a tooth, place loudspeaker squarely on top of it. DO NOT TREAT METAL FILLINGS. Move to the neighboring location and repeat. When jawbones are both done on three surfaces, continue on all soft areas of mouth.

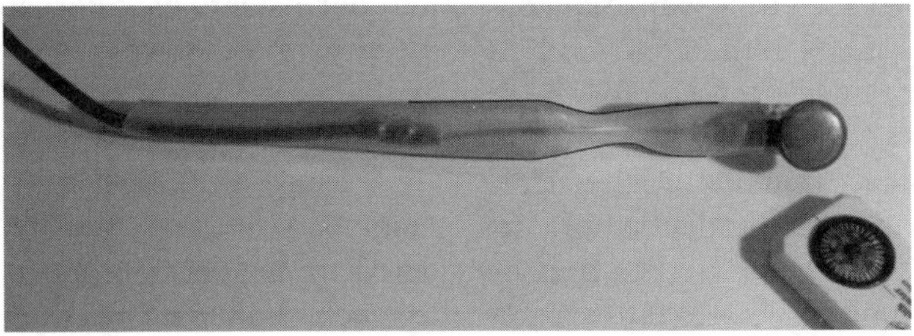

Fig. 105 Tooth zappicator and compass

Divide the whole mouth, roof, sides, and back into imaginary little squares. Treat each square for 5 minutes. Leave no surface unzappicated. Don't miss the inside of the cheeks and the tonsils as far as you can reach. Drink water several times to help with excretion. Be sure to take a dose of hydrangea, selenite and vitamin C first. Be prepared for some detox symptoms.

You are returning immune power to your mouth.

For years, ever since you had amalgam put in your mouth, the 40 metals you were sucking on have been dissolving and moving into the rest of your body in tiny deposits. I can estimate, by extrapolation from Syncrometer® tests, there are about 1000 such deposits in cancer patients, mostly in the brain and spinal cord. Some of these also have polonium and uranium, setting the stage for cancer and its metastases. If you are terminally ill with these, you can still save yourself by quickly removing all metal and plastic teeth by extraction.

But gum trimming and socket cleaning will still be necessary for good results. You must reach the result of zero radioactivity in the mouth.

Summary – Chapter 16

1. As an industrialized nation, our leaders have lost their cautious attitude toward radioactivity. They have promoted commerce for it as for any regular chemical.
2. Industry is now spreading uranium throughout our planet thinking it is relatively safe because of its long half-life and lesser production of large mutations.
3. What has not been considered are the decay products of uranium whose half-lives can be much shorter and biological damage much greater than the uranium itself. Included are radon, lead, polonium, bismuth, radium. Each does serious, irreversible damage.
4. All this new radioactivity in our environment is raising our parasitism while lowering immunity.
5. Our protective agencies should not allow dispersion of radioactivity in water as buffers, in fertilizer as phosphate source, in softener salts and bleach as phosphate pH buffer, in potassium as potash, in dental supplies and in building supplies.
6. The result of dispersal of radioactivity is seen in much increased birth defects, increased cancer rates and new diseases.
7. A step-by-step procedure to remove and replace radioactive dental repairs is given to make the mouth radiation-free.
8. Each malignancy has its Po supplied by several repaired teeth along permanent routes. The cancer becomes benign within a day of cutting such a supply line

9. A Dental Aftercare program leads you from Day 1 of dental work through the first week when healing should be carefully nurtured while the uranium and polonium, dislodged from your teeth, should be spit out continuously.

10. Tooth zappicating can harden a new filling so seeping stops, but radioactivity cannot be stopped this way. Radioactive teeth must be removed from the mouth, and with great care, not to spread the polonium and uranium along the way.

11. A beginning **Home Dentistry** is proposed to improve dental health of US citizens. It prevents cavities and uses early detection to reduce the incidence of tooth damage. Many hidden cavitations can be cleared up with these methods.

WANTED DEAD—OR DEADER

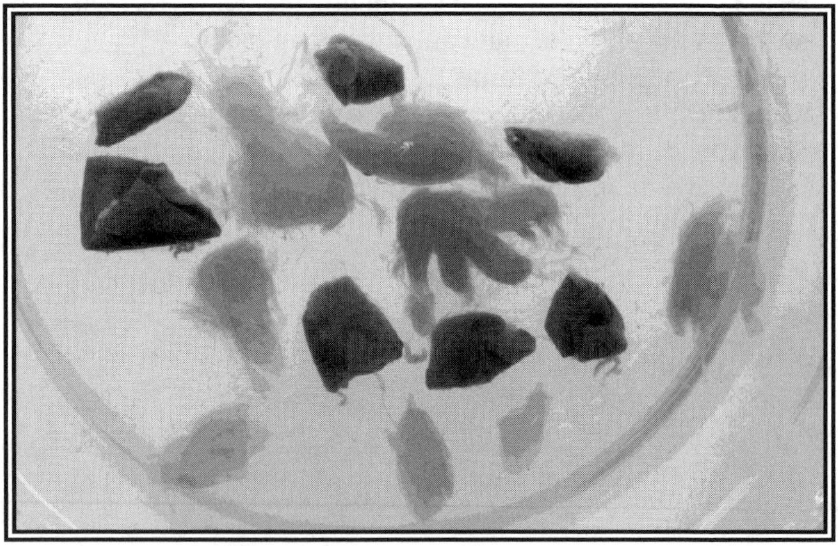

More odd-shaped segments show how they draw their ends shut like purse-strings might, to stop loss of eggs from open ends. Center proglottid was damaged.

WARNING: DO NOT EXPERIMENT ON YOURSELF to remove tapeworm. The recipes were not complete at time of publishing.

CHAPTER 17

TESTER'S GUIDE

A set of tests has been arranged so any Syncrometer® tester can follow the path to a cure for each patient with cancer. The first one was printed in *The Prevention of All Cancers* book, called *The Syncrometer® Tester's Flow Sheet*. The second one, with updated tests is now printed separately and included in the *Syncrometer® Science Laboratory Manual*. A short set of tests is given here so even a novice tester* can get a cancer victim started on the curing path. How to correct each problem in detail is found in the *Flow Sheets*.

When a new person sits before you or has sent a fax, water sample and a homeographic copy of their saliva, try to comfort them in a realistic way. Clinically, it is still a death sentence to be diagnosed with cancer except a few varieties. You can save them, by helping them to comply with this program. It is a cause-and-effect process, not dependent on good luck, or even attitude. When your client has corrected each problem, their cure is essentially guaranteed. Only mistakes or inability to correct their problems can bring failure. Hopefully, people will try to cure themselves and each other long before they are advanced and clinically ill.

Use these ***Questions*** and **Answers** to arrive quickly at useful conclusions and know what to do next. Each ***Question*** represents a test to be done.

Q1. *Does this person have cancer?*

---

* Testers, putting a metal tube around bottles being tested makes the test much more sensitive. They are identical to bottle-copy shields. The results described in this chapter were all obtained this way.

A1. Test for OPT at a saliva sample. If *Positive*, the answer is YES. If *Negative* test at lymph. The cancer is not at clinical level, but may lurk somewhere. Test at locations where the client has complaints. Also test from a list of body organs for men and women.

For men, test at prostate, colon, bone, lung, liver.

For women, test at breast, lung, ovary, liver, bone.

Test both left and right organs. Make your own combination test bottle in this way: first make a right side organ, then make a left side. To combine the two, place a blank bottle at the center. Place a left organ on one side and the right organ on the other side. They should be in a straight line. Give each bottle its metal shield. Copy for 20 seconds at the highest voltage your battery can produce, not less than 9.4.

Make a list of organs with cancer.

Q2. *Flu – If* Positive*, this person is in a detoxifying state already. Native health or perhaps other treatment has allowed the body to kill a F. buski parasite without special help. It indicates strength of immune power.*

A2. As soon as your client has switched to safe water and clean house, start them on the protective herbs and supplements, along with WBC supplements and kidney cleaning drops. Without these, the person can become ill, spontaneously, from detoxifying into the liver or kidneys which then get blocked and start edemas and infection.

> The simple act of switching to safe water, food, and house has a tremendously stimulating effect on the immune system. Immediately, the body starts to kill its parasites.

Various organs show their distress in the blood test results which get worse instead of better. The avenues of excretion must be opened in time for this automatic detoxifying.

Q3. *3 Salmonellas – (this is a combination of 3 Salmonella varieties as listed on page 302). If* Positive, *this person already has parasite-killing capability. It shows immune power better than average. Occasionally, people "pick up" Salmonella from food, a very different experience. Salmonella always emerges from killed F. buski and probably from Fasciola and others.*

A3. Start your client on the WBC supplements, sets of kidney cleaning drops, plus ginger and uva ursi, and protective herbs and supplements. Do not start without the drops, if available, but second best is the *Kidney Cleanse.* They should have done 3 weeks of this program before starting the cancer program. They should continue 8 more weeks of the *Kidney Cleanse* along with the cancer program. Start them on the projects and also the apricot suppository as their first activity.

Q4. *3 Clostridium – (this is a combination of 3 Clostridium varieties: C. tetani, C. botulinum, C. perfringens). If* Positive, *this person has already been killing their F. buski parasites and is allowing these bacteria to multiply in them. They spread throughout the body, producing very toxic chemicals while feeding on parasite refuse.*

A4. Check the latest blood test results to see if this has been going on for a long enough time to lower the uric acid level. Make sure they take oregano oil, 10 drops in a capsule, 2-3 times daily, before meals, until the saliva test is *Negative* for Clostridium. Also start them on betaine HCL, 3 capsules with each meal, to kill Clostridium bacteria in the intestine. The action is complete in 3 days. Teach them that killing a buski always leads to a clostridium attack so it can be used as evidence that you killed a F. buski and a malignancy may have disappeared, too. It is welcome news.

Q5. *Chlorox bleach – This is for completeness only. A Negative answer has never been found if OPT is* Positive, *namely, cancer is present. Testing for the individual ingredients of the bleach may also be important for the patient's understanding.*

A5. PCBs, benzene, asbestos, azo dyes of many kinds, heavy metals of many kinds, malonic acid, motor oil, wheel bearing grease, isopropyl alcohol, MUSTARD oil, potassium ferrocyanide and polonium will all be *Positive* for each cancer patient, coming from chlorox bleach. Demonstrate resonance with chlorox.

Q6. *Search for major toxins in the home using their dust sample. Search for asbestos, arsenic, Freon, formaldehyde, fiberglass, vanadium, and radon. Since radon would not last long due to its short half-life (3.8 days), it is recommended to test for bismuth, lead, thorium, uranium, and radium as well. If all of these are present, it follows that radon, the radioactive parent must be constantly present in rather high amounts. To find which elements are radioactive place a test bottle of alpha, beta, or gamma radiation beside (touching) the element.*

A6. Asbestos implies that some material is in use that should not be present but, actually, it comes in huge amounts from chlorox-bleached water. Arsenic implies the use of pesticide <u>inside</u> the house and it should not be here. Freon implies leaking refrigerator or air conditioner. Formaldehyde implies new clothing, or furniture which should be removed to an outside location; also stacks of old newspapers. Fiberglass implies open insulation which should be sealed off or fiberglass curtains. Vanadium implies fossil fuel presence, such as gas can or auto exhaust. Radon implies that radiation from underground is reaching the human air space. It always includes polonium. If cerium is present it implies that the lanthanide elements are rising to the earth surface, as well. Cerium may be already in a complex, PoCe. In fact, they may both be missing unless you search for PoCe-complex.

All these toxins must be removed from the home before the cancer patient goes home, besides cleaning out chlorox contamination.

Q7. *Polonium (at saliva) – If* Positive*, it shows there was enough to be testable. If it is* Negative*, it may be combined with other elements, or just not high enough at this time to be detectable.*

A7. Polonium in free form in the air has not been the cause of cancer in any of our past patients. Experiments are needed to see if Po chemistry occurs in the body from inhalation and whether it is significant.

Q8. *Cerium – If* Positive *there is a large amount present, coming from underground sources or artificial sources.*

A8. When artificial sources are cleared away in the patient (from rubber and plastic absorbed through skin, besides teeth) there will never be any free cerium leftover. It will all be in the form of a polonium-cerium-promethium complex, or polonium-promethium-cerium and vv.

Q9. *PoCe – The 2 test substances touch each other on the plate. If* Positive*, it would appear to be the partly formed cancer-complex and, therefore, quite dangerous. Actually, it acquires promethium at the cerium end in Nature and in our bodies, which apparently blocks access to cerium and prevents cancer-complex formation.*

A9. Both *Positive* and *Negative* answers are normal. If *Negative*, there is very little polonium or cerium rising to the earth's surface or available in the body, which is good.

Q10. *Potassium ferrocyanide – If* Positive *it will lead to cancer-complex formation. It comes only with chlorox varieties of bleach and bleached water or food.*

A10. It should be *Negative* after treatment with oxidizing agents like the quinone set used for malaria treatments, or a shot of benzoquinone (which is not currently in use). Several other things can oxidize it, too, turning it into potassium ferricyanide but methylene blue should never be used because it is reversible. In fact, methylene blue should be carefully excluded from detergents, water and food.

Q11. *Potassium ferricyanide – Can be* Positive *or* Negative *depending on whether chlorox bleach (ferro) or NSF bleach (ferri) was used in the water.*

A11. If *Positive* in a cancer patient it is the result of using both kinds of water. It is detoxifiable by Rhodanese, but is not normal for the body so a chronic cyanide toxicity develops in sick and "well" people. The ferricyanide is very harmful too, because it supplies the critical link between different parasites and your DNA. The parasite excretes its own kind of alkylating agent that causes mutations which form the basis of disease. The ferricyanide combines with the different alkylating agent and the combination gets pulled right into your DNA by cerium and polonium. The damage is done at close range, so large, repeatable, "site-selected" mutations are produced.

Q12. *Isopropyl alcohol – If* Positive, *it came from chlorox bleach or from a commercial product, or cosmetic or even food. It should be Negative.*

A12. Isopropyl alcohol plays a role in the cancer-complex. Test for these complexes:

- PoCe isopropyl alcohol
- PoCe — ferrocyanide

  |

  isopropyl alcohol

Both the ferrocyanide and isopropyl test bottles should touch the cerium bottle but not each other. The addition of isopropyl alcohol to the complex leads to the HCG mutation. Place the HCG sample on opposite plate. Find the resonance in this chemical simulation.

Q13. *Malonic acid – If* Positive, *it implicates chlorox bleach, but also other industrial products. It is detoxifiable along a route that leads to D-malic acid, a "universal antigen" that combines with the B-cells of the blood to increase the globulin level. It is very prominent in malaria.*

A13. Malonic acid can make a variety of combinations with the other ingredients of the cancer-complex. Search for these using simulated chemistries. Place the saliva sample on L plate and possible mutagen constructions on R plate.

• PoCe-ferrocyanide
|
malonic acid

isopropyl alcohol
|
• PoCe-ferrocyanide
|
malonic acid

Q14. *Allyl methyl sulfide and allyl alcohol – If* Positive, *the ONION group is involved as source of alkylating agents. GARLIC and MUSTARD oils also share these compounds. There are many more, forming part of a large group of mutagens. This means they combine with DNA, causing mutations. They are so toxic they can be used to kill cancer cells as well. Read about them as chemotherapies on the Internet. It is common practice to "fight fire with fire" in the case of cancer, by using the cause of cancer in a very high dose to kill cancer cells. It is quite short-sighted, but is justified when the life left in the patient is so short that there is no need to think of the future. Our goal is to secure the future.*

A14. These can be removed with MSM and also with vitamin D3. Take up to 3 X 5 MSM till all alkylators are gone. You will know the alkylators are gone if MSM can be found in the free state. The body also makes it normally. Take about 10 times the regular 400 unit dose of vitamin D3. Beware of lead pollution. Test each lot.

Q15. *MUSTARD compounds (test any jar of mustard) – If* Positive*, they will be attached to the cyanide as the alkylating agent. Search for Po/Ce/ferrocyanide /mustard, each bottle touching the previous one.*

A15. The MUSTARD oils can be removed with MSM, too. When all is removed it should be *Negative*. Don't believe it when a journalist or agency states: 'This does not mean the ONIONS, GARLIC and MUSTARD you eat'. We should definitely not be eating them. You can go down to taking 2 X 3 MSM eventually.

Q16. *PoCe/ferrocyanide/F. buski – If* Positive*, F. buski has combined directly with ferrocyanide. It is probable that the ONION and MUSTARD compounds are inside the parasite, too, still linked to the ferrocyanide.*

A16. MSM can remove the alkylating end of the complex and also the iron cyanide. That should make it the most powerful single-item cancer protector.

Q17. *PoCe-ferricyanide – If* Positive*, it will not form the cancer-complex, nor attach to F. buski so does not lead to OPT formation.*

A17. This form of complex is found in the non-chlorox bleaches and waters. It is a toxin that also requires detoxifying by the enzyme Rhodanese to thiocyanate. Without Rhodanese the ferricyanide will build up till acid conditions develop turning it into free potassium cyanide, the poison. Several more parasites make mutagen complexes that cause absence of Rhodanese. Search for a parasite that is attached to the ferricyanide. See if Rhodanese disappears in the simulation.

Q18. *PoCe-ferrocyanide – If* Positive*, it is a partly formed cancer-complex and will lead to OPT formation in the body.*

A18. It can be oxidized to the ferri form by quinone-type compounds like malaria medicines. The copies alone are quite effective in a few days.

Q19. *Methylene blue dye – If* Positive*, it implicates both bleaches, among other sources, which are not all known. Although it can change ferricyanide to the cancer-causing ferrocyanide, I have not seen a cancer case produced this way. (Also test leukomethylene blue).*

A19. Methylene blue can reduce the ferricyanide form to the ferrocyanide form, thereby making it eligible as a maintainer of the cancer-complex. All sources of mixed dyes would contain methylene blue and should be avoided in dentalware, filtration materials, chlorinated food and detergents. Leukomethylene blue is the reduced, colorless form. Always test for both. Make your own leukomethylene blue test substance from methylene blue by adding vitamin C and sodium bisulfite until it is colorless and keeping it in a closed bottle away from air.

Due to the hygroscopic (water loving) nature of Po, Ce, and the cyanides, they can be separated from each other by flooding with water. Once separated the complex no longer functions as a mutagen. But the components should be removed as rapidly as possible from the body to prevent them from combining again. Even polonium alone, if it attaches to DNA will produce the OPT mutation as seen by Syncrometer® simulation. This is the logic behind the numerous hot showers in the curing program with sweating and washing and copious urination. But OPT alone has never started cancer in our experience. It must be accompanied by chlorox-water and the living F. buski parasite.

Q20. *PoCePm – If* Positive, *this is normal. Evidently the cyanides compete against promethium. This could result in the loss of a shield from cancer development. Pm is plentiful and need not be supplied. It will appear as soon as the cyanides are gone.*

A20. Promethium is a radioactive lanthanide…the only one in Nature. It may have many more interesting properties.

Q21. *Paper bedding – This is a "bed sheet" made of paper that cancer patients sleep on for 2 weeks. It soaks up the sweat and chlorox chemicals from the skin. It also picks up the carcinogen components after they have become separated by copious water drinking. They also react with our supplements. In the morning the paper sheet is rolled up tightly and placed in a plastic bag for testing. It will be* Positive *for whatever is still in the body. When testing paper bedding instead of saliva sample, OPT* Positive *means there is still a malignancy present. It must be searched for if not known. If* Negative, *it does not mean there are no more malignancies. Make smaller and smaller body wipes till you can be certain nothing, not even the inner ear has been missed.*

A21. The paper has probably missed quite a few skin areas, particularly on the head, at the lower abdomen, at the genital area and lower back. These should be emphasized by making body wipes here, making sure no tiny area is missed in the final OPT search.

Q22. *Body wipes – Divide the torso into convenient areas, numbered or labeled. At each area test for:*

1. OPT – If Positive, *find a slide of an organ at that location, although it is not essential. There will be a polonium-containing tooth or tooth location supplying polonium to this malignancy. Search for "tooth" (generic) even if it is "missing". Then search at tooth numbers from #1 to #32 even if they are missing. If one is* Positive *search at the gingiva, gingival margin, sulcus (canal), papilla, medullated nerve, bone and cerium of this tooth The cerium represents composite or plastic. Place these special sites so they touch the tooth number. The Po will be in contact with U, probably reflecting the source, such as amalgam (Hg) or chlorox. The canal can be cleared of Po by mouthwash in about 2 days. The other* Positive *gum sites are surgically removed by the dentist. It is very minor surgery. Finding that a tooth site has Po touching the nerve or Po touching bone means that a tiny crumb of the old filling material fell into the hole as the tooth was extracted. It is now resting at the bottom near the nerve or along the side which is bone. It is not too late to clean this socket as should have been done right after extraction. Bur-type drills can loosen the crumbs, throwing them against the mouth tissues. Hopefully they get suctioned up by the dentist.*

If OPT is Negative, test for Clostridium, which would mean the malignancy had just recently been there.

2. Chlorox – If still Positive *after a week, search for an ongoing source of chlorox bleach in food, medicine, supplements, products such as dentures, wig, unwashed hair, eyebrow pencil, skin cream, shoes, slippers, unwashed clothing, or due to walking barefoot in their room. It could be a root canal, already removed, but with the socket still not cleaned. Find the old root canal teeth to test for residual chlorox and cerium (rubber).*

A22. The Po, Ce, ferrocyanide, and alkylating agents can be washed away in 1 week using the hot shower and sweats technique. But certain malignancies will be very resistant to your efforts. This is due to Po arrivals from the teeth. Polonium from a dental location is resonating with each surviving F. buski, somehow providing protection from all attempts to kill the parasite. WBCs at such a location always lack vitamin C, regardless of amounts recently taken, although not lacking germanium and selenite. We must look into the possibility that vitamin C has been captured in the reducing chemistry of methylene blue at the DNA where the cyanides are involved. The F. buski will promptly disappear as soon as the dental location is cleared of polonium (within 12 hours), although far away. In its place will be Clostridium, as usual, when a buski has been killed.

Q23. *Radon – If* Positive, *the residence or local lodging is suspect. Test a dust sample from your client's home residence for radon. If* Positive, *move patient's bedroom immediately to one without radon or its daughters. Discuss the importance of moving to a safer residence with your client. Radon "mitigation" as described in pamphlets or the Internet is seldom useful enough. Although different rooms in a house have different radon exposures the only security for the client comes from moving to a radon-free residence.*

A23. The patient should not return home to rooms with radon. Nor should they be given lodgings with radon. Any radon in the saliva sample could be gone in a few days. If the patient's radon persists, search for an ongoing source, such as bottled water. If water is *Negative*, search for the rest of the decay series: lead, bismuth, thorium, uranium and radium, all of them being radioactive. Track them till they are gone (several days).

Q24. *Alpha, beta, gamma radiation – If Positive search for radioactive teeth containing U, Po, or UPo. UPo is a duplex; the test bottles touch each other. Since Po is a decay product of U, it would be natural to expect them still together. To find the Po-tooth, search the body wipe for tooth/Po, giving each tooth its turn, from 1 to 32. Removal of radioactive dentalware should follow the sequence given in The Advanced Dental Program Step-by-Step, page 413.*

A24. As soon as uranium and Po are out of the mouth, the malignancies they support wane and disappear in about 24 hours. This applies to uranium dust and crumbs in the sulcus (dental groove) as well as that saturating the gums. There is no malignancy without a stationary Po source.

If one polonium or uranium bit has moved to a different location along the canal the symptoms are different. Different nerves have been reached which transport them to different organs. New metastases can be expected. With more mouthwashes you could dislodge it, even if you have a tooth at this site. Both missing tooth locations and pristine tooth locations can harbor chips of polonium or uranium. Non-stop EDTA mouthwashes are most useful. Dental washing does not help because it does not move the radioactive chips to the outside of the body.

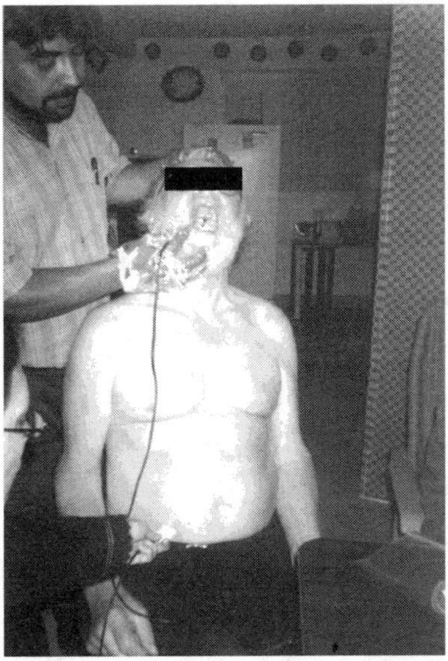

Searching for teeth with polonium or uranium connected to a right lower abdomen tumor.

Fig. 106 Using a Dental Probe.

If the polonium or uranium crumb is not in the gums, nor canal, nor papilla, you can test the plastic filling, represented by cerium. Place cerium between the tooth number and Po. If such a tooth is *Positive* for U or UPo it should be extracted, not replaced. If the filling is quite small, so the dentist can saw or drill around it without touching it, it may be possible to save the root and apply a safe crown later. Before refilling or crowning, the tooth it must be retested. When clear disinfect it with *Dental Bleach* or *Lugol's* iodine (6 drops in a teaspoon of water) and apply an earplug of compressible foam (see *Sources*). Trim away the entire associated gum, as well as the gum margin and papilla. Later, remove the plug before suturing over. If polonium does get trapped inside the socket you could find it two days later by Syncrometer®. It is not difficult to open the wound and do dental wash with added suctioning action. You will not know you removed the trapped radioactive particle till next day's Syncrometer® test finds it missing at tooth/bone/Po.

Continue testing the body wipes for malignancies and then for tooth/polonium at *Positive* locations. Identify the exact locations, whether gum, gum margin, papilla, dental canal, bone, or plastic filling.

It is not too late to do a socket cleaning at a root canal or other "missing" teeth, even decades old. Any repaired tooth could be contributing to your malignancy in this powerful way. Any <u>missing</u> repaired tooth could still be contributing to your cancer. Repeat tests at all tooth locations for every malignancy till it is found.

With the removal of radioactivity, the body spontaneously begins a massive parasite-killing. Protect the patient carefully. Oregano oil, zapping, and protective teas are all essential now. Follow up plans should be made to review the dental work in the future (in 6 to 10 weeks). There should be no alpha, beta, or gamma radiation in the saliva. We must be alert to any new pain and run-amok radioactive particles arriving in the gum canal for several months.

While the dental work and cancer-complex removal are proceeding, you can complete the general survey of the patient's health.

Q25. *15 parasites – including Strongyloides, Paragonimus, Onchocerca, Dirofilaria, Fasciola, Fasciolo-*

psis buski, Clonorchis, Eurytrema, Ascaris megalocephala, Ascaris lumbricoides, Echinoporyphium recurvatum, Echinostoma revolutum, Macracanthorhynchus, Acanthocephala, Gastrothylax. Teach your clients how to find their own parasites, find the parasites' essential foods and minerals from tables in the books and begin to starve them.

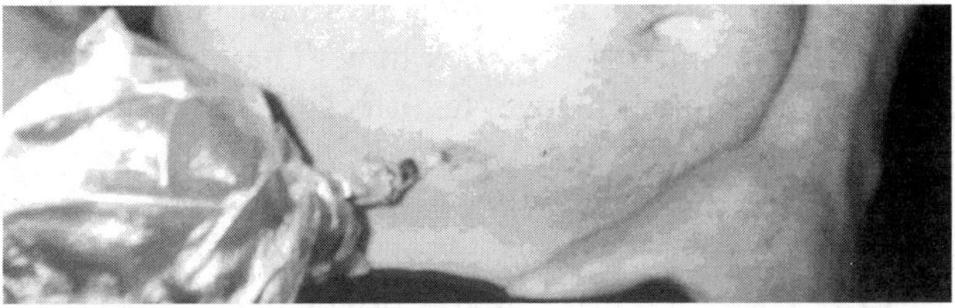

A second probe at the tumor site detects resonance from tooth location. The third probe is in the hands of the tester nearby.

Fig. 107 Dental probe search for linked teeth

A25. Many parasites cause diseases by producing mutations in a similar way to F. buski. This time the Po and Ce make a complex that attaches to ferricyanide found in NSF bleach. The alkylating agents are usually taken from mustard in the diet. Again, cerium does the recruiting of iron cyanide, alkylating compounds and the parasite to make a mutagen that firstly disables Rhodanese enzyme. This is followed by other mutations characteristic of that disease.

Q26. *E. revolutum – also a fluke, always found in neuromuscular disease. Search for them in the brain, spine, and "motor endplates". See photo on page 185.*

A26. This parasite, like F. buski, is protected by the prevailing radioactive elements such as thorium, besides polonium. When it is killed abscess bacteria become the "undertakers", analogous to Clostridium for F. buski. They are Streptococcus pyogenes. The fungus, **Claviceps**, claims the dead parasites first, though. Its mycotoxin is

ergot, which prevents any neurotransmitter from appearing. Give niacinamide, 500 mg., 1 x 3, to detoxify ergot. With both acetyl choline and epinephrine missing, the organ cannot function. Ergot removal is necessary for neuro-transmitter function.

Q27. *Acanthocephala – an amoeboid parasite with no predictable structure. See page 120.*

A.27 They are rather easy to eliminate and to observe physically, being 1-1½ inches long. They are most easily seen during a liver cleanse. Its effects are unknown.

Q28. *Malaria – You will only find it where benzene still remains. Test for Plasmodium falciparum, because this is the variety that causes most serious illness.*

A28. Test for PGE2 at the organ that has malaria. If *Positive*, search for the food allergy at this organ. Start killing the parasites with the quinone drop set. Use the cancer location table to find the related food allergy or test with the foods being served. There should be no resonance with food. This brings the swiftest (most life-saving) improvements.

Search for PGE2 at the RBCs and liver, their main "home" organs. Search for fructose (honey), ASA (aspirin) and limonene at the RBCs. Remove these from the diet, using the *Food Table*.

The picture will change each day as the patient stops eating the allergenic foods. Improvement comes quickly, even if transfusions were already part of treatment.

Q29. *Po/Ce/ferrocyanide/malaria – If* Positive, *notice there is a parallel development as with the cancer parasite, F. buski. It is not clear whether this is a mutation-causing-complex. If we assume it is, what mutations might there be? Drug resistance could be one, but this could also be due to a sudden big increase in subtype varieties. We might expect this from the polonium radioactivity so intense and so near the parasite body.*

A29. Notice that the malaria goes wherever the F. buski goes and where benzene is *Positive*. My interpretation is that the malaria parasites are inside the buski parasites and perhaps in other parasites as well. In a week of diligently removing allergenic food, the symptoms are very much reduced, including pain.

The benzene may already be gone from the water but still coming from a mycotoxin, **zearalenone**. This is made by Potato Ring Rot fungus, found in potatoes.

Intense pain, especially of legs, is said to be due to torn bits of red blood cells sticking to the capillary walls, making them spasm. RBCs are the malaria parasites' primary food, namely, the hemoglobin inside. But they only attack those RBCs with benzene in the membrane. This can be nearly all of them, resulting in life-threatening anemia.

Search at platelets and B-cells (CD37) for PGE2, malaria (stages), and benzene. Search for the food allergen to be avoided. The B-cell count and globulin both have a tendency to rise

Q30. *Bacteria tested should include Strep pyogenes, Strep pneumoniae and Strep pneumoniae/gold, Strep G, E. coli, Staph aureus and Staph aureus/gold, the Shigellas, and bread Yeast and Yeast/nickel, which is a fungus. If pyogenes is Positive search in the teeth, or soft tissue of the jawbones. It does not cause pain to alert you. These are seldom found clinically before an organ is destroyed. The gold attached to these pathogens is a new development. Only draining out gold by take-out drops at kidneys and lymph can clear away these mutants.*

A30. Clean the teeth that test *Positive* for abscess bacteria with *Dental Bleach* first, then radioactivity removal and repair of cavities. Afterwards keep mouth disinfected with *Dental Bleach* and oregano oil tooth powder, alternating once a day, after flossing. Stop the

Dental Bleach after 1 month, to reduce chlorine intake. Substitute "peroxy" (17½% hydrogen peroxide). There are no symptoms even after it infects the brain. Because S. pyogenes is so silent, research is needed to see if Alzheimer's patients all have brain abscess bacteria.

Q31. *The virus (oncogene) test should include EBV, RAS, MYC, mumps, JUN, Adenovirus, hepatitis B, hepatitis C, CMV, measles, NEU, FOS, SRC, SV40, Papilloma or common warts.*

A31. Each virus has a parasite or bacterium host. Destroying the host is the fastest way to remove the virus or oncogene.

CHAPTER 18

EMERGENCIES

Emergencies happen and they always surprise us. We are accustomed to thinking immediately of the ambulance, the emergency room, a babysitter, a neighbor. And all these serve us well, for which we can be very grateful.

But we could get ready for them ahead of time because every terminal cancer case leads right to them. If you or a loved one with cancer see a dropping RBC or hemoglobin you can get ready long before there is an emergency. Maybe you could even persuade them to do the necessary dental work or move to another house and cure themselves instead.

The symptoms that will lead to an emergency are not so many, or so difficult, that it takes special training. They only require a common sense approach. **Anemia** is one. If you do nothing to cure it, and rely only on quick clinical treatments it will lead to transfusions. Then you will need the transfusions closer and closer together. You obviously need enough good red blood to supply the heart. The emergency will be heart failure. Start curing it as soon as you read this.

- Stop eating honey. Honey is made of FRUCTOSE sugar. As cancer advances, you get allergic to fructose. In fact you get more and more allergic—to anything. Radioactivity makes this happen. Radioactivity makes us allergic. The liver can't digest fructose efficiently, as well as many other things, so they linger in your blood…where all your precious red blood cells are. Fructose is <u>their</u> allergen. They get inflamed from being given their allergen. "Inflamed" RBC's let the "doorways" in their membranes stand open. Many things are now allowed in.

It is surprising that something so **natural** as honey could become an allergen. But what is **unnatural** is the excessive radioactivity in our bodies.

Soon the red blood cells burst because so much water and so many invaders have entered; the pressure on the inside gets too great. Red blood cells, by the million, can burst, giving you a steep drop in RBCs. Now there are fewer RBCs to carry oxygen to your cells; the heart and brain will suffer most.

Changing your water to be unchlorinated and changing dentures to non-radioactive will help most to stop these attacks on your RBCs.

Internal bleeding is another cause of anemia. Even a very tiny spot that bleeds chronically will cause anemia.

- Stop eating Acetyl Salicylic Acid: It is the chemical name for aspirin. It causes very tiny "bleeds" anywhere and everywhere in your body. Choose a different painkiller; ask your pharmacist to read the ingredients of the common painkillers to you so you can choose those without aspirin. Also check the *Food Table* to make sure you are not eating ASA-foods every day. Many foods have it.

Possibly, the biggest cause of internal bleeding starts as benzene (see page 305). As soon as you have switched your water to the NSF disinfected variety (free of chlorox) this cause will end and you should see the benefit on the next blood test report.

Stomach cancer is still another cause. Actual hemorrhage and sudden death is always an anxiety in stomach cancer. An old ulcer does not heal well here, not enough to be strong again. When your serum iron keeps slowly dropping you should have the stomach checked inside with a scope; it could be treated by cauterization to stop chronic bleeding. Make sure the serum iron is included in your blood tests.

A stomach cancer patient should avoid alcohol because this makes the stomach twist and turn. If alcohol causes pain in the stomach, do not use the Black Walnut Hull tincture. Use the freeze-dried form even though it is slightly less effective.

Parasites themselves cause bleeding. Wherever there is a parasite that attaches itself to you, like flukes, there is chronic bleeding. Bleeding invites the pain bacterium, Streptococcus pneumoniae. That is how we get our chronic widespread pain as we age. Killing parasites regularly and keeping a good digestion is the easiest solution.

The bleeding problem is made worse by lanthanides entering your house. They come in with dust particles along with radon and inhibit blood clotting.

I suspect you may be told you have a "blood disease" or "dyscrasia" or a bad gene that misbehaves when you get foreign protein into yourself so the RBCs "precipitate". We need not be convinced by such "glamorized" explanations, even if your mother and grandmother had the same problem. You may all have been living near to each other at some time and even shared your diet, water, and dentist. It seems best not to be fatalistic over genes, but to improve yourself in the most obvious way you can see. Get more calcium to help your blood clot by adding bones to every soup and having soup nearly every day with 2 or 3 drops of hydrochloric acid or a teaspoon of safe vinegar (see *Sources*) added rather than taking supplements. Calcium requires acid in the stomach to dissolve. When there isn't enough acid, bacteria grow and calcium will not dissolve. Then the calcium precipitates, mainly in the liver and kidneys. Calcium supplements are mostly contaminated with chlorox bleach and lead, besides. Check your liver enzymes (ALT and AST). If they are moderately elevated, such as 40 to 70 it is most likely due to lead in the liver. Lead in the liver is almost certainly due to a supplement (check your vitamin A, D, and calcium first). But it can only be found by Syncrometer® testing. Start using goat milk for vitamin D_3, genuine butter and green vegetables for vitamin A, and the dyscrasia may soon disappear.

- Do not put HCl or vinegar into a stainless steel saucepan; it will dissolve chromium from it. Add the acid drops after serving the soup **complete with bones**.
- Ventilate your house from the ground up so the radon and lanthanides do not get in and fill your air. They travel so fast that they can be everywhere in seconds because they ride on dust particles. If you can light a match at the door and smell it upstairs in seconds, you can tell what path these earth elements are taking through your house.

There are 15 lanthanides that you inhale throughout the day. The less the better. They compete with your calcium so your blood can't clot quickly. They land on your ATP so you have much less fuel to burn as energy. They land wherever a tissue is sticky, namely inflamed. They land on your thrombin and prothrombin so your blood can't clot. Any little bruise or bump gives you a bluish spot under the skin where the blood leaked out of its vessels; it couldn't clot quickly enough. It will help your anemia significantly not to get these bruises any more. You can watch your blood improve on your blood test. Ask for the PT (prothrombin time) test and get it closer to 100%.

To get further away from radon and lanthanides, move to a house without a below ground "level". Put a fan in the crawlspace. Use radon-proofing techniques to keep out the lanthanides, too. Read about them on the Internet but do not believe the reassurances given.

Taking vitamin E makes the red blood cells' membranes (skin) tougher, so they can't burst so easily. Start with 100 units, not more, tested for chlorox.

All these tactics can help to reverse, namely cure, your anemia and avoid an emergency trip for a transfusion.

Malaria parasites are the most important cause of severe anemia. They can be controlled rather easily by avoiding benzene in the drinking water. They only attack RBCs with a weakened membrane, after an allergen or benzene is present. Benzene is found in the chlorox-containing water, but is not detectable in the NSF varieties. Malaria follows benzene closely.

Kidney failure is another emergency just waiting to happen. When the creatinine level on your blood test is at the top of the range you are headed in this direction and should already fix it.

Remove all the filters and softeners from your water pipes. The kidneys are very susceptible to the malonic acid coming from these.

Whether you have kidney cancer or blocked kidneys, or just swelling of the legs or have a huge abdominal effusion that must be drained regularly, you can start to cure it.

Measure your urine output first and then set your goal on 2 quarts (liters) in 24 hours (without use of a diuretic).

Doing A 24-Hour Urine Test

Find a 1-gallon water bottle. Buy a plastic funnel to fit it, and a roll of tape to write on it. Use a plastic food container to urinate in; then pour it into the gallon jug. Put a strip of tape on the jug to write the time of beginning on it. Collect it all this way till next day at the same time. It does not need to be precise. Eyeball the amount you made. 1 gallon holds 4 quarts/liters.

Curing The Kidneys

• First remove the malonic acid blockade in your kidneys. It turns into methyl malonate, which is the culprit. Take 2 herbs to remove the methyl malonate: ginger capsules, 2 three times a day, and uva ursi capsules, 2 three times a day. This unblocks them after 5 days and you will see a surge in the 24 hour urine amount. It can't continue to work for more than a few days if you have plastic teeth because they all seep malonic acid. Zappicate the plastic teeth 3 times to harden them enough to stop seeping. Or harden them with the recipe on page 602. Then repeat the 2 herbs. You should not stay on the 2 herbs all the time. Go off after 5 days. You could repeat it every 2 weeks until your dental metal or radioactivity is gone. Then the cure can be permanent.

• Remove the metal from your teeth. Lead, mercury, cadmium, uranium are kidney blockers all coming from amalgam fillings. Be careful not to replace amalgam with plastic that also has uranium in it. This would happen if the composite or other dental material had chlorox disinfectant in it (over half do; ask your dentist to give you samples for testing). Only a Syncrometer® tester can test for alpha, beta, and gamma radiation or chlorox disinfectant or uranium in trace amounts.

• Do the *Kidney Cleanse* program on page 592.

• Take baking soda in a small amount (1/4 tsp.) at bedtime and upon rising. This helps the kidneys excrete phenols, which are acids and quite difficult to get out of the body. We all make them from our food.

• Make kidney drops for yourself out of rainwater and take them for 2 weeks; see page 204.

• Sterilize all your food, so no Salmonella or E. coli invaders can live in your kidneys. If you can't sterilize, cook all herbs into teas instead of taking them as raw capsules. You will get less bacteria.

Kidneys need organic vitamin C, such as in rose hips or in fresh fruits. They also need vitamins B_2 and B_6, folic acid, and pantothenic acid. Feed them well.

Liver failure is another emergency you can prevent. It leads to coma, but often jaundice comes first. Whether you have hepatitis C, beginning jaundice, or very high liver enzymes on your blood test, you can take immediate steps to cure it.

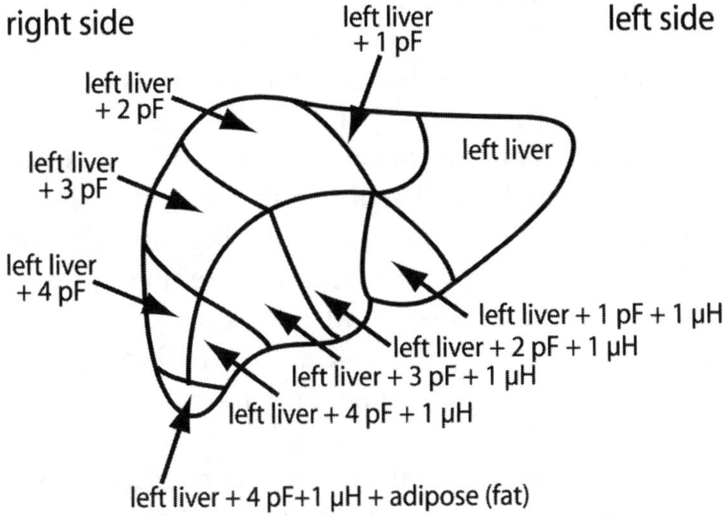

The left liver is just to the left of your midline, each picofarad (pF) moves you to the right; each microhenry (µH) moves you a few inches down.

Fig. 108 Drawing of divided liver

Hepatitis C is easily cured by removing metal and radioactivity from the teeth. This takes the burden of detoxifying these off the liver. It begins to recover immediately (in days). If the **total bilirubin** is already climbing, even very slightly over the top of the range, you should jump into action. Fungus is trying to grow in the liver, spreading itself, and producing **aflatoxin**. This poisons the liver's ability to detoxify your hemoglobin for excretion. At the same time, the mercury from your teeth is poisoning the enzyme that should help to keep your bilirubin low…it is your **bilirubin oxidase**. You may have already changed your amalgam to plastic. Unfortunately, a large part of it still resides in the gums and gum canal where all the tiny pieces collected during removal. Start the mouthwash and gargle routine (see page 420) to get loose bits out yourself. Make it a daily habit like brushing teeth. In a few months you could be much better. The gum-clearing must be done by a dentist.

In all hepatitis C as well as jaundice cases getting the metal out of your mouth more completely is the key and the cure, specifically copper, cobalt, chromium, nickel, and mercury. You can have this done in 2 days. Do not replace the dental metal with anything till the bilirubin is down. Otherwise you could be covering up a tiny missed bit that would never be found later. Getting "most" of it out won't help! It must be all out. If survival is at stake you should extract amalgam-teeth, not replace. Then clear the gums while doing the chelating mouthwashes on page 419.

- As soon as the metal is out of the mouth, take the set of drops called "heavy metals-out-of kidneys and lymph".
- This can be followed by "heavy metals-out-of liver"; this means "out-of each part" of the liver, as shown in the drawing, page 462.
- This can be followed by "heavy metals-out-of-blood" and then "mercury-out-of-blood".

Removing metals <u>always</u> saves a **jaundice** patient since this program is effective in 2 days. Watch the total bilirubin level on your blood test; it should get down to 1.0 before you can relax.

The fungi, Penicillium and Aspergillus, depend on the specific metals mentioned; when these metals are gone the fungi stop making aflatoxin. The missing mercury stops inhibiting the bilirubin oxidase enzyme. Hepatitis C disappears in days, almost too quickly to be able to study it.

• Take milk thistle seed capsules to help the liver (1 capsule 3 times daily). Disinfect by freezing after testing for chlorox and contaminants.

• Take thioctic acid capsules, 1 capsule 5 times daily, to do the exotic kinds of detoxification the liver is normally capable of. Test for contaminants and freeze.

• Take herbs to kill Salmonella and E. coli in the liver. You are getting these from your daily foods, products and supplements and also as detox-effects. Take 6 Lugol's drops 4 times daily (10 drops if you have 2% diluted iodine) and burdock for Salmonella. The herbs to kill E. coli are turmeric and fennel, 6 capsules of each, 4 times daily for 2 days. If you do not get the good results expected you are still eating these bacteria. Search for the source.

• Sterilize all your food, products, and supplements.

The next 2 emergencies should be treated one after the other, not together. Symptoms can occur, but none are serious. One is when the **alkaline phosphatase level** is over 500 on the blood test. It means the dye DAB is trapped in all your white blood cells! Your liver, lungs and bones are immediately affected. The major source is chlorox bleach in your water, food, and teeth. It is an azo dye, also seeping from plastics.

• Stop all processed foods because they probably have this dye.

• Zappicate your plastic teeth and harden any denture pieces to stop seeping dyes (see page 602).

• Start the drops called "dyes-out-of kidneys and lymph". Stop after 2 weeks.

• 5 days after starting these drops start taking DAB-out-of-WBCs for 5 days (only).

This whole program can be repeated every 3 weeks till alkaline phosphatase is normal.

A parallel emergency, just as deadly, is when the **LDH level is over 500** on your blood test. It means the dye,

Sudan Black B, is trapped in your red blood cells. Your body is filling up with lactic acid, but little more is known about this emergency. Sudan Black is a biological stain and presumably it could also come from a fabric manufacturing plant or dye factory.

The major source is chlorox bleach in food, water, and your plastic teeth.

- Stop all processed food.
- Zappicate your plastic teeth and harden your denture pieces.
- Start the drop set called "dyes-out-of kidneys and lymph" for 2 weeks.
- 5 days after starting "dyes-out" start Sudan Black B-out-of RBCs for 5 days. Expect side-effects the first day. Stop after 5 days.

You can repeat this every 3 weeks till the LDH is normal.

New RBCs and WBCs that your body makes will not fill up again with dyes, if you do not use chloroxed-water. We may assume you stopped using commercial cosmetics, hair dye, nail polish and regular body products, all of which will be disinfected with chlorox bleach. See recipes for homemade cosmetics in earlier books.

- Take vitamin B_2 in large amounts to detoxify dyes, such as 2 capsules 5 times daily; the urine should be yellow.
- Take Coenzyme Q10 in large amounts, such as 1 capsule 5 times daily.
- Take thioctic acid, 1 capsule 5 times daily.
- Take milk thistle seed, 1 capsule 5 times daily.

Repeat the blood test 10 days after the first one. If the alkaline phosphatase and LDH are not down substantially, you are still getting these dyes! And the liver enzymes may be <u>up</u> significantly from <u>accepting</u> these dyes. If so, go back to a 6 times daily routine of taking dyes out of kidneys and lymph. Most of all, stop the source of them.

Can't Eat

Not eating is a very neglected emergency.

This kind of emergency should only be tolerated for 1 day. Once your weight begins to slide downward it may not stop till 20 lbs. are lost. It is fortunate if you had it to lose. Never try to lose weight when you are sick. Your fat and muscle are your Bank of Survival for such times. The higher the better (within limits)!

If you have not eaten at least half of the usual amount, rush to avoid the **weight loss emergency**. It is not completely understood, but 2 procedures can stop it: killing YEAST and clearing the hypothalamus of metals, particularly cobalt and gold.

Invading yeast is doing what all yeast does when you give it exactly what it needs: sugar, water, and warmth. Once it is in your blood you cannot stop its growth, it has found your "pantry". But it needs an essential element, chromium. If it is deprived, it slows its growth immediately. It can live on mere molecules of chromium, though. The rule that works is: Touch no metal, eat no metal, wear no metal (this implicates a watch, necklace, ring, eyeglasses and tooth fillings). Remove the metal from teeth completely: this means extraction, not replacement of amalgam. Yeast can live on any tiny grindings that slide under the gum line as the dental dam is removed. Be sure to clean the dental canal yourself with mouthwashes and gargles. Have the gums trimmed by your dentist. Eat and drink nothing commercially processed; use no dishes or cutlery except HDPE and boiled plastic spoons. Fortunately, no natural food contains chromium metal. Yeast growth is the cause of CEA production and AFP, both cancer markers of long standing. Yeast actually participates in the tumor growth. It plays the same role as a parasite in donating its DNA to the cancer complex to make cancer mutations (CEA, AFP). Yeast takeover has always been a result of cancer advancement, it grows faster as our defenses fail. It is the terminal stage of all cancers, but it starts much sooner in breast cancer.

Removing chromium by EDTA chelation is very useful, too. This may be available in your area.

Clean the hypothalamus. Make bottle copies of both the right side and left side of the hypothalamus. Take them as drops in the usual way: 6 drops, 6 times a day for 2 days. Then 6 drops, 3 times a day until no longer needed.

Also make drops for heavy metals-out-of R hypothalamus and heavy metals-out-of L hypothalamus. Take these the usual way.

In 2 days the hypothalamus will make a special substance for you, called hydrazine sulfate. It will be found in every organ after that. Then you (or your loved one) will say, "I am hungry". This is the turning point. Be sure to provide natural, home cooked, chlorine-free, bromine-free, fluoride-free food. Search for such food ahead of time. Cooking pans should have been tested for chromium as well as supplements. Make sure the WBCs are fed.

Until the appetite improves, give drops of hydrazine sulfate with the usual dosage and frequency.

Gain It Back

You can gain back your weight much faster by **blending** your food with a safe blender (see *Sources*). It will not be possible to identify the food! You will eat more automatically by trying to taste its identity. In a few days you can begin to enjoy your new food, it is so effortless! Switch back to unblended food when you have gained back your weight.

If you can't eat for the simple reason that there is too much pain in the stomach immediately after the meal, search for cancer in the stomach. Kill the parasites there with the apricot suppository method or Green Black Walnut method. Avoid alcohol. Then kill all bacteria there with oregano oil if tolerated. If not use pomegranate (2 capsules, 3 times daily), moose elm and alginate, see recipe page 588. Start each meal with moose elm and alginate, then heavy whipping cream. Then white rice or potatoes or pasta. Don't be tempted to eat anything that could scratch, like popcorn, cornflakes, whole wheat baked goods, fruit peels, nuts.

Empty all capsules and mix them in heavy whipping cream or pudding.

Taking digestive enzymes of any kind gets more food value out of your food.

If you can't eat because there is too much "water" in the chest and it presses against your heart and lungs and stomach, arrange to get drained and get a drainage tube installed. It should be easily removable.

Water accumulation is not a cancer problem. It is a dye and malonic acid problem, both coming from chlorox bleach. You can clear this by removing the problems, see page 474.

Time is on your side. Your stomach is very hardy and "wants" to heal as soon as toxins are gone.

Can't Sleep A Minute

Insomnia is another emergency. To get cured you must sleep; it is not a luxury. Sleeping pills are fine if they do not contain chlorox bleach, but over 90% do! You cannot take such a risk.

It is always caused by bacteria. They are always Salmonella and E. coli. You have more bacteria than the average patient and must find the most useful recipe to kill them. Taking 6 capsules turmeric and 6 capsules fennel before supper and again before bedtime is the most helpful. These bacteria escaped through a thin and bleeding spot in your intestines, made by the larger parasites. You also got them from unsterile food and supplements. Everything edible is contaminated with them. Mixing so many sources of bacteria lets them all hybridize and get extra virulent. Carrying radioactivity on themselves makes bacteria extra hardy.

The pineal gland in the middle of the brain controls sleep. It should be making melatonin. Often there is a beginning malignancy there—too small to get attention by the oncologist.

Start curing it with 9 wormwood capsules 3 times daily for 2 days. Very few people are "allergic" to this but stop if you get an important symptom. Wormwood is one of the few herbs that can get into the brain, so is extra valuable.

At the same time take pineal drops and heavy metals-out-of-pineal drops.

If you typically wake up in a few hours, repeat the turmeric and fennel in the night.

If you have repeated bouts of gas and indigestion in the night you can be sure it is E. coli. Next day search for the culprit food or supplements. (Remember to sterilize and test the turmeric and fennel).

It helps to assist the liver and digestion at bedtime, with 1 milk thistle seed capsule, 2 digestive enzymes of any kind and 1 rose hips capsule or vitamin C. Others can keep you awake.

Do not drink liquids after supper unless you are detoxifying, nor eat your supper later than 7 p.m. It delays your liver metabolism (workload) and ability to sleep.

If you absolutely must sleep "right now", take 12 ornithine capsules plus 3 melatonin, each 3 mg. Do not take more. These, too, must be sterilized.

You may open capsules and stir into a beverage.

Constipation is a semi-emergency. It, too, is caused by Salmonella and E. coli. Be sure you are not eating them in unsterilized food or supplements. Then kill them with the herbal supplements and teas. As a last measure take **Epsom salts**; the magnesium is good for both you and your heart. But note the rule: your stomach must have no food for 4 hours before taking Epsom salts or you will feel quite ill.

Also, double the magnesium supplement, taking it 5 to 10 minutes before meals to avoid interfering with digestion.

The Biggest Emergency...PAIN

The most acute pains can come from the simplest sources—the allergy to gallic acid. It is often just a muscle spasm, but the pain is horrendous and we, the sufferers believe it is mysterious, came out of the blue and is completely undeserved. Gallic acid comes from food. List the gallic acid-containing foods (see food table page 97) and remove them from your house; They are often very tempting and we yield again when pain is gone!

If you are on a pain patch or other addictive painkillers you must solve your pain problem quickly. Staying on them will soon start killing you. They constipate you, they don't let you thrive or gain weight, they give you a casual attitude to life as though it mattered not if you chose death or life. This demoralizes your family and caregiver, too. You must somehow be serious about wanting to live.

All cancer related pain is caused by bacteria—one and only one variety, Streptococcus pneumoniae. They will be where the chronic muscle spasms are. They must surely have some very special ability to open the pain-channels in our nerves. By studying them we would have a chance to find pain stoppers that could put an end to the narcotic-consumption. Strep. pneu (noo) appears to be a blood eater. So stopping bleeding should stop pain. Formic acid causes this bleeding and is made from benzene in the body. So it is actually benzene that brings our pain. Benzene comes from chlorox bleach, so, again, we must change our water to cure it. It will take 5 days to detoxify the formic acid. The bleeding stops within hours after formic acid is gone. Pain leaves a few hours after bleeding stops. Hurry to get rid of benzene sources and allergy sources of your pain.

All cancerous tumors start to bleed as the benzene turns to formic acid there. Then they are painful. Tumors only form at allergic places, so the "stage is set" for pain.

Start to neutralize the formic acid with baking soda, ½ tsp. morning and night till pain comes down. Reduce it to ¼ tsp. morning and night as pain lessens. There will be good days and bad days that tell you mistakes are being made. Till you get relief use the least amount of painkiller necessary to let you eat, sleep, and get your cancer program started. Never choose an aspirin variety because it prolongs bleeding.

Zapping pain can be very helpful too. Zap the exact location of the pain with a plate zapper. The north pole field produced by the zapper's *Positive* offset current has pain-relieving effects all its own. This is besides activating the white blood cells to destroy the bacteria that cause pain.

Starving Pain

Taking away the metals that are essential for the Streptococcus bacteria is more powerful than taking an antibiotic that blocks their metabolism. Sometimes more powerful than zapping…all living things need to be fed! Streptococci are dependent on chromium. Stop using all pots, pans, bowls, cutlery, and dishes until you have tested them for chromium seepage (see page 614). There may be little left—not even cups and saucers (see temporary place setting, page 364.)! Test your food and water. Remove metal from your mouth. Remember to clear the dental canal and trim the gum at each tooth, too. Amalgam could always be expected to contain chromium. After this, making homeographic bottles that take out chromium will be effective in 2 to 4 days. Make these, using your own zapper and a plain piece of aluminum sheet metal, about 3¼ inches square (see *Bottle-copying*, page 189).

Take out chromium by itself from kidneys and lymph so it will be drained from the whole body slowly and steadily, and eventually deprive the bacteria. This could take 5 days. For a stronger effect take out the heavy metal mixture, too.

<u>It does no good to *"take-out"* the bacteria themselves</u> because you are feeding them blood and chromium. Feeding while fighting bacteria never works.

Pain Lurks Nearby

There are hazards to avoid that will certainly bring your pain back! If you drink or eat more benzene, even one polluted tablet (such as the <u>painkiller</u> itself), will make more formic acid. The pain will be delayed because it takes time to reach the formic acid stage. All this obscures the cause, the one polluted tablet or an untreated toothbrush or "high quality" china cup. Do not take such risks. Do not risk a dab of lotion, an untested spice or a tea bag. Commercial products are being manufactured more and more with chlorox bleach disinfectant, spreading benzene everywhere.

Killing Pain With...Herbs

How could pain be stopped by herbs? Quite simply, by killing Streptococcus pneu bacteria.

But knowing which ones to use must have been kept a secret of the deepest kind. Nowhere in herbal books have I seen a chapter or paragraph called: Pain-Killing Herbs. Maybe such herbs were said to have magical or dangerous powers in order to keep prying hands and eyes away and written records never made. Only aspirin, morphine, and codeine escaped suppression, but became worthless to average citizens. Aspirin makes you bleed more and the narcotics bring addiction.

Use the recipe on page 264 to get yourself off painkillers. Be patient with your own mistakes. Give yourself excellent grades when you succeed.

Prescription Painkillers

You can, of course, use prescription painkillers. The hazards are rather serious, though. Well over half of all pills I have tested were themselves bringing chlorox bleach disinfectant, namely polonium and chromium. Their dyes are usually obvious, but even white pills contain numerous dyes that are invisible. When forced by emergency to take them, try to wash some dye off under the faucet. Let the washed pills dry on a paper towel. Alternate brands, if possible, so not so much of one pollutant accumulates. Take extra vitamin B_2 and coenzyme Q10 to help detoxify these dyes. Painkillers usually contain aspirin also, so bleeding and pain are worsened 5 days later, but not suspected because it is delayed. A pharmacist can help you get aspirin-free painkiller. The morphine/codeine varieties slow down the intestine so much that constipation results. Then bacteria levels skyrocket, especially E. coli, greatly reducing your chance of recovery. Taking stool softeners and bowel activators helps but each brings its own chlorox bleach hazards. Sodium alginate is a stool softener (see *Sources* and *Recipes*) without this risk. The narcotic painkillers also disturb weight gain and general thriving. Try to switch to substitutes, even if you have to double or triple the amount.

In spite of all this, emergency need for pain relief has first consideration. Do not feel bad or guilty about needing it. Just be sure to zap your pain all day, take small amounts of baking soda for 2 or 3 weeks, and remove all your malignancies as fast as you can.

Permanent Pain Relief

It may take several tries before pain stays away because there are unsuspected benzene sources and mistakes must be made.

Every source of benzene or heavy metals that you find can lead to a permanent improvement for your health, not just for pain. You may have a dozen unsuspected sources. Finding them and eliminating them will help cure your other illnesses, too, besides the cancer.

Making Your Own Painkillers

Taking drops of a copied pain medicine gives you about ¼ of its action, but gives it to you must faster (5 to 10 minutes).

There is no toxicity to worry about so you can take it over and over till you get relief.

Choose several varieties, up to 4 or 5, taking all of them one after the other in one session.

This is an example:

1. Copy several Advil tablets, tested for chlorox and sterilized, writing the total dose on the label, with the name NOT-ADVIL (check for aspirin first).

2. Copy a few morphine-containing tablets the same way.

3. Copy Indomethacin or Indocid.

4. Copy Tylenol (check for aspirin first).

5. Find a codeine variety, tested for chlorox bleach. Place several pills in a small, ½ oz. bottle, so they add up to about 4 times a real dose. Put this dose on the label. Add pure water to cover them. Place a similar bottle, almost full of water, beside the bottle with the pills. Place a metal pipe around each one on the copy plate and zap 20 seconds. See copy making instructions on page 189. Label the new bottle NOT-CODEINE or FAKE-CODEINE. Copy the copies immediately into bottles without rubber droppers. Then dump the real originals for safety from accidents by children.

Take 6 drops of each, 1 minute apart. Repeat every 15 minutes till pain is tolerable*. No addiction or side-effects have been seen. Do not combine these into a single bottle. (The frequencies interfere with each other.) Keep copying your copies to make more. Be sure to dump the originals for safety.

Effusions Can Be Emergencies

"Water holding" is a common problem for cancer patients. Of course, it isn't really water. It is your precious lymph, full of body proteins and other important things your body made. Now you will throw them away as you drain it. But drain it you must until you can stop it from forming. If you don't, it will put pressure on neighboring organs till they can't do their work. We are very fortunate to have a clinical method available to drain…putting in a drainage tube…and sometimes "patching" an effusion site. It buys you a little more time to find the causes.

This time the causes are malonic acid and dyes.

* Testers, an organ in pain shows loud resonance with both acetyl choline and epinephrine at the same time. Many painkillers can "turn off" acetyl choline resonance. Morphine can "turn off" epinephrine, though more slowly, to give deeper relief.

Dyes

We are inundated in dyes—not only the legal and accepted kind, but the illegal and unacceptable kind. How could DAB, formerly used to color margarine, but long ago banned, be everywhere in our environment now? How could Sudan Black, a tissue dye, never made legal, be so prevalent now that you can see its effect on nearly every cancer patient, even in their blood test? Fast Red and Fast Red Violet cause all the effusions in cancer patients. This makes them very dangerous. Why is there so much in our environment? We know, of course, that anything in the water supply becomes very prevalent. These dyes are in the chlorox bleach water only.

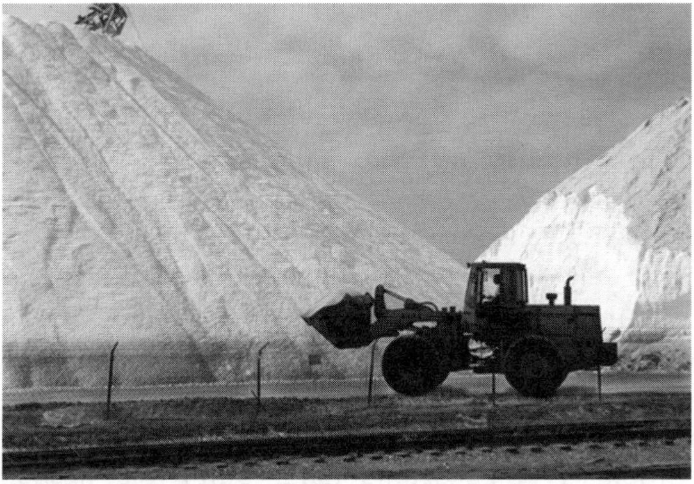

This salt pile goes to half the dairies and other markets in the USA, we were told. It is "sea salt" or "mineral salt". The ocean flats where this salt is harvested had a pink period during the summer for two years. The salt has pink stripes running down the length of it and pink patches here and there. Will your dairy herd get this dyed salt?

Fig. 109 Sea salt pile, a bearer of red dyes

These 2 red dyes do not act alone to cause the effusion. They seem to block an enzyme that we all have that can detoxify maleic anhydride. Maleic anhydride is the real cause of effusions. It comes from malonic acid.

Malonic acid is an industrial chemical, used so much that you can find residues of it in almost anything made by industry (amalgam, food spray, plastic teeth, chlorox bleach, glassware, ceramic items, for instance). We eat and drink large amounts every day in chlorox bleach water, sprayed food, and from seeping dishes. The body uses several steps to detoxify it, found by Syncrometer® in 1993. The steps are:

Malonic Acid Diagram

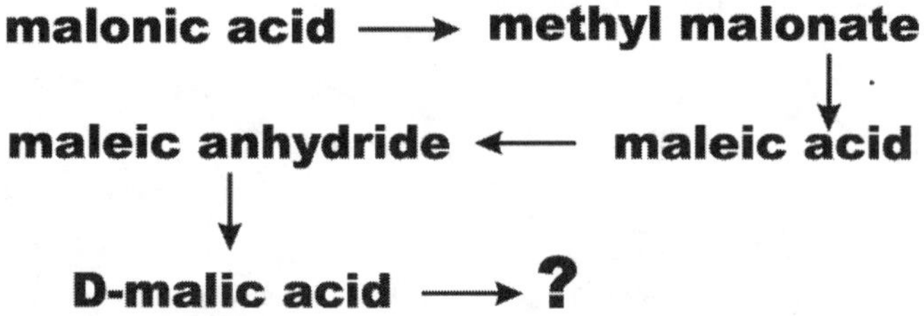

Learn this sequence the medical student way: Mabel met a male malingerer doing a Main Street dance.

Fig. 110 Malonic acid detoxification pathway

Each step depends on having enough of the necessary detoxifiers. The first two require B_{12} and folic acid. The last three steps are the hardest, requiring a lot of vitamin C, particularly the organic parts, rutin and hesperidin. Maleic anhydride will often stay backed up for long periods, waiting for more organic vitamin C to become available. Where it is backed up it develops a porous spot in the tissues where fluids can pass through. Thin tissues like linings of the lung or abdomen will seep fluid if a thin spot develops in them. The fluid has no way to drain out again, so it fills up the lung space or the abdomen space. We call them effusions or "water holding" and need to drain them if we can't stop them.

The 2 red dyes are found wherever maleic anhydride builds up. Presumably, they are blocking an enzyme that could detoxify it further.

We can treat the problem with vitamin C in large doses; somehow this bypasses any enzyme that is needed. But treating a problem without removing the cause does not last. You will have to get IV treatments of 50 gms of vitamin C again and again unless you get rid of your malonic acid source and dyes.

Finding and eliminating the source of the dyes and the malonic acid is the permanent solution. Of course, that is made easier when they both come from the same source and they often do. Then the body drains itself with a little help from potassium, boiled parsley water, and vitamin C supplements.

The causes can be very hard to find. For example, your mashed potatoes! A cooked, peeled, organic tomato! Your beautiful, superior-rated toothbrush! A plastic strainer! Your hair dye and cosmetics!

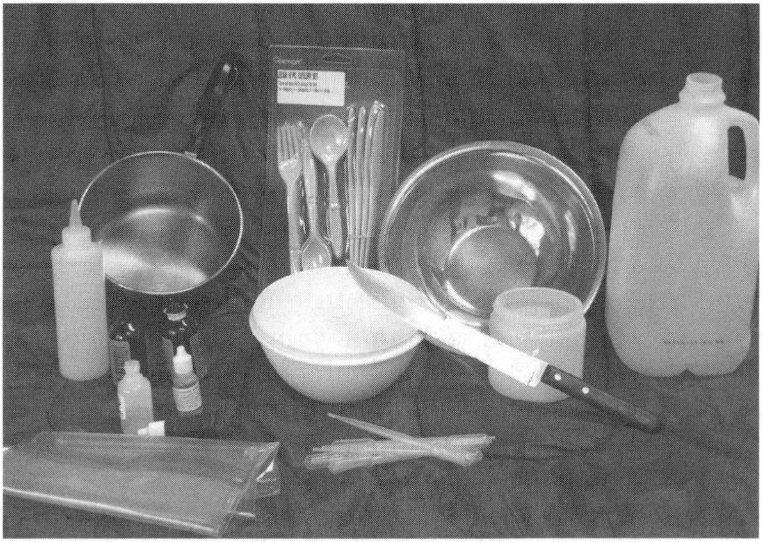

Fig. 111 HDPE utensils and stainless cookware

The dyes and the malonic acid are deep inside the potato, too deep to come out with hot-washes. The potatoes were sprayed with anti-sprouting chemicals. You can hardly find a potato that is not so sprayed! Tomatoes and carrots have the same problem. The colorful plastic toothbrush is made so soft, the colors and malonic acid diffuse into your mouth immediately, every time you use it. These doses are much too great for the advanced patient, *or for anyone*.

If you have an effusion, switch to farmers' market produce, not store bought. Freeze it yourself for the winter so no glass or cookware is involved. Switch to a temporary place setting (see page 367) and stainless steel cookware till you have tested all other kitchenware.

This may be all that is needed for an early effusion—less than a year old. The dental clean up, water change, environmental clean up, and new diet can bring so powerful an immune recovery that the kidneys can drain it all without help. If not, help them with the methods that cure kidneys (page 459). Then the thin spot heals and an x-ray shows a lung full of beautiful black (on the x-ray) air. Your body can still do miracles for you.

A New Lump

It is demoralizing and panicking to see a new lump appear or an old one grow again after you have been shrinking several others. It brings home the painful truth that you still have something arriving at your tumor when you thought you had found it all and removed it. The chance is best that a new crumb of radioactive tooth filling has entered the dental canal or has been moved along it. The <u>location</u> in the canal decides on the location of the new lump. This is so because the conduction of the Po is along the tooth nerve, which is permanently situated. Making a body wipe is the fastest way to find out. Fold ½ of a paper towel 3 times and wet it slightly. Wipe the skin over the lump in the morning before taking a shower. Place in a small plastic bag and test for chlorox, OPT, polonium, and uranium. Immediately start the chelating mouthwashes and gargles as described on page 419 without letup for 2 or 3 days to remove any loose bits of Po or U in the dental canal.

> About half of all new lumps start with loose bits of Po that have been herded into the dental canal and are stuck there. You can get rid of these yourself with EDTA mouthwashes. There will be loose polonium bits arriving at the dental canal for <u>months</u>. Be prepared.

If there is no OPT in the body wipe over the lump, it is not malignant and does not have Po, but you must still get rid of uranium there.

If you have never trimmed your gums, arrange to do this for all your teeth, whether they are missing or not. You will be removing heavy metals, uranium, polonium, and abscess bacteria at the same time.

If the new lump has mercury, you still have amalgam in your teeth. Ask your dentist to remove more from the teeth that had them. But if the body wipe has uranium, not polonium, search for U/Po. This is uranium and polonium combined. It is a more sensitive test for polonium. If this is present you are finding a particle of uranium that came with amalgam or chlorox bleach. The <u>uranium has broken down further into polonium and started a new malignancy</u>. Even though uranium has a very long half life, there are enough molecules in any sample to increase the odds for making polonium. <u>Routing out all the polonium from your teeth stops all metastases</u>. Leaving uranium behind will only delay the return of metastases. Search for traces of old amalgam or of a plastic filling that had chlorox in it when it was placed there by the dentist. Tumors that are not shrinking are still receiving either uranium or polonium. If the new lump has chlorox it means you very recently got a dose of it, in a pill or food or dental treatment. Track it down immediately.

When some tumors refuse to shrink*, or new ones grow, jump into action. Not to zap, take drops and otherwise obliterate the new growth, but to find the source of allergens for that organ and the source of the cancer-complex. Chances are best that your food has phloridzin, chlorogenic acid or gallic acid in it to supply tumor nuclei. Or that a piece of uranium is still left in your mouth from previous porcelain, plastic, veneer or amalgam. Or that a bit of polonium is still trapped in a tooth, in a leftover plastic filling that was originally disinfected with chlorox. If this is so, the new lump will become malignant. Extract any suspicious tooth with radioactive residue.

ALL problems are current.
NO problems date only to the past.

If the new lump shrinks in a day or two you guessed right. Notice that you have more power in your hands than the finest cancer institute. Use it to detect these simple causes. Soon there will be more patients with experience like yours to help you.

* Testers, search for SCF, HGH, gallic acid, chlorogenic acid, phloridzin, Fasciolopsis cercariae, CEA, Yeast, HCG, heavy metals, chlorox bleach, polonium, ferrocyanide in the saliva.

CHAPTER 19

HOW TO READ YOUR BLOOD TEST RESULTS

Knowing how to explain your own blood test results gives you insights that no doctor of the past was ever taught. There will be optional interpretations that can be settled with a Syncrometer® and can help you choose the best path.

In earlier books, many blood tests were discussed in detail. Please refer to them for greater understanding of their meaning. In this chapter I will show you how to use your blood test to find your health problem instantly and correct it.

People in the best health have results near the middle of the lab range. Values very close to the ends show that there is a health problem developing. If you can catch it, find its cause and remove it, you can prevent disease. Our working range shows you the limits we used to decide if a problem should get immediate action. You can set narrower limits. To protect your own health, you should search for the same causes when a test even begins to show an unhealthy direction.

For example, if your RBC is below 4.3 you could consider yourself anemic, although a therapist or clinic might not. Start to search for the same causes as would drive it down to 3.1 (see page 484).

To be useful for the very sick person, needing quick answers, a flow sheet format is used here.

First find the problem in your blood by seeing if the result is too high or too low. Then find possible causes in the alphabetized list that follows. When a cause is found, go to the *Tester's Flow Sheet* to find its source and its correction.

NOTE: The *Tester's Flow Sheet* was printed in *The Prevention Of All Cancers* and is now found included in the *Syncrometer® Science Laboratory Manual*, 2007.

Blood Test Results

		Our Working Range	Our Lab Range	Units
a	RBC	3.1 – 4.8	4.5 – 6.5	MIL/mm^3
b	WBC	5 – 15,000	4.0 – 10.0	thous/μL
c	Plts	150-400,000	150 – 450,000	thous/μL
d	BS (non-fasting)	80 – 140	65 – 115	mg/dL
e	BUN	8 – 22	5.0 – 26.0	mg/dL
f	creatinine	.9 – 1.4	0.60 – 1.4	mg/dL
g	uric acid	3 – 4	2.2 – 7.7	mg/dL
h	cholesterol	200 – 250	130 – 200*	mg/dL
i	triglycerides	100 – 200	30 – 180	mg/dL
j	T.p.	6.5 – 7.5	6.3 – 8.3	gm/dL
k	albumin	4 – 5	3.9 – 5.1	gm/dL
l	globulin	2 – 3	2.0 – 5.0	gm/dL
m	GGT	10 – 45	0 – 57	U/L
n	AST	5 – 40	0 – 55	U/L
o	ALT	5 – 40	0 – 55	U/L
p	T.b.	.1 – .9	0.1 – 1.8	mg/dL
q	i.b.	.1 – .6		
r	d.b.	.1 – .3		
s	alk phos	75 – 95	39 – 117	U/L
t	LDH	120 – 140	91 – 250	U/L
u	calcium	9.0 – 9.7	8.5 – 10.4	mg/dL
v	phosphorus	3 – 4	2.2 – 5.6	mg/dL
w	chloride	100 – 110	95 – 111	m Eq/L
x	sodium	135 – 144	133 – 145	m Eq/L
y	potassium	4 – 4.5	3.3 – 5.6	m Eq/L
z	serum iron	30 – 100	30 – 170	μg/dL

Fig. 112 Checking your blood test results

* Cholesterol range is set by corporations, not scientists.

The lab range depends on which test is used by the individual lab. If your range is different, use the top figure to compare the two and make an adjustment in your interpretation. For example, if <u>your</u> range for LDH is about twice as high as ours, you should double the working range, too.

Common Abbreviations

RBC	red blood cells
HGB	hemoglobin
WBC	white blood cells
plt	platelet
BS	blood sugar/glucose
BUN	blood urea nitrogen
creat	creatinine
Chol	cholesterol
trig	triglycerides
T.b.	total bilirubin
d.b.	direct bilirubin
i.b.	indirect bilirubin
T.p.	total protein
	albumin
	globulin
alk phos	alkaline phosphatase

LD or LDH	lactic dehydrogenase
ALT	alanine amino transferase
AST	aspartate amino transferase
GGT	gamma glutamyl transpeptidase
Ca	calcium
Na	sodium
K	potassium
Cl	chloride
CK	creatine kinase
P	phosphorus
CO2	carbon dioxide

<means “less than”
> means “more than”

Blood Test Flow Sheet

Spotting Your Problem From Your Blood Test

a	if RBC < 3.1	Give transfusion of packed RBC with plasma as needed. Search for causes of anemia (see page 455), Sudan Black dye, cobalt.
	if RBC>4.8	Search for vanadium in RBC, bone marrow, reticular tissue. Search for hypothalamus or pituitary-free cells attached to RBC.
b	if WBC< 5	Search for lead, cobalt, other heavy metals, DAB in bone marrow, WBCs.
	if WBC>15	Search for copper in lymph, bone marrow, WBCs, liver, cancer (leukemia), infection.
c	if plts< 150	Search for dyes, antigen (limonene), wheel bearing grease in plts, malaria.
	if plts> 400	Search for HGB in saliva, lymph (bleeding).
d	if BS< 80	Search for yeast, chromium in saliva, lymph.
	if BS >140	Search for Eurytrema, Echinoporyphium recurvatum, limonene, phloridzin in pancreas and islets of Langerhans*.
e	if BUN< 8	Search for azo dyes in saliva, lymph, WBCs.
	if BUN >22	Search for Clostridium in saliva, kidneys. Search for cobalt, heavy metals, E.recurvatum in kidneys.
f	if creat< .9	Search for dyes in saliva, lymph.
	if creat > 1.4	CHALLENGE! avoid KIDNEY FAILURE; search for methyl malonate at kidneys; E. recurvatum.
g	if uric acid< 3	Search for Clostridium, yeast at saliva, lymph.
	if uric acid >4	Supplement folic acid, 1 mg. 3 times daily.
h	if chol < 150	Eat butter, cream, do liver cleanses, parasite program.
	if chol > 250	Do liver cleanses every 2 weeks, take milk thistle seed. Search for thallium; kill parasites.
i	if trig < 100	Eat butter, cream.
	if trig > 200	Supplement pancreatin-lipase, do liver and kidney cleanses, do parasite-killing program till normal.
j	if T.p. < 6.5	Do parasite program (search for cobalt, vanadium, malonate set in liver).
	if T.p. > 7.5	Search for cobalt, vanadium, other heavy metals in liver, B-cells.
k	if albumin < 4	Search for cobalt, other heavy metals in liver.
	if albumin > 5	Search for heavy metals and dyes in liver.

* Testers, to locate islets, put insulin sample touching pancreas.

l	if globulin < 2	Search for dyes, cobalt, vanadium at B-cells, malaria.
	if globulin > 3	Search for dyes and heavy metals in B-cells.
m	if GGT > 45	Search for DAB at WBC, liver; do liver cleanses, search for strontium, CMV.
n	if AST > 40	Search for lead at liver, bone marrow, and in supplements, also radon.
o	if ALT > 40	Search for lead at liver, bone marrow, supplements.
p	if T.b. > 1.0	EMERGENCY! Avoid jaundice and liver failure; search for copper, chromium, cobalt, nickel, aflatoxin at liver; remove with homeographic drops at each liver location.
Search for bilirubin oxidase in blood. If Negative search for mercury in blood, lymph, liver. Make take-out –mercury- from blood drops.		
If aflatoxin is Positive, search for Aspergillus, Penicillium at liver locations.		
If Aspergillus is Positive, search for chromium, cobalt, nickel in liver.		
If Penicillium is Positive, search for copper in liver.		
q	(d.b.)direct bilirubin	Is the detoxified portion of bilirubin. It reflects on liver function.
r	(i.b.) indirect bilirubin	Is the undetoxified portion of bilirubin.
s	if alk phos < 75	Search for cobalt, Sudan Black, Fast Garnet dye in liver, WBCs.
	if alk phos > 95	Search for DAB dye in WBCs.
t	if LDH < 120	Search for cobalt at saliva, lymph, liver, kidneys.
	if LDH > 140	Search for Sudan Black B dye in RBCs, kidneys. Search for Fast Green in WBCs.
u	if calcium < 9.0	Search for toxins in parathyroids.
	if calcium > 9.7	Search for toxins in thyroid.
v	if P < 3	Supplement vitamin D_3 tested for lead; search for vitamin D_2 in bone, lymph.
If vitamin D_2 is Positive, search for Ascaris in bone marrow, lymph.		
	if P > 4	Search for toxins in bones.
w	if Cl < 96	Supplement hydrochloric acid with meals. Search for toxins in adrenal glands.
x	if Na < 135	Search for toxins in adrenal glands.
	if Na > 145	Increase fluid intake till urine output = 2 L.

y	if K < 4	Supplement potassium gluconate. Search for toxins in adrenal glands.
	if K > 4.5	Search for toxins in thyroid gland.
z	if iron < 30	Supplement with liquid chlorophyll, 1 Tbsp., twice daily. Take hydrochloric acid and safe vinegar with meals.
	if iron > 100	Search for heavy metals in liver. Take EDTA 1 x 2

CHAPTER 20

CURING CANCER IN PETS

Our pets suffer in silence when disease strikes. It is heartbreaking to keep your pet company in the last weary days and hours when nothing more can be done, but wait. Instinctively, we humans know it is our fault. We did not provide. But what? What did we not provide? If only we knew. We all agree our animal friends deserve wellness. Then why are we letting them get our diseases? It must have something to do with our lifestyle…what we eat and the way we do things.

Animal cancer has been increasing along with human cancer. Are the same forces at work? If so, we could apply our new knowledge and begin to prevent their cancers, too.

Searching for similarities and differences from the human species was my first pet project. It seems promising. Animal saliva can be used the same way as human saliva to give us a window into their well being. It can be copied electronically, made into a homeopathic or homeographic form and studied with a Syncrometer®.

Cats, **dogs** and **horses** have remarkably similar blood to ours (see next page). Also notice how complete their testing is, thanks to a responsible veterinary profession. Clues to their condition can be read in it as easily as in ours. They too, have been struck by the immunity-destroying toxins in chlorox bleach. They now get new diseases as a result of the cyanides, polonium, lanthanides and alkylating agents in their water, like we do. The cyanide pipe-protectors and methylene blue dye interact with their parasites and parasite excretions like ours, to induce large numbers of mutations. They are the same mutations for any one parasite. The "syndrome" that F. buski is inducing in them is cancer like in us. But there is a big difference between animals and us. They recover much faster! If you are gazing with long glances at your terminally ill pet, given up by your compassionate vet, and would like to give it one more try, here is how you would do it.

Dog Blood Test Results

CHEM 25	Results	Range	Units
Alk phos	322 (H)	10 – 150	IU/L
ALT (SGPT)	137 (H)	5 – 60	IU/L
AST (SGOT)	62 (H)	5 – 55	IU/L
CK	100	10 – 200	IU/L
GGT	9	0 – 10	IU/L
Albumin	3.0	2.6 – 4.3	g/dL
Total Protein	6.0	5.1 – 7.8	g/dL
Globulin	3.0	2.3 – 4.5	g/dL
Total Bilirubin	0.1	0.0 – 0.4	mg/dL
Direct Bilirubin	0.1	0.0 – 0.1	mg/dL
BUN	14	7 – 27	mg/dL
Creatinine	0.7	0.4 – 1.8	mg/dL
Cholesterol	156	112 – 328	mg/dL
Glucose	81	60 – 125	mg/dL
Calcium	9.1	7.5 – 11.3	mg/dL
Phosphorus	3.9	2.1 – 6.3	mg/dL
TCO2 (bicarbonate)	16 (L)	17 – 24	mEq/L
Chloride	110	105 – 115	mEq/L
Potassium	4.4	4.0 – 5.6	mEq/L
Sodium	146	141 – 156	mEq/L
Indirect Bilirubin	0.0	0 – 0.3	mg/dL
WBC	15.4	6.0 – 17.0	thous./uL
RBC	6.17	5.5 – 8.5	million/uL
HGB	13.4	12 – 18	g/dL
HCT	40.9	37 – 55	%
MCV	66	60 – 77	fL
Neutrophil Seg	85 (H)	60 – 77	%
Lymphocytes	6 (L)	12 – 30	%
Monocytes	9	3 – 10	%
Platelets	427	164 – 510	thous./uL
Absolute Monocyte	1380 (H)	150 – 1360	/uL
Remarks: Slide reviewed by technologist. WBC and RBC morphology appears normal. No parasites seen.			

Fig. 113 Checking your dog's blood test.

Notice that the alk phos is too high in the dog's blood test, like very many cancer patients', due to the dyes that were drunk in the chlorox bleach water. The WBCs have picked up DAB dye but can't detoxify it and let it go again, quite like peoples' predicament.

The liver enzymes are high, both SGOT and SGPT; it is due to lead in the liver, as in people.

The protein picture is the same, as well as bilirubin and the kidney tests. Blood sugar and calcium are the same. The CO_2 level is slightly low, no doubt from panting or having a fever that makes us breathe faster. The chloride, potassium and sodium levels are similar to ours, too.

The WBC is normally higher than for people. This means immunity is better. The RBC is higher, meaning energy and strength are greater. The platelets are higher so blood could clot sooner than for people.

As soon as you have decided, JUMP into action. Prepare many small wastebaskets to collect rainwater by inserting a large, zippered bag inside each one. Do not filter or strain. Later, zip shut and store as is, in a cool place. While you wait for rain, order the supplements and other items you will need. If you can't expect rain in a day, have it shipped from a friend or relative. Next, order the two ingredients for Lugol's solution (see *Recipes*) or ask your neighborhood pharmacist to order them for you. Do not buy ready-made Lugol's solution. Do not believe the pharmacist who promises to make it from scratch. You must see the dry ingredients yourself from which it will be made. All ready-made solutions have significant amounts of wood alcohol and isopropyl alcohol, now, as 10 years ago. Buy inexpensive diet scales, plastic cups and spoons to do it yourself. Use the recipe on page 584.

As you rush about, give your pet meaningful glances and a few words telling it to hang in there; something marvelous is going to happen. Communicate with a very light touch, not to be oppressive. Promise it that if he or she gets well you'll do something for its **cat cousins** or **dog** or **horse family**. Its eyes may be closed, but this promise will keep you both strong. You will be the natural doctor and **cat** or **dog** or **horse** will be a good patient. It is a subtle bargain they both understand after the vet has offered it eternal sleep.

We will treat a horse first. Success is nearly certain. But I have not written down the details for the latest changes yet, and not for cats and dogs either. Pattern them after the horse. Feedback will be much appreciated.

Horse Cancer

This was some of the email written from recall:

Hulda,

Does your method work for horses? We are a stable. Can we zap for chronic fatigue? Another vet took a look at her recently and thought I had nothing to lose, considering it's a young horse and she might have one of these new viruses. Do you recommend zapping or a parasite program?

Kathy F., Vet

Dear Dr. Kathy,

I appreciate your interest in true causes of ill health. Although zapping can't hurt, I consider it a treatment and not sufficient to truly cure. It's best for all horses to remove causes. I would be willing to search, as a courtesy, if you are able to implement the changes needed. Are you willing to make changes? You can find people on the Internet who cured their horses by older methods. This is new, more direct, and faster.

Hulda,

This horse "Honey" was originally in training for racing and there are others being seen with similar symptoms. We could not find EBV, CMV, and many more.

Dear Dr. Kathy,

We are a research clinic so I think we can find the causes, but not necessarily a new pathogen unless you send it on a slide. Please send a small amount of drool, picked up with paper towel (also send control). Stuff in plastic bag and pass under UV for safe shipping. Or do homeopathic treatment as on page 584 in The Prevention Of All Cancers. I don't suspect cancer, HIV or Lyme's so any suggestions you can give me would be welcome. Please send samples of barn dust (where Honey sleeps), trough water, city source water, direct from water meter or the outside faucet of the house. If there are 2 outside faucets send both, also samples of daily feeds.

The package arrived. There was also a photo of the 3 children with Honey. They had written: "Please help Honey get up in the morning. She only likes her treats. Please help her run."

Abbreviations and definitions

Neg: = *Negative*, meaning absent
Pos: = *Positive*, meaning present
: WBC = white blood cells
: lymph is the clear fluid in the body
: saliva used for testing is systemic in scope for an animal, as is blood.

A sample of saliva (drool) was received for testing. The owner said Honey was chronically fatigued and didn't want the children to ride her.

All tests are done by Syncrometer®, which is a 1-transistor audio oscillator that resonates with a loud sound when identical items are placed on the 2 testing plates. Can be built from a kit or purchased already assembled. These were my tests:

At saliva (drool):

1.) OPT – *Pos* (I'm so sorry Dr., your Honey is in the early stages of cancer. OPT is orthophosphotyrosine, our cancer indicator, from years of experience, not by medical definition. When you see what the true cause is, you will be able to clear it up in a few weeks.) Please read one of my cancer books for background and many helpful tips.

Bacteria test at saliva:

1.) Clostridium – *Pos* (These bacteria would only be present systemically if dead flukes were available to them. It shows that Honey is strong enough to kill some but not all Fasciolopsis buski.) F. buski is the cancer-causing fluke parasite in people and several animal species.

2.) E. coli – *Pos* (This bacterium is most common in human cancer patients, too.) I think this is because bacteria carry the body's radioactivity and make it difficult for the WBCs to catch and kill them. Here we see the bacteria with 2 kinds of radiation attached.

2a.) E. coli with alpha radiation (α) – *Pos*

2b.) E. coli with beta radiation (β) – *Pos*

This is excessive radiation for any animal, in my experience. We will find the source of this radiation and eliminate it for a cure.

3.) Salmonella – *Pos* (This adds more digestive problems to Honey and feelings of illness. They come from the killed F. buski flukes, not the living ones. They carry radioactivity, too.)

Since the WBCs are Honey's immune system and they are not managing to keep the body clear of E. coli, Clostridium and Salmonella bacteria, we need to help Honey by killing these for her. The best, 2-day treatments for people are TURMERIC and FENNEL for E. coli, and Lugol's iodine for Salmonella. Could you check your veterinarian references for any contraindications for these treatments? An herb called burdock is next best, then eucalyptus. Is there an herbal literature for animals? Perhaps you could cautiously experiment.

4.) Shigella – *Neg*

5.) Streptococcus G – *Neg*

6.) Streptococcus pneumoniae – *Neg* (This is so fortunate. She is not in pain yet; to be sure and prevent pain, you need to avoid chromium, even the supplement variety. These bacteria need this metal but Honey does not need it.)

7.) Strep pyogenes – *Neg*

Virus Test at saliva:

1.) Flu (Influenza A and B) – *Pos* (When Flu and Salmonella are present together it is evidence that the body has just killed F. buski flukes.) The symptoms, together, are called "Detoxification Symptoms or Syndrome". The symptoms are varied; maybe fatigue is her main symptom at this early stage. It requires constant treatment, though, since we are planning to kill all remaining F. buski. Honey needs to stay well enough to endure it all without getting too sick. A very sick horse could die from over deparasitizing; please check your references since I do not have enough experience with horses yet on these new herbs. For people we use epazote, boneset, eucalyptus, and burdock, birch bark, and Reishi mushroom, as well as a homeopathic called Oscillococcinum. Do you have animal references regarding any of these? If yes, could you suggest a dose? The dose for people is on page 404.

Oncovirus (Oncogene) Test: I will search for these later.

Parasite Test:

1.) Strongyloides stercalis – *Pos* (In people this parasite requires potatoes in the host diet, namely, ours.) Horses are known for their high levels of Strongyloides. Are there wild plants that are related to potatoes, and eaten by horses (perhaps nightshade)? Or is Honey getting potatoes in some form in a food supplement?

2.) Onchocerca – *Pos* (depends on corn in the host, namely our diet.) This grows into a thread, many feet long, as thin as silk. It gets itself tangled up around a lymph node in people, growing into a fairly large mass. It is called a non-Hodgkin's or a Hodgkin's lymphoma or just abdominal or chest mass. In people it can be eliminated with vinegar in the diet (but not in colon or prostate cancer).

3.) Dirofilaria – *Neg* (dog heartworm)

4.) Paragonimus – *P*os (lung fluke)

5.) Eurytrema – *Pos* (pancreatic fluke)

6.) Fasciola – *Neg* (This is very fortunate because they can consume the body easily and need only wheat for food…partly digested into gluten and gliadin.

7.) Clonorchis – *Neg* (liver fluke)

8.) Ascaris megalocephala – *Pos* ("horse variety")

9.) Ascaris lumbricoides – *Neg*

10.) Fasciolopsis buski – *Pos*

Meanwhile…

Dear Dr. Ashcroft (vet for Kathy's stables),

Your veterinary office serves the Felascez Stables. Dr. Felascez suggested I go directly to you with questions I was asking her. I am trying to show her how to salvage her once highly-prized horse "Honey". Enclosed are parasite test results.

I have not tested for other parasites that might, more specifically, belong to horses. But if you would like a particular one tested in Honey and have a sample or slide of it, I would be glad to test for it using my electronic equipment.

She seems to have excessive parasitism. This is caused in people by radioactivity lowering the immune power of white blood cells. By this I mean the WBCs are not active. They do not contain bacteria when bacteria are all around them. And they do not empty out their bacteria soon after filling up on them. I have never watched a live blood sample from a horse with cancer to see the macrophages barely moving. Is such a service available to horse owners?

In people, I believe this immune power drop is due to ingesting radioactivity in the common household bleach contaminating the drinking water, of a variety called chlorox. It contains polonium and a cyanide compound, called potassium ferrocyanide that are directly responsible. If I find these in Honey's tissues and saliva, I will be recommending well water, unchlorinated, and stopping all feed and supplements with chlorox disinfectant. Chlorox bleach disinfects about 75% of all items in a supermarket. Can you support this change and help them find the non-chlorox ones if a medicine or supplement is advised? I will be glad to do the testing.

Dr. Clark,

I have watched this horse deteriorate for no good reason, by all clinical standards. Honey is on my regular rounds and I would welcome new information on her behalf. I know nothing about alternative horse care.

D. Ashcroft V.M.

Testing of horse drool continued for Dr. Kathy F.:

Tumor Nucleus Test At Saliva:

1.) tumor nucleus (TN) – *Pos* (This is the same as in people!)

2.) tumor nucleus / SV40 – *Pos* (This means the SV40 virus is touching or inside the tumor nucleus, as indicated by the slash.) The Syncrometer® testing device cannot distinguish between adhering or internal items.

In people the tumor nucleus is made of 3 kinds of cells: from the hypothalamus, the pituitary gland, and pancreas.

Testing at Honey's lymph (body fluid):

1.) freely floating hypothalamus cells – *Pos*
2.) freely floating pituitary cells – *Pos*
3.) freely floating pancreas cells – *Pos*

Honey has all 3 kinds and can now make tumor nuclei, in large numbers. It means these organs are inflamed. I believe it is equivalent to the "somatic cell count" for cows' milk which is due to an inflamed udder.

People have Strongyloides at the hypothalamus, Clonorchis at the pituitary, and Eurytrema at the pancreas. But your horse did not have Clonorchis!

Let us see what is disturbing these 3 glands in Honey.

At the hypothalamus:

1.) Strongyloides - **Pos* She has very high levels (indicated by asterisk), literally crawling with these. It is the expected one.

2.) PGE2 – *Pos* (This is prostaglandin E2, a sign of inflammation. Several things could cause inflammation. I find PGE2 only if the cells have nickel or radioactivity inside themselves. These are the only 2 causes of allergies, too. Knowing this could help people to get rid of their allergies. But note that if people eat their allergenic food anyway, PGE2 will continue to be made, even without nickel or radioactivity. They have to be off this food a short time, like 1 week to lose their allergy and the PGE2.

Dr. Ashcroft,

Would you be able to find references on allergies or PGE2 in horses? It would be very much appreciated. Thank you.

At the hypothalamus (continued):

3.) chlorogenic acid – *Pos* (This is the allergy for this gland, in humans, too.)

4.) raw and cooked potatoes – *Pos* The chlorogenic acid allergen comes from potatoes, but not all potatoes.

Dr. Kathy,

This raises more fundamental questions than it answers, but we can see that Honey should not eat potatoes.

At the pituitary gland:

1.) PGE2 – *Pos* (There is inflammation here too.)

2.) phloridzin – *Pos* (This is the allergy here for the pituitary.) It is in oats. It is not necessarily present in all oats, only the unripe grains.

3.) oats – *Pos* (This is in one of her feeds you sent me.)

4.) Clonorchis – *Pos* (Honey has these liver flukes here even though they are not so numerous to be *Positive* systemically in the test at the saliva.)

At the pancreas:

1.) PGE2 – *Pos* (Allergic inflammation)

2.) Gallic acid – *Pos* (The allergy is due to this.)

3.) Eurytrema – *Pos* (This is the parasite here.)

4.) SV40 – *Neg* (These viruses are not infecting the pancreas yet.)

5.) Eurytrema / SV40 – *Pos* (The pancreatic flukes are infected with SV40, bringing it into Honey's body. You can stop letting the virus spread by stopping gallic acid in her feed. That is the viral trigger.

Dr. Kathy,

You can stop all these parasites by starving them. Stop feeding chlorogenic acid, phloridzin, and gallic acid. All these might be in her RATIONS but surely not in her NATURAL feed. These allergens will not be on the label. Gallic acid would be in the preservative of oils and grains.

For dogs and cats I recommend natural feed, too, even when they beg for their commercial food. Maybe you can "doctor it up" with natural goodies from a farmer's market or kosher store. Apples from a supermarket would be the worst choice because these are full of cancer-causing chlorox spray. Even organic food is washed with chlorox bleach-containing water, not intentionally, of course.

Your instincts were correct, namely, turning Honey loose in a luscious pasture.

We will switch now to searching in Honey's water sample for the carcinogen responsible for all human cancers.

Analysis of water from trough:

1.) chlorox bleach – *Pos* (This is what you were advised to pour into the trough to clean it and even leave a residue to disinfect it.) This has numerous carcinogens but it also has the specific cancer-complex that causes all people's cancers.

2.) PCBs – *Pos*

3.) benzene – *Pos*

4.) asbestos – *Pos*

5.) heavy metal set – *Pos*

6.) azo dye set – *Pos*

7.) malonic acid – *Pos*

8.) motor oil – *Pos*

9.) wheel bearing grease – *Pos*

10.) POLONIUM – *Pos* This is the radioactive element in all human (100%) cancer victims.

11.) cerium – *Pos* This attaches to polonium.

12.) polonium-cerium-duplex – *Pos*

13.) isopropyl alcohol – *Pos*

14.) potassium <u>ferro</u> cyanide – *Pos*

15.) potassium <u>ferri</u> cyanide – *Neg*

16.) methylene blue – *Pos*

You will recognize some of these as known carcinogens. She will have all of these in her organs and fluids because she is drinking them. They will also be in her commercial feeds and supplements because the manufacturers are using non-food-grade bleaches to sanitize their equipment.

But which of these is part of the cancer process for Honey? We will soon see, as we examine an organ where cancer is developing.

ORTHOPHOSPHOTYROSINE (OPT) cancer test at saliva:

1.) at lip – *Neg*
2.) at nose – *Neg*
3.) at eye – *Neg*
4.) at colon – *Neg*
5.) at bone – *Pos*
6.) at skin – *Neg*
7.) at tendon – *Neg*
8.) at skeletal muscle – *Pos*
9.) at left liver – *Neg*
10.) at Right & Left lung – *Neg*
11.) at a chest mass – *Pos*
12.) at an abdominal mass – *Neg*

OPT is a mitosis stimulant of an extreme nature. The tests were made using microscope slides of organs in series (electrically) with the drool sample.

Dr. Kathy,

Other locations were not tested. Perhaps you could be interested in this new technology yourself. I would gladly help if you take initial steps.

You might call this cancer a sarcoma based on its muscle location in people. In dogs it is often attached to the bone, like it seems to be here. We do not need to be precise with a biopsy when the tumor is located. We will not need chemotherapy, x-rays, or surgery, so don't need to discriminate between different cancers.

The curing method we use is based on the experience with people that if polonium or F. buski is removed, preferably both, and the body's needs met nutritionally, the body's immune system removes the cancer and heals itself, especially when still young.

Honey is quite young so I think she can mobilize a lot of her healing forces, if we can kill her F. buski parasites and stop her practice of drinking polonium in her water. I don't know if the polonium in her air space contributes to the cancer-complex by providing for a higher turnover rate, but it seems wise to move her sleeping space above ground level.

Dr., we will next examine the cancerous tissues, beginning with bone.

Bone test:

1.) PGE2 – *Pos* Inflammation and allergy are at a bone. It is caused by nickel or radioactivity or both. It is perpetuated by a food reaching the bone before it is digested. For this reason I will next test a set of about 60 food antigens, called phenolics, so you can avoid feeding her this. I won't list them here.

2.) MELON – *Pos* (This is not actually the name of a food phenolic, though. I searched for a list of foods after my phenolic set had no *Positives*. I suspected MELON because it is the allergen for muscles. Muscles and sarcomas are always allergic to melons.)

3.) PIT – *Pos* (This is a food phenolic, phenylisothiocyanate, found in the cabbage family.) Does Honey like to eat broccoli, collards, or wild mustard? Could she be eating anything in the wild she should be protected from?

4.) Polonium – *Pos* (The most dangerous of radioactive elements for people is also in her bones. It comes up from the ground, is in her water, and probably her commercial feeds due to the disinfectant used, chlorox, which has it.)

5.) Cerium – *Pos* (This is the lanthanide element that comes up from the ground beside polonium.) Polonium and cerium will attract each other and combine into a little complex. **Cerium is attracted to chromosomes and genes**, especially in those places where they are multiplying quickly. This includes bacteria, viruses, and parasites that make thousands of eggs. Cerium also attaches to isopropyl alcohol and to malonic acid. These are 2 very reactive chemicals found in chlorox bleach. Cerium is attracted to the ferri and ferrocyanides. Cerium even appears to be attracted to F. buski flukes possibly because they metabolize ONION, GARLIC and MUSTARD chemicals from their food, leaving waste products that contain ONION oils, GARLIC oils, and MUSTARD oils. These are all very mutagenic.

6.) PoCe-duplex – *Pos*

7.) PoCe/isopropyl alcohol – *Pos*

8.) PoCe/malonic acid – *Pos*

9.) PoCe malonate/isopropyl – *Pos*

10.) PoCe/buski – *Pos* (This includes stages of the buski parasite.)

11.) PoCe/ferricyanide – *Neg* (found in NSF bleached water)

12.) PoCe/ferrocyanide – *Pos* (found in chlorox-bleached water)

13.) PoCe/ferricyanide/buski - *Neg*

14.) PoCe/ferrocyanide/buski – *Pos*

The slash stands for direct contact.

Dear Dr. Kathy,

Can you see how reactive cerium is with many items that are always present in the body, and in chlorox bleach? Can you see how cerium is always pulling the polonium element along with it? Cerium will take all these items to the DNA with itself. Huge mutations will result from the polonium, even direct chromosome breaks.

Honey and humans share all 5 ingredients in the **cancer-complex**. Many cancer-complex variations are possible.

The importance of seeing all these details is that you can devise your own prevention method for Honey. Maybe you can see a cure, too. Both prevention and cure methods work well for people and should be even better for animals since they don't have the extra dental complication.

Honey has a body full of the PoCe-complexes. They come from the earth besides her water, but the earth source cannot **start** a cancer. These can only support or maintain a cancer-complex. By getting rid of the cancer now, she cannot get it again without the chlorox water. The further away from the ground she is the less Po and Ce she'll have to support the cancer. Her bed location is important. Could you raise her bed?

The only way she can get ferrocyanide and MUSTARD oils is from common chlorox bleach and that can be stopped.

We can see that the whole cancer would stop if she stopped accumulating the things that make the mutation OPT and got rid of those she already has. Here we are very fortunate. For people we can take the supplement MSM. It combines with the ONION, MUSTARD and GARLIC oils so they break free of the big complex. We can also take a supplement that has a quinone structure. That oxidizes the ferro to ferricyanide and makes it impossible for the ONION and MUSTARD oils to attach themselves to F. buski. There are other oxidizers, too. But iron supplements, which are mostly ferrous compounds, have the opposite, reducing, effect. We stay strictly away from them now. The way to get the iron level up is to take away the poisonous cyanide. It is the cyanide that complexes the iron.

We can take **hematoxylin** to combine with lanthanides, especially cerium. Then it breaks free of the big complex.

We can remove Po itself with IP6, inositol hexaphosphate, or a chelator like EDTA.

All in all it is fairly straightforward for people and should be even easier for pets.

Of course you must kill F. buski. As long as it is alive, it will make alkylating agents from ONIONS, MUSTARD and GARLIC. I don't know which fluke-killer is best for horses. There is considerable hearsay being discussed but it is too important to leave to chance. Can you find any literature that can be trusted?

Once you have broken up the big cancer-complex with the supplements you should not let the pieces regroup. They are very hygroscopic (water loving). Get her to drink a lot more water so the different pieces of the cancer-complex float apart. Read the properties of each segment in the Merck Index or chemical catalog. For people it takes about twice as much water drinking, twice as much urination and much more sweating than they were used to. We wrap people in paper for the night and give them 3 hot showers during the day to help them take up water and sweat out the complex.

If all this is making her sick with aching muscles, a fever, and sweats, you will know that <u>the cure is working</u>. If you could test her for Flu and Salmonella it would be more reassuring. But she should be treated clinically for Flu and Salmonella, in addition to herbally. She could die from it if her body kills its parasites too vigorously, just from health returning.

By day 2 and 3 we already see all the pieces of the cancer-complex separated and absorbed in the paper for humans. Most important is not getting the pieces anywhere near the skin again. The skin absorbs them all again and starts a metastasis right there. This is how we get our metastases...our hair, the furniture, our teeth.

Dear Dr. Felascez,

Does this tell you what to do? Do you think you can come up with a horse-solution as quick and easy as our human solution? We can virtually guarantee the cure now.

In short, I would recommend:

1.) Finding a horse bed location with low background radiation using a Geiger Mueller counter. Higher off the ground would be better. 6 foot higher would get her right away from both Po and Ce! Aim for that.

2.) Make a ramp and a very warm place to bed down on so she can sweat.

3.) Give her unchlorinated water to drink so she will get neither ferro nor ferricyanide. Collect rainwater in wastebaskets or barrels lined with garbage bags. You may store it in a HDPE 100-gallon tank with spigot. Do not filter. Add nothing. If you are concerned about water quality, ozonate it with a small (not commercial) ozonator. I would not recommend it, though. The trade-off with ozonator toxins (nickel, thallium) is not worth it.

4.) Give <u>only</u> native feed if she can still graze. If not, feed her only with items tested for chlorox, ferri and ferrocyanide, gallic, phloridzin, chlorogenic, onion, garlic, mustard, melon, cabbage. Make your own feed mix for her. Find a Syncrometer® tester by Internet. Do not be tempted to give supplements. Grass is better than hay. Hay should not be moldy.

5.) Get her to urinate twice as much by drinking twice as much. Keep her covered so well she must sweat, but not be chilled. Wipe the sweat off with paper towels you throw away. Are there ways you do this to a horse? If people can do this in 5 days, a horse should only take 3. Don't give medicine to lower temperature unless extreme. Test all medicine for chlorox.

6.) Keep drying her with paper towels and throwing them away.

7.) Without polonium stuck in her tooth fillings like people have and without cerium in plastic teeth, nor mercury in her kidneys, she stands an excellent chance of cure.

If you get her cooperation with eating, drinking, urinating and sweating, she will recover. For her immune system she can be given germanium and selenium in the form of nuts in the shell (you crack them). Peanut butter is fine (see Sources). Stir 20 drops Lugol's iodine into a spoonful. Also any dried fruit, chopped fine and frozen to disinfect, like rose hips, blueberries, juniper berries, only 1 Tbsp. at a time for extra vitamin C. Detoxifying Po and U consumes large amounts of vitamin C.

Dear Dr. Felascez,

The cancer was a surprise. I did not pursue a pathogen after that finding. I made an electronic copy of her saliva so we can keep it for future testing if you have a different suspicion. I have not applied my new research findings to a horse yet; please give me some feedback if possible.

Notice that we have not killed her parasites yet. It is best to do Part I first where we correct her water, diet, and air. This will strengthen her immune system so much, her body will make its own parasite-killing effort. If so she will be ill with Flu and Salmonella symptoms. Be ready to help with clinical methods at such a time.

It has been rumored that Black Walnut is specifically toxic to horses. But at the same time, many persons have cured their horses, I presume with it. Is there any reliable knowledge? Which herbs do you know of that have been used for horses? Hopefully, you can tap into some accumulated experience on the Internet. Please send a second drool sample after making all the changes for Part I.

I did not bring up zapping because it may not be needed. But certainly it should not be an embarrassment for you now *that a group of Israeli scientists has proved beyond a doubt that zapping works**. *Best Wishes*

Wild and free our pets once were
But suffer now our lot
Our sincerest wishes
with their pain is fraught

For outcome, see page 514.

A Cancer Mutation Family

Hundreds of cancer mutations are possible, including the different "cancer markers" produced by different organs*. The mutagen always starts with polonium.

Polonium is no ordinary toxin. It is to be feared and never risked. People were never skilled and equipped enough to exterminate themselves in the past. It was simply too complicated. But now we could do it in 1 generation.

Polonium could do it. Simply putting it in our water; simply in our food, so nobody is left out of massive genocide could do it. It is happening on a small scale in Africa now. We must make it impossible again.

Notice what is happening to this horse. It is the same as for people. But the horse is trapped in our environment and we are not…unless we choose to be.

---

* *Disruption of Cancer Cell Replication by Alternating Electric Fields*-Department of Biomedical Engineering, NovoCure Ltd., Haifa, Israel; B. Rappaport Faculty of Medicine, Technion-Israel Institute of Technology, Haifa, Israel; Department of Molecular Cell Biology, Weizmann Institute of Science, Rehovot, Israel; and Elisha Medical Centre, Haifa, Israel http://cancerres.aacrjournals.org/cgi/content/full/64/9/3288

* Testers, arrange mutagens on left plate and search for the mutation or "cancer marker" on right plate.

A horse is majestic and beautiful. It deserves as much of its true heritage as is possible for a human to give it. A horse roams; it does not settle down in one location. With a roaming lifestyle, it could never pick up too much radon or cerium from resting, or sleeping above a radioactive air current coming up from the ground.

A human CAN do this and characteristically does.

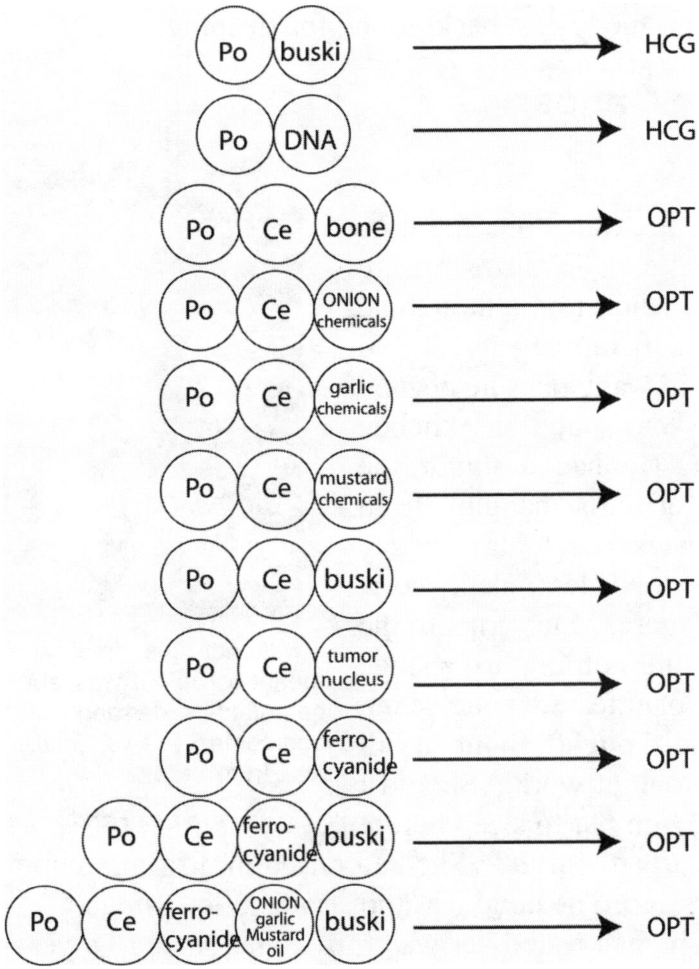

Many cancer mutations are possible, starting with OPT, HCG, HGH, absence of Rhodanese, p53, CEA, AFP, etc. Many variations of mutagen cause them.

Fig. 114 Cancer Mutation Family

Lanthanides, like cerium, come up at the same places as radioactive elements so you will be avoiding this at the same time if you relocate to a low-radon region. The amount of radiation coming up from the ground and down from space is called the "background radiation". That is all you need to compare from place to place. While you are at it compare your bedroom to the other rooms and choose the lowest background for sleeping.

Dog Cancer

Luke

Luke was a big, big dog. Age and arthritis were taking their toll, although he was still moving about and his tail wagged as he begged for "out" at the kitchen door. He had a tumor the size of a fist hanging from his neck. Each day he ate less, drank less, slept more, hurt more. Many trips to the vet did nothing to change that one feared conclusion. Leila thought about it all day long at work. "Should I have him put to sleep before he starts to suffer?" She had raised him from a puppy, 12 years ago. The bond was too strong to let him go.

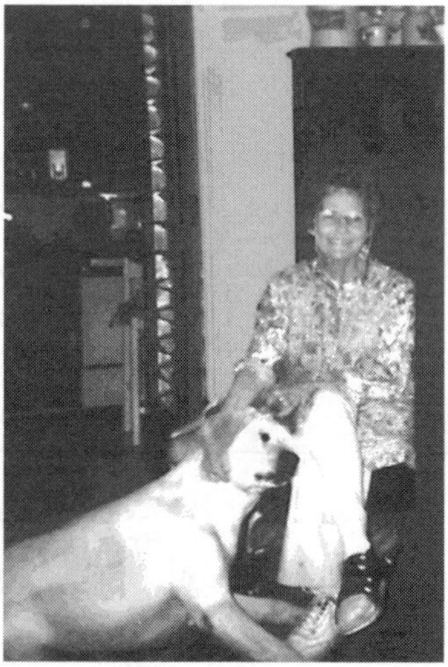

It was not "his time" and not "meant to be". It was abuse of the potable water and water-for-food-contact laws that took Luke from Leila.

Fig. 115 Leila and Luke

She had tested her water, by Syncrometer® a year ago, just before Luke came down with this lump at his throat. It was fine—no chlorox bleach, no water softener. Now his drool (saliva), though, had PCBs, benzene, asbestos, heavy metals and dyes, the exact recipe for cancer. It must be his dry dog food, Leila thought, and switched him to home cooked ground meat and liver.

She fed him the parasite program without hiding anything; he loved it. He got his Lugol's; that was easy, too. But his lump did not loosen or shrink. Getting IVs seemed too burdensome. Time passed.

Suddenly, he did not want to get up. His eyes half-closed. Leila helped him to his favorite spot under a shady tree and went to work, sending out samples of water, feed and saliva for testing.

The water had NSF bleach now but she recalled that her water pipes from the city had been worked on most of the previous year. Nobody had thought much about it. Would the workmen have used regular chlorox bleach, she asked?

Most certainly, I answered. No workman would want to deal with the hazard of 12% bleach (twice as strong as the laundry varieties) in difficult circumstances of underground trenches. Generously sloshing about the high quality NSF bleach would go against the grain of expense-conscious supervisors, too. And anyway, if "bleach was bleach", wouldn't you rather pick up a couple of gallons as you needed it, rather than head for the pool store to get a 4-pack to stand around in the bed of your pickup truck? It loses potency with time. And hazardous chemicals in such large amounts are a constant worry.

This time Luke's saliva was full of chlorox bleach and dyes, asbestos, PCBs, benzene and heavy metals. Nothing had been cleaned up in half a year in spite of the home cooking. And in spite of the "good" bleach coming to her kitchen faucet. Leila now suspected the meat. Every kind of meat he had eaten was full of these same things. It was meant for humans. She saw the "Beef Blood" it was dipped in. Its very name disguised its real intent, to keep the meat looking <u>red</u>. It tested *Positive* for chlorox bleach and all the dyes in my collection. She quickly bought different meats from all the markets for miles around to find one good store. Only turkey giblets and beef bones for soup were free of dyes. She quickly cooked some during her lunch hour, and got the supplements ready. At 5 p.m. she zoomed home, with drops, zapper and all. Her neighbor met her. It was all over. Time had run out*.

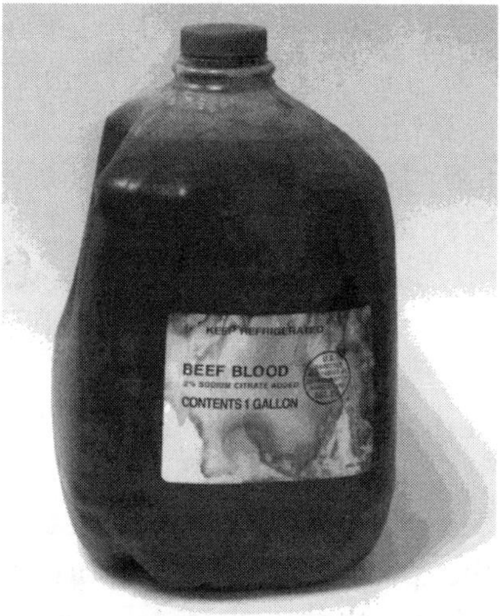

In reality beef blood is a red dye mixture, keeping meat looking deceptively red.

Fig. 116 Beef blood or hoax?

Frankie

Frankie was a big dog, too. He lived in an affluent sector of town with multi-level homes that served him badly. Better to lap water from ponds and ditches in a plain farm setting than the sparkling faucets that bring chlorox bleach in a high radon area. But he was stuck, as we all are. He was old, and arthritic, just lying around and moving himself from basement bedroom rug to front porch to "out" and back again. His lump was hanging from the ribs, somewhat floppy, but not loose. It was the size of a fist. The vet, very sincerely, told Susan that all treatments would be a waste. There was nothing…but Susan got to work. His bed was moved to the second level kitchen and the lower level door was closed. His water was changed to a laundermat's from the part of town

---

* Special thanks to Leila who wanted to know the real cause of Luke's failure to recover. She found the beef blood, to educate us all, a fitting tribute to true love.

where no water softener was added and certainly no filter. The Syncrometer® said it had NSF bleach. Two drops of Lugol's were added to each bowl of his water. No new bowls or special plates were used.

His expensive Health Food Store chows were changed to Health Food Store ground round—ground before Susan's eyes. It had not been dipped in "Beef Blood" and had only NSF bleach remnants. After Syncrometer® testing, Susan went back for pounds more. She made round meatballs and put most of them in the freezer.

Immediately she fixed one up for Frankie. It had ¼ tsp. green Black Walnut Hull tincture in the middle. He swallowed it whole. Another, small one had 3 drops of straight Lugol's solution in the middle. A third one had ½ capsule wormwood. This was breakfast. He drank nothing and went to sleep. He didn't want to go for a walk with Susan, otherwise his favorite activity. At suppertime he went "out" briefly. When he came in he sniffed the cupboards for his favorite chow. His pleading half-closed eyes brought tears to Susan's eyes. Could she deny him his only pleasure in these last days? She went to the refrigerator and split open a meatball. It got ½ capsule cloves in one spot, 2 drops Lugol's in another, and ½ capsule wormwood in another. He took it standing and flopped down on his rug. Susan's daughter came and zapped him. Then he wanted "out" again. He was barely dragging his hind legs along, but she gave him no arthritis medicine till it could be tested for chlorox bleach and water softener pollution. He hid under the porch steps a while then vomited and had diarrhea. Would he ever take another meatball? Susan cleaned him up.

Next morning Susan did exactly the same thing. This day she gave a capsule of vitamin C, too, in a separate meatball. Frankie stood now to take his meatballs in single gulps. He slept all day. He drank his "doctored" water, with 2 drops Lugol's in the bowl, without noticing the smell or taste. That evening he started working at his fur, gnawing and licking his rib region. He started to get up and bark several times at the front doorbell when it chimed, but felt too wobbly, too full of pain to meet the stranger. There was no pain medicine for him. He must lie still.

The third morning Susan and her daughter felt terribly sorry for him. They asked if they could break his mono-diet. They thought each day could be his last. He seemed to have taken a turn for the worse. He staggered as he walked. His eyes teared and he panted as if he was hot. Just "steer the ship; you're the natural doctor; he counts on your wisdom" was my answer. Susan did exactly the same thing. The water was from an east end gas station now. He didn't mind drinking it with Lugol's. He took all his meatballs and slept. But in the evening he wanted to go for a walk. Susan felt his lump, it seemed to be dangling. He wasn't dragging his legs so much.

Days 4 and 5 saw more tiny improvements.

On day 6 he suddenly jumped into the car to go shopping with her. Later, he went for a short walk, without much pain, it seemed. He wasn't missing his chow (a good time to throw it all in the garbage cans). His lump had come free from the ribs and was getting smaller. He was obviously digesting it or having the WBCs remove it.

That final downturn must have been detox-illness!

At that point I was not getting status reports anymore.

One half year later he was back on arthritis pills, but the tumor had disappeared and Susan felt it was divine intervention. She had her companion back and I could fade into the background.

GiGi

There are no two cat cures alike in my collection. My suggestion would be to kill no parasites at first to avoid early detoxification illness; only correct her cancer-causing water, food and radioactive atmosphere. This could activate the white blood cells so much that the body does a moderate amount of parasite killing on its own. Giving the herbs and supplements should reduce the detox-symptoms to manageable. If not, find a vet quickly.

For Gigi, these are the highlights of her encounter with the "big C". The water, food and air were corrected. The water was from a gas station, no filtering, distilling or processing. The food was cooked turkey, tested for chlorox, minced finely, without salt, made into small portions and frozen to -20°F for 24 hours. The fat was frozen too. No other food was given till she was cured.

Her bed, in a cardboard box complete with toys was moved to the upstairs bathroom (just outside). The "cat box" went, too, and her water bowl. Her food bowl stayed downstairs. She got one drop of Lugol's solution, delivered by plastic dropper straight into her mouth twice a day. She got a pinch of wormwood taken from a capsule and mixed in water to be delivered by dropper. If she hates this and gags on it, try mixing with catnip tea or heavy whipping cream. She got cloves, too, by tiniest pinch from a capsule. She was zapped for 7 minutes 3 times a day. It took 3 weeks till she became her old self.

Seeing this, her family fixed their water, changed bedrooms to family rooms, did their computering upstairs, and thanked Gigi on Thanksgiving Day for bringing them wisdom that special way.

Summary – Chapter 20

Notice that for Frankie nothing heroic was done. No IV's, no homeography or medicines, no enemas. He was strong enough to heal himself with just a little help for his immune system—real help! Taking away his toxic water, food, and air.

Frankie was zapped, once a day, through his front paws and his back paws. Soon after, he would run a bit or try jumping. Was zapping essential? We cannot know.

If your dog has cancer, be sure to get these basics done that were done for Frankie. Clean, native food and water…and a bed where the radiation level is low.

> If you do succeed and your dog had been marked by the vet for his eternal sleep-shot, remember your promise and tell your vet. Show him or her what you did. Dogdom will thank you forever…and so, too, for horsedom and cat land.

As for Honey, several months passed. Then an email came: …looks better …gained some weight …lets the children ride …does not seem sick anymore, but not what she should be yet. Can we continue?

Answer:

Please send drool sample to see what progress has been made and what the next step is.

CHAPTER 21

ZAPPERS

Being able to kill your bacteria and other invaders with electricity seems like a panacea, especially when you can do it all in three, seven-minute sessions. But killing things that your body should have been able to kill itself, or things that should not have gotten into the body in the first place, should make us think: "Why did this happen to me? Could I have prevented this?" Prevention is infinitely better than treatment, and is the true goal for us all. Nevertheless, zappers are a superb help when the complete picture is kept in mind. This means respect for the immune system, understanding our extreme dependence on it for survival of our species.

The evolution of the zapper from the earlier frequency generator is described in *The Cure For All Diseases*. The advantage of not needing to know the frequency of the pathogens you wish to kill makes it exceptionally useful.

No matter what frequency your zapper is set at (within reason), it kills large and small invaders: flukes, roundworms, mites, bacteria, viruses and fungi. It kills them all at once, in seven minutes, even at 5 volts. But the current does have to reach them and there are certain hard-to-reach places: for instance the eyes, the appendix, the testes, the inner ear bones and most of the contents of the intestine.

How does it work? I suppose that a *Positive* voltage applied anywhere on the body attracts *Negatively* charged things such as bacteria. Perhaps the battery voltage tugs at them, pulling them out of their locations in the cell doorways (called *conductance channels*). But doorways can be *Negatively* charged too. Does the voltage tug at them so they disgorge any bacteria stuck in them? Perhaps it just closes these doorways. How would the *Positive* voltage act to kill a large parasite like a fluke? These questions cannot be answered yet, although the evidence is clear: a sudden release of parasite eggs into the blood, bits of parasite in the white blood cells, and later, the appearance of mold just where the flukes had been. Killing action is also suggested when a large fluke can no longer be heard on the Syncrometer® (meaning its frequency cannot be heard) in seven minutes.

Another earlier question has a clear answer, now. Is the killing effect due to immune system stimulation? The answer is "*Yes*". The empowering effect on white blood cells is seen when they suddenly possess parts of the fluke and bacteria, when minutes before zapping they did not.

Other fascinating possibilities are that the intermittent *Positive* voltage interferes with electron flow in some key metabolic route, or straightens out the ATP molecule disallowing its breakdown. Could it pull off course the electrons headed for RNA to make DNA? Such biological questions could be answered by studying the effects of *Positive* electrical pulses on pathogens in a laboratory. Some research of this kind has already been published and has shown good results (see footnote on page 506).

The most important question, of course, is whether there is a harmful effect on you. I have seen no effects on blood pressure, mental alertness, or body temperature. It has never produced pain, although it has often stopped pain instantly. This does not by itself prove safety. Even knowing that the voltage comes from a small 9-volt battery does not rigorously prove safety although it is reassuring. The fact that thousands of zappers are in use suggests safety, too. And finding that one of its mechanisms is through the immune system, makes it even more appealing. Viruses and bacteria disappear in three minutes; tapeworm stages, flukes, roundworms in five; and mites in seven. People who are not ill need not go beyond this time, although no bad effects have been seen at any length of treatment.

The first seven-minute zapping is followed by an intermission, lasting 20 to 30 minutes. During this time, bacteria and viruses are released from the dying parasites and start to invade you instead. Such releases form the basis of “detoxification-illness”, which must be controlled and counteracted. Each parasite has its own bacterial and viral escapees.

The second seven-minute session is intended to kill these newly released viruses and bacteria. If you omit it, you could catch a cold, sore throat or something else immediately. In fact, if you do, you know you killed some serious parasites. Again, viruses are released, this time from the dying bacteria. The third session kills the last viruses released.

A fourth and fifth session may be very beneficial, too, especially when we see bits of protein called “prion protein” streaming from the parasite Macracanthorhynchus, and killed Salmonella bacteria. But not enough experiments are completed to be sure these are their origins or that everyone needs extra sessions. Remember, cancer patients will be plate-zapping for 20-minute sessions anyway. So, the need for more regular zapping sessions is not yet certain.

That is all there is to it. Almost all. The zapping current travels best through blood and lymph, two rather salty (conductive) fluids. But it does not reach deep into the eyeball or testicle or bowel contents. It does not reach into your gallstones, or into your living cells where Herpes virus lies latent or Candida fungus extends its fingers. To reach deeper, the herbal parasite program (page 154) and homeography should be added to the zapper treatment.

Do Not Zap if you are Pregnant or Wearing a Pacemaker.

These situations have not been explored yet. Don't do these experiments yourself. Children as young as eight months have been zapped with no noticeable ill effects. For them, you should weigh the possible benefits against the unknown risks.

Cancer victims have many nerve endings covered with motor oil and wheel bearing grease, which bring PCBs and benzene with them. You cannot pass enough electricity through your hands or wrists due to these insulators, nor will it penetrate the tumor effectively.

To reach specific organs electrically, with a significant effect, you will need to do plate-zapping (see page 528) and use foot electrodes. You merely need to put a sample of similar organ tissue on the zapping plate.

For cancer victims, copper pipe electrodes are placed under the feet just in front of the heels. The choice of copper is important because it is the most conductive metal, besides silver. The pressure of your feet on the pipes helps the current penetrate. Hand pressure is hard to keep up. A flat electrode provides too little pressure under the foot for good penetration.

Blood and lymph are still the most important locations to zap. These are reachable by regular zapping (without a plate). Using foot electrodes helps greatly, for both plate-zapping and regular zapping.

The circuit with this surprising health benefit produced a totally *Positive* electrical field at all times, called "*Positive* offset". But many zappers were built with small substitutions when the exact components were not available. This often brought the resulting electrical field too close to *Negative* so that brief excursions into the *Negative* field were inevitable. Even very brief "*Negative* spikes" are undesirable. For this reason the circuit given here has an additional component, a *Positive* offset resistor. With this addition, it is easy for the builder to measure the *Positive* offset on an oscilloscope. It will be ¼ volt. **Anyone purchasing a zapper should ask for this measurement. The consumer should also request copper electrodes of tubular design and plates of correct dimension (3¼ to 3½ inches square) and composition (aluminum).**

Although wrist straps are convenient, not enough research has been done to accurately compare effectiveness with the tubular design of electrodes. A very ill person should use the copper tube electrodes, of correct dimension, correctly placed and not risk poor conduction.

Zapping once a day is now a common routine for many persons. The elderly seem to be keeping more alert for their years. For many it is a daily pain-reliever, fatigue-lifter, or mystery-helper. For the ill, zapping all day, continuously, for a month or more has often brought significant improvement. Only further research can shed light on how all this happens.

Just as amazing as its action is the simplicity of the circuit design. Even a complete novice could build one.

Building A Zapper

You will be given two ways to build a zapper: the **shoebox** way and the **breadboard** way. The breadboard way for a 1000 Hz (1 kHz) zapper is on page 533.

Both have ¼ volt *Positive* offset. You will be able to test your zapper (or any commercially made one) for its *Positive* offset feature simply by observing it on an oscilloscope.

Parts List for 30 kHz Zapper Circuit Shoebox Way	
Item	**Radio Shack Catalog Number**
Shoebox	
9-volt battery	
9-volt battery snap connector	270-324 (set of 5, you need 1)
on-off toggle switch	275-624A micro mini toggle switch
If not available, choose any toggle switch with holes in the contact points or Radio Shack 275-612	
1 KΩ resistor, brown-black-red-gold	271-312 (500 piece assortment) use 2
3.9 KΩ resistor, orange-white-red-gold	Use 2 from the 500 piece assortment
39 KΩ resistor, orange-white-orange-gold	From 500 piece assortment
low-current red LED	276-044
.0047 uF capacitor	272-130 (set of 2, you need 1)
.01 uF capacitor	272-131 (set of 2, you need 1)
555 CMOS timer chip(TLC 55)	276-1718 (may wish to buy a spare)
8 pin wire-wrapping socket for the chip	900-7242
If only 16 pin sockets are available, cut one in half OR leave half empty.	
short (12”) alligator clip leads	any electronics shop, get 10
If not available, use 14” length from Radio Shack, 278-1156	
Micro clip jumper wires	278-017 (need 2 packages of 2)
If not available, use mini-clip jumper wires 278-016	
2 bolts, about $^1/_8$” diameter, 2” long, with 4 nuts and 4 washers	hardware store
2 copper pipes, ¾” diameter, 4” long	hardware store
sharp knife, pin, long-nose pliers, tape, 4 twist ties or rubber bands	

Hints for absolute novices: Don’t let unusual vocabulary deter you. A “lead” is just a piece of wire used to make connections. When you remove a component from its package, label it with a piece of tape. A serrated kitchen knife is useful, as well as a large safety pin. Practice using the micro clips. If the metal ends are L-shaped bend them into a U with the long-nose pliers so they grab better. Chips and chip holders (wire wrap sockets) are very fragile. It is wise to purchase an extra one of each in case you break the connections. The "555" timer is a widely used component; if you can't locate this one, try another electronics shop or see *Sources*.

The Shoebox Way

This circuit has been improved since the one given in earlier books.

A resistor has been added that gives every pulse an added *Positive* offset of ¼ volt. You no longer need to operate your zapper so daringly close to a *Negative* voltage.

To build your zapper you may take this list of components to any electronics store (Radio Shack part numbers are given for convenience). You may also order a kit, see *Sources* or enquire.

Assembling the Zapper

1. You will be using the lid of the shoebox to mount the components. Save the box base to enclose the finished project.

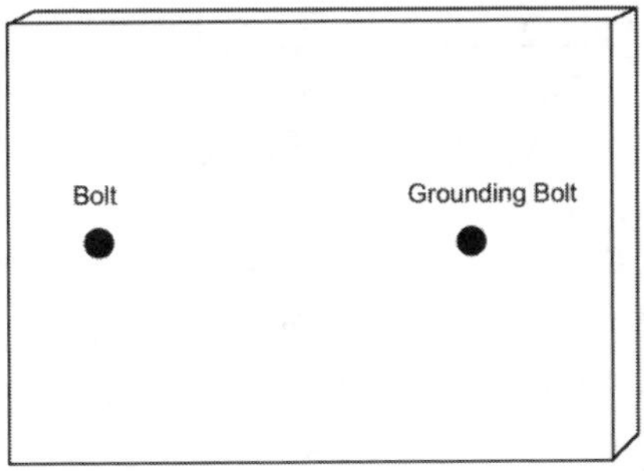

2. Pierce two holes near the ends of the lid. Enlarge the holes with a pen or pencil until the bolts would fit through. Mount the bolts from the outside about half way through the holes so there is a washer and nut holding it in place on both sides. Tighten. Label one hole "grounding bolt" on the inside and outside.

3. Mount the 555 chip in the wire wrap socket. Find the "top end" of the chip by searching the outside surface carefully for a cookie-shaped bite taken out of it or an imprinted dot. Align the chip with the socket and very gently squeeze the pins of the chip into the socket until they click in place.

4. Make 8 pinholes to fit the wire wrap socket. Enlarge them slightly with a sharp pencil. Mount it from the outside. Write in the numbers of the pins (connections) on both the outside and inside, starting with number one, near the "cookie bite", as

seen from outside. After number 4, cross over to number 5 and continue. Number 8 will be across from number 1.

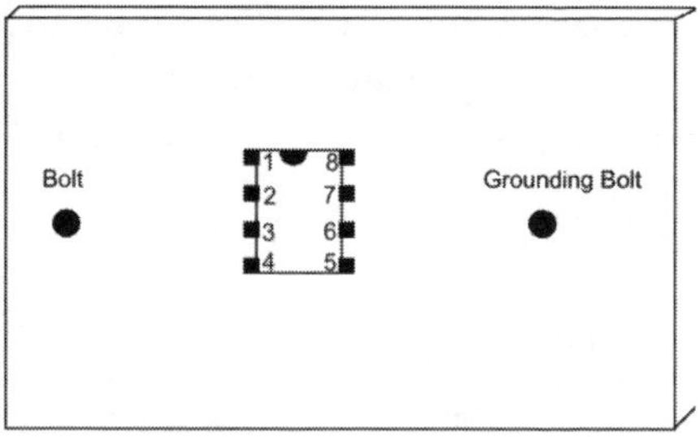

5. Pierce two holes ½ inch apart very near to pins 5, 6, 7, and 8. They should be less than $^1/_8$ inch away. (Or, one end of each component can share a hole with the 555 chip.) Mount the .01 uF capacitor near pin 5 on the outside. On the inside connect pin 5 to one end of this capacitor by simply twisting them together. Loop the capacitor wire around the pin first; then twist with the long-nose pliers until you have made a tight connection. Bend the other wire from the capacitor flat against the inside of the shoebox lid. Label it .01 on the outside and inside. Mount the .0047 uF capacitor near pin 6. On the inside twist the capacitor wire around the pin. Flatten the wire from the other end and label it .0047. Mount the 3.9 KΩ resistor near pin 7, connecting it on the inside to the pin. Flatten the wire on the other end and label it 3.9 K. Mount the 1 KΩ resistor and connect it similarly to pin 8 and label it 1 K.

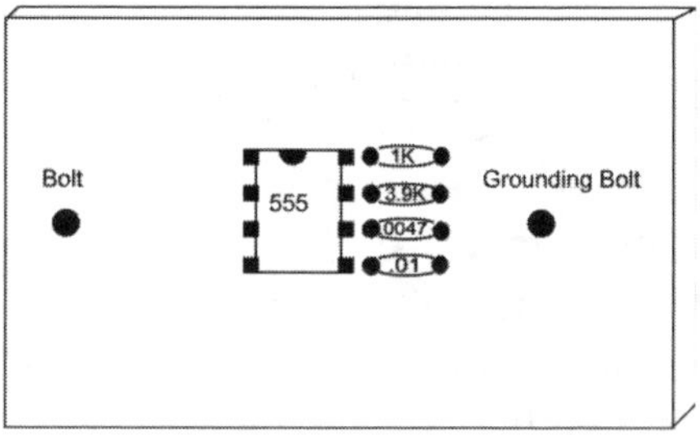

6. Pierce two holes ½ inch apart next to pin 3 (again, you can share the hole for pin 3 if you wish), in the direction of the bolt. Mount the 1 KΩ resistor and label inside and outside. Twist the connections together and flatten the remaining wire. This resistor protects the circuit if you should accidentally short the terminals. Mount the 3.9 KΩ resistor downward. One end can go in the same hole as the 1 KΩ resistor near pin 3. Twist that end around pin 3 which already has the 1 KΩ resistor attached to it. Flatten the far end. Label.

7. Next to the 3.9 KΩ resistor pierce two holes ¼ inch apart for the LED. Notice that the LED has a *Positive* and *Negative*

connection. The longer wire is the anode (*Positive*). The flattened side of the red dome marks the *Negative* wire. Mount the LED from the outside and bend back the wires, labeling them (+) and (-) on the inside.

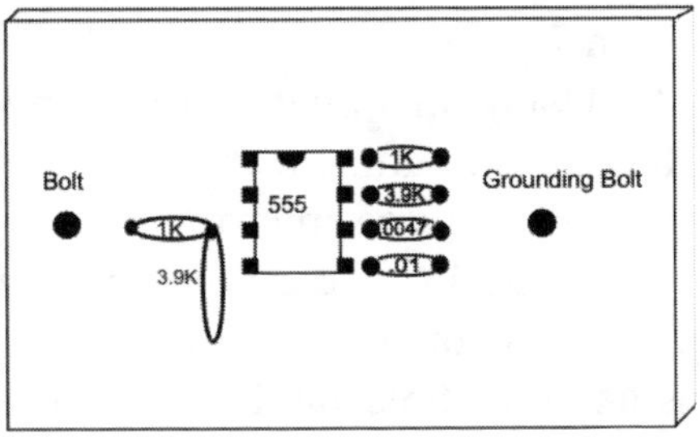

8. Near the top pierce a hole for the toggle switch. Enlarge it until the shaft fits through from the inside. Remove nut and washer from switch before mounting. You may need to trim away some paper with a serrated knife before replacing washer and nut on the outside. Tighten.

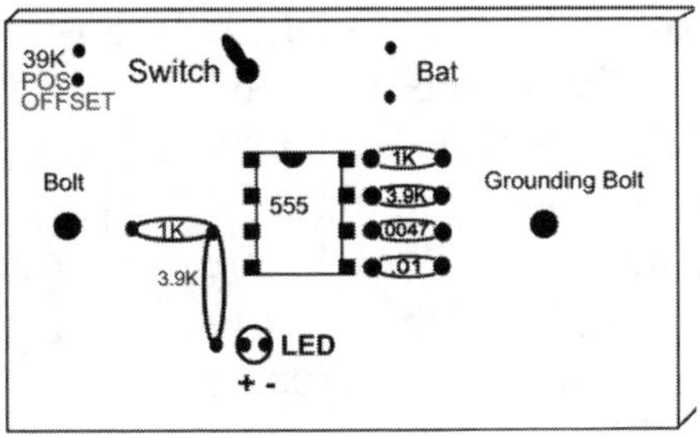

9. Next to the switch pierce two holes for the wires from the battery snap connector and poke them through from the outside. Do not attach the battery yet.

10. An inch away from the switch pierce two holes ¼ inch apart. Mount the 39 KΩ resistor from the outside and label it inside and outside as "39 K, *Positive* offset." Flatten the wires on the inside.

Now to Connect Everything

First, make slits at each corner of the lid with a knife. They will accommodate extra loops of wire that you get from using the clip leads to make connections. After each connection gently tuck away the excess wire through the most convenient slit.

1. Twist the free ends of the two capacitors (.01 and .0047) together. Connect this to the grounding bolt using an alligator clip.

2. Bend the top ends of pin 2 and pin 6 (which already has a connection) inward towards each other in an L shape. Catch

them both together with an alligator clip and attach the other end of the alligator clip to the free end of the 3.9 KΩ resistor by pin 7.

3. Using an alligator clip connect pin 7 to the free end of the 1 KΩ resistor attached to pin 8.

4. Using three micro clips connect pin 8 to one end of the switch, pin 4 to the same end of the switch, and one end of the offset resistor to the same end of the switch. (Put one hook inside the hole and the other hooks around the whole connection. Check to make sure they are securely connected.) Connect the free end of the offset resistor to the bolt using an alligator clip.

5. Use an alligator clip to connect the free end of the 1 KΩ resistor (by pin 3) to the bolt. It is the output resistor.

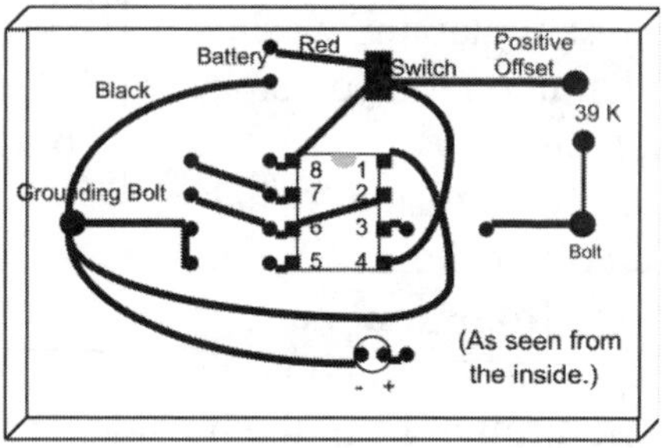

6. Twist the free end of the 3.9 KΩ resistor by pin 3 around the plus end of the LED. Connect the minus end of the LED to the grounding bolt using an alligator clip.

7. Connect pin number 1 on the chip to the grounding bolt with an alligator clip.

8. Attach an alligator clip to the outside of one of the bolts. Attach the other end to a handhold (copper pipe). Do the same for the other bolt and handhold.

9. Connect the minus end of the battery snap connector (black wire) to the grounding bolt with an alligator clip.

10. Connect the plus end of the battery snap connector (red wire) to the free end of the switch using a micro clip lead. Attach the battery <u>very carefully</u>. Before attaching the battery to its snap connector, cover one terminal with tape. After snapping in one terminal, remove the tape to attach the other terminal. This is to prevent accidental touching of terminals in a backwards direction. If the LED lights up you know the switch is ON. If it does not, flip the switch and see if the LED lights. Label the switch clearly. If you cannot get the LED to

light in either switch position, double-check all of your connections, and make sure you have a fresh battery. Even if it does light up, check every connection again.

11. Finally tie up the bunches of wire pushed through the slits in the corners with twist-ties or rubber bands and replace the lid on the box. Slip a couple of rubber bands around the box to keep it securely shut. For safer storage, place it inside a larger box.

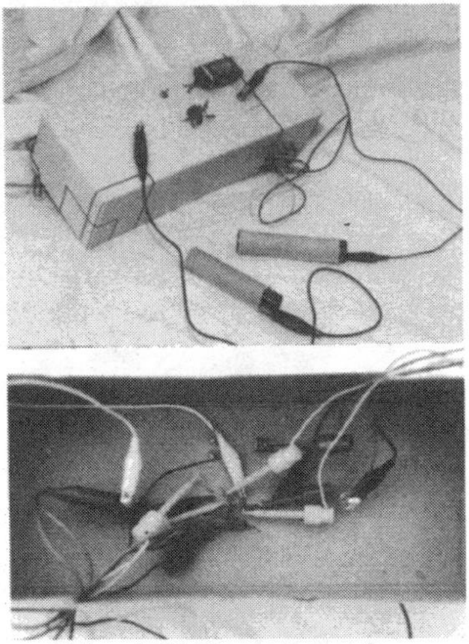

Fig. 117 Zapper under construction

***NOTE*:** Having gained this much experience, you may prefer to build your next zapper on a piece of cardboard folded in the shape of a bench, ⎍, and able to fit <u>inside</u> a shoebox for more protection.

- Optional: measure the frequency of your zapper by connecting an oscilloscope or frequency counter to the handholds. Any electronics shop can do this. It should read between 20 and 40 kHz. (The shop can also read the voltage [peak to peak] and the amount of *Positive* offset [on the .5 volt-per-division scale]). The voltage output should be about 8 volts when you are holding the handholds.
- ***NOTE***: a voltmeter will only read 4 to 5 volts because it displays an <u>average</u> voltage.
- Optional: observe the square wave pulses without holding on to the handholds. They begin to rise from a base voltage of about ¼ volt. This is the "*Positive* offset". The tops and bottoms of each pulse are flat, each lasting about the same time (50%) called the duty cycle. The rise and fall of each pulse is vertical, without a spike in the *Negative* direction (down). When you grasp the handholds (called "under load") the peak-to-peak voltage drops considerably, and the shape has rounded instead of square corners for each pulse. This is a reflection on your body's capacitance; it is normal.

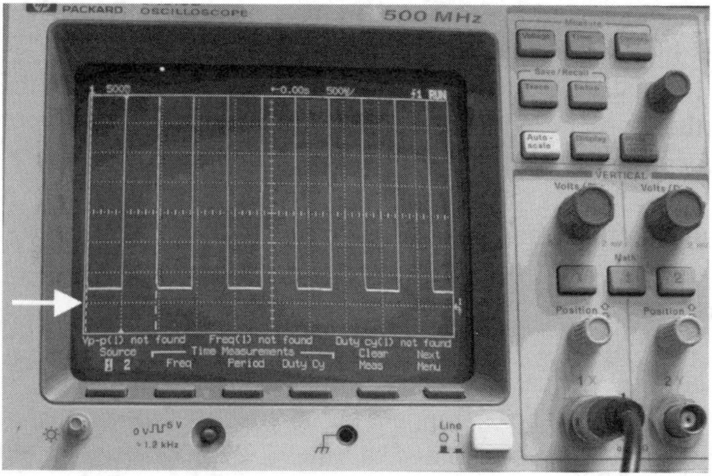

At a range of .5 volts per division, it is easy to see the offset. Before the unit is turned on, the zero line is found at arrow on left side of oscilloscope screen. (Also see arrow at right side). Turning the zapper on shows the elevated bottom edge of each pulse. Also, no spikes go below the zero line into the *Negative* field at any time.

Fig. 118 Zapper output with ¼ volt Positive offset

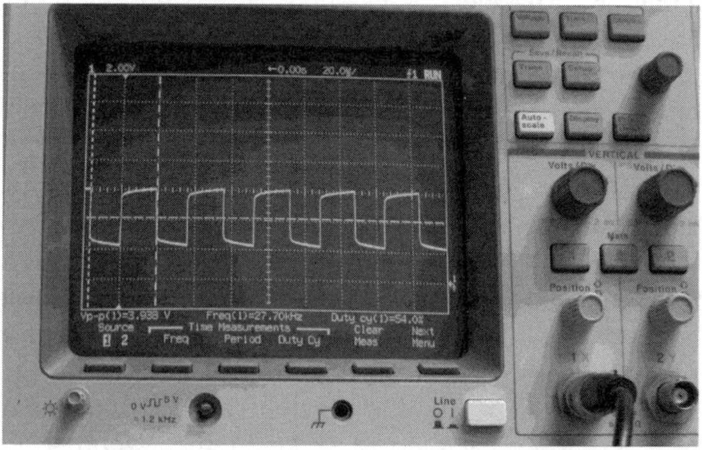

Duty cycle, voltage and frequency are less important than absence of *Negative* spikes and presence of the extra ¼ volt *Positive* offset.

Fig. 119 Zapper output under load shows effect of body capacitance.

- Optional: measure the current that flows through you when you are getting zapped. You will need a 1 KΩ carbon resistor and oscilloscope. Connect the grounding bolt on the zapper to one end of the resistor. Connect the other end of the resistor to a handhold. (Adding this resistor to the circuit decreases the current slightly, but not significantly.) The other handhold is attached to the other bolt. Connect the scope ground wire to one end of the resistor. Turn the zapper ON and grasp the handholds. Read the voltage on the scope. It will read about 3.5 volts. Calculate current by dividing voltage by resistance. 3.5 volts divided by 1 KΩ is 3.5 ma (milliamperes) of current.

Could you build this zapper the breadboard way? Yes, see page 533, and use the 30 kHz parts list.

If Someone Else Builds your Zapper

PARTS LIST

R1	1 K
R2	3.9 K
R3	1 K
R4	3.9 K
R5	39 K
C1	.01 µf
C2	.0047µf
U3	MC1455
LED	2 ma LED red

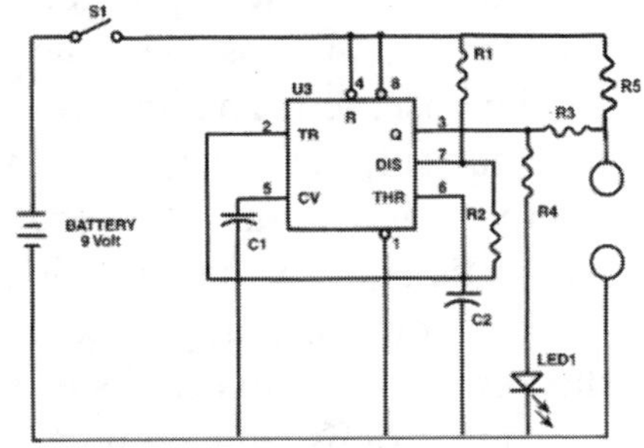

Give this to an electronics person to build in a project box.

Fig. 120 Zapper schematic

Using The Zapper

1. Wrap handholds in <u>one</u> layer of wet paper towel before using. More will reduce the current. Grasp securely and turn the switch on to zap. Keep a bottle of water handy to keep them wet.
2. Zap for seven minutes, let go of the handholds, turn off the zapper, and rest for 20 minutes. Then seven minutes on, 20 minutes rest, and a final seven minutes on. This is the routine for regular zapping.

3. For plate-zapping stay connected for 20 minutes at any one tissue location, and move on to others after that.

Testing the Zapper

Trying the zapper on an illness to see "if it works" is not useful. Your symptoms may be due to a non-parasite. Or you may reinfect within hours of zapping. The best way to test your device is to find a few invaders that you currently have. (This is described in the *Syncrometer® Science Laboratory Manual*, Exp. #13). This gives you an exact starting point. Then zap yourself. After the triple zapping, none of these invaders should be present. If they do survive, especially the larger ones like Fasciola flukes, they are undoubtedly saturated by an insulating substance such as PCBs, Freon or benzene. For this reason, plate-zapping is chosen.

Plate-Zapping

By passing the zapper current through a capacitor plate in the same manner as the Syncrometer® current, a similar effect can be observed. The item placed on the plate directs or invites the current; in fact, nothing else will be zapped. My interpretation is that the capacitor plate on the resonance box has a "standing wave" relationship to an identical capacitance in your body (actually, a capacitance-inductance unit), making the resistance between them essentially zero. For this reason the dimensions and composition of the capacitor plates are important. Nearly all the current will go to this location in your body. The standing wave relationship can be seen for the Syncrometer® where the addition of two picofarads capacitance to the plate destroys resonance, but the further addition of two microhenrys inductance restores it again.

Only make plate-zappers as described below. Other shapes, sizes and compositions have either not been tested or not been found useful.

Making A Plate-Zapper

I have experimented and gotten good results from two configurations. One uses two sardine can lids to form a single plate. The second uses two pieces of aluminum as separate plates. The advantage of the first configuration is that it is easy to make from items around your home. The advantage of the second configuration is you can zap two locations at once. Theoretically, a three-plate, or four-plate, or fifty-plate configuration would increase efficiency even more, but it would also bring a proportional increase in detoxification-illness.

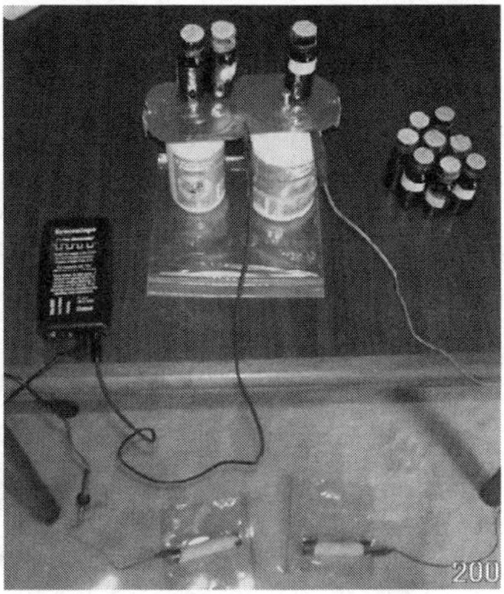

Using a homemade or purchased zapper, connect the *Positive* output to your sardine can plate. From there another lead goes to a foot electrode (copper pipe). The *Negative* output goes to the other foot. One location and a few bacteria are on the plate.

Fig. 121 Homemade plate-zapper

Single Plate-Zapper

The easiest plate-zapper to build uses sardine can lids (not other cans). After careful washing and unrolling to make the surface as flat as possible, you mount them on the LIDS of empty vitamin bottles (the kind with plastic caps). Make a nail hole near the center of each lid and bottle cap. Find sheet metal screws to fit the holes. Tighten the can lids to the bottle caps just enough to be still movable by finger touch.

Place your two lids so they overlap slightly. They are held together tightly by the grip of an alligator clip lead, making a single plate out of it. Fasten the other end of the alligator clip to the bolt of your homemade zapper (***Positive*** side). Now attach a second alligator clip lead from this plate to a copper pipe. A third alligator clip lead goes from your zapper grounding bolt to the second copper pipe as usual.

The two can lids must be very securely connected at all times. Use copper pipes for best contact to your body. The high frequency and single layer of wet paper prevent the copper from penetrating your skin.

Double Plate-Zapper

Get two $^1/_{32}$ inch (1 mm) thick aluminum plates. They should be 3¼ to 3½ inch (8 to 9 cm) square. Drill a hole in the center of each one and mount on a cardboard or plastic box with bolts. Place them about 2-3 inches (5-8 cm) apart.

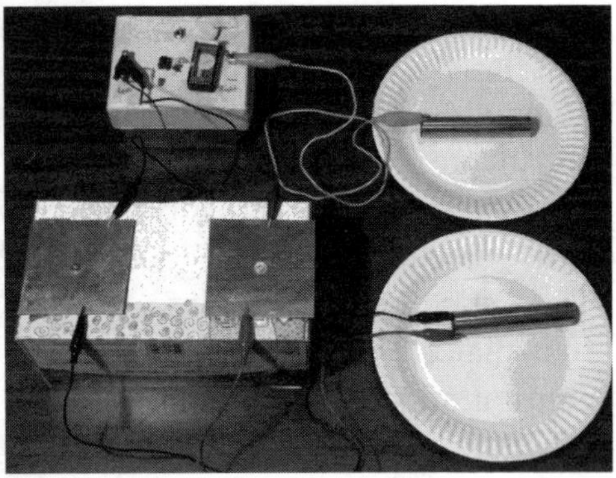

Fig. 122 Double plate-zapper

Run a lead from the *Positive* output of your zapper to each of the plates (two leads altogether, clip them directly onto the edge of each plate). Then run a lead from each plate to one of the copper pipes. There is a lead from the *Negative* output of the zapper to the second copper pipe as usual. You will need five alligator clip leads altogether.

Plate-Zapping Tips

Because you should use your feet to zap, you may wish to put the copper tubes on the floor. The tubes should be wrapped with only one layer of wet paper towel. To protect your floor, shove paper plates inside plastic bags underneath the tubes.

With plate-zapping, a 9-volt battery will wear out even quicker than for other arrangements. Of course, your body is benefiting from this greater energy input by converting it, in some way, for itself. You need to check the battery voltage after every zap at first. If the battery voltage ends up at 8.9 or lower, you will have to repeat the last zap. Start each zap at no less than 9.4 v. Expect to drain about .4 volts from the battery for each zap using this dual plate arrangement. Get rechargeable batteries, a battery charger, and a voltmeter all of which will save you money and delays.

For detailed instructions see the *Plate-Zapping Schedule* on page 173.

The Zappicator

Attaching a zapper to a loudspeaker brings the electric pulses to the magnet that makes the speaker's paper cone vibrate. The paper cone vibrates the air at the same frequency. We can hear this if the electric pulses are at the correct frequency for our ears, which is from 20 Hz to 20,000 Hz (vibrations per second).

If we attach a zapper to a speaker we would not hear any sound, because the zapper outputs a frequency of about 30,000 Hz (too high), although the vibrations continue. Each pulse is shorter now and might reach the molecules themselves, the way a passing train can rattle the dishes in your cupboard. If the correct frequency is found you could "rattle" a specific molecule and perhaps destroy it without harming the neighbors. That was the theory. But experiments showed that the incoming pulses had to be totally *Positive* (100%) and the circular magnet around the speaker had to be producing a north pole magnetic field to have such an effect. Moreover, if an actual current was running through the loudspeaker, the whole phenomenon vanished!

I experimented with other frequencies, hoping to find one that not only destroyed bacteria and viruses, but "bad molecules" like phenolics (allergens) in food. I found 1,000 Hz worked well, which surprised me because I expected a much higher frequency.

I could not understand the physics involved, but there were no exceptions. Only the single lead attachment worked, from the (+) output of the zapper to the (+) end of the speaker. If the (-) end was used at all, this unusual chemistry does not occur. The loudspeaker must be acting as if it were an antenna, suggesting that resonance is involved in finding and destroying the "bad molecules." Fortunately I did not find evidence that "good molecules" like vitamins and organic minerals were affected. They let the pulses pass through unnoticed, like open gates letting through the traffic. But "bad molecules," like food allergens, PCBs, benzene and phenol were destroyed. In fact, phenol appeared after benzene disappeared reminding us of the benzene-detoxification pathway. After this, wood alcohol appeared as if phenol molecules had broken in half. With longer zappication even this wood alcohol disappeared, producing formaldehyde, and this broke down further to formic acid. Some significant "chemistry" is going on during zappication.

Zappicating food is so beneficial you are encouraged to build this device. The circuit is just like the zapper, but with a few component changes to lower the frequency to 1000±5 Hz.

There will be no sound because no current is flowing. But a very tiny voltage and the 1 kHz frequency are affecting all the food that touches the plate or touches other food that is touching the plate. That is easy to see on a frequency counter.

The zappicator circuit will also have the *Positive* offset feature, namely, a special resistor to produce a ¼ volt offset, so no *Negative* voltage could ever be delivered accidentally. It will produce a frequency of 1000 Hz, instead of 30,000.

Building The Zappicator

The zappicator has two parts:

- a speaker box (with one or two loudspeakers) where food is placed and
- a 1 kHz zapper to supply power to the box

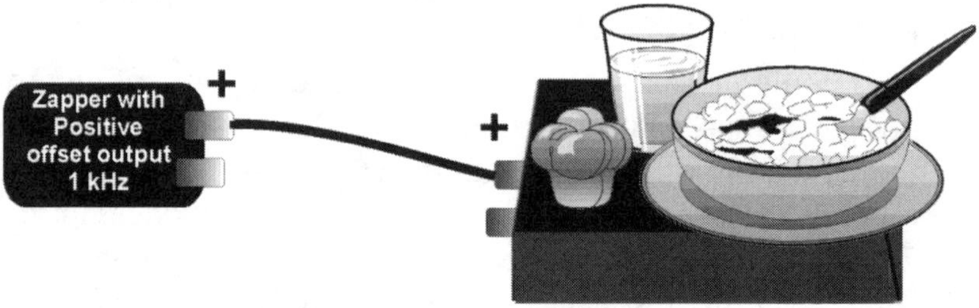

Fig. 123 Zappicator with speaker box & 1 kHz zapper

First we will build the 1 kHz zapper. We will build it on a breadboard to avoid the tangle of wires, clip leads, and the soldering of other methods.

The Breadboard Way

Instructions for making a 1 kHz zapper:

Parts List for Zappicator Circuit	
Item	**Radio Shack Catalog Number**
9-volt battery	
9-volt battery snap connector	270-324 (set of 5, you need 1)
on-off toggle switch	275-624A micro-mini toggle switch
if not available, choose any toggle switch with holes in the terminals, OR Radio Shack 275-612	
1 KΩ resistor, brown-black-red-gold (2)	271-312 (500 piece assortment)
2.2 KΩ resistor, red-red-red-gold	use one in the assortment
4.4 KΩ resistor	use one of the 4.7 KΩ resistors in the assortment (yellow-violet-red-gold)
144 KΩ resistor	use two of the 270 KΩ resistors in the assortment (red-violet-yellow-gold)
39 KΩ resistor (for *Positive* offset) orange-white-orange-gold	use one in the assortment
low-current red LED 2 ma	276-044
.0047 uF capacitor (2)	272-130 (set of two)
555 CMOS timer chip (TLC 555)	276-1718 (you might want to buy a spare)
*alligator clip leads (2)	any electronics shop
or use Radio Shack 278-1156 (set of 10)	
breadboard	276-175 (called Experimenter Socket)
breadboard wires	276-173
*2 copper pipes, ¾ inch diameter, 4 inches long	plumbing store
long nose pliers, scotch tape, wire stripper	

**you won't need these while you are zappicating with this circuit.*

The total cost, as of 2007, was about $35.00 not including the copper pipes.

A breadboard is a plastic pad with holes in it. If you look closely at the Radio Shack "Experimenter Socket," you can see the rows are lettered A through J, while the two outermost rows are X and Y. The columns are numbered 1 through 23. Any other breadboard will work, too. The components connect by contacting a metal board under the holes. Here are some tips for the novice builder:

If the end of a wire is not bare, use a sharp knife to scrape off about ¼ inch (1 cm) of the plastic insulation. When stripping wire, if you accidentally cut some of the wire strands off, then cut them all off and start fresh. Hopefully you will succeed before you run out of wire!

If the wire is solid, great, but if it is stranded then twist it with your fingers to help keep the strands together.

When you push a wire (either solid or stranded) into a hole in the breadboard, you should feel it go in securely. If you tug the wire gently it should not come free. If you turn the breadboard upside down and shake it, nothing should fall out. Sometimes (especially with stranded wire, which is flexible), the wire will bend instead of going in. Just straighten it out and try again. Hold the wire as close to the end as possible to prevent bending, or grab it with long nose pliers.

You don't need to know this, but if you are wondering how the rest of the breadboard works, holes A1 through E1 are connected internally, A2-E2 are connected to themselves, A3-E3, and so forth. Also F1-J1, F2-J2, etc. Finally, X1-X23 and Y1-Y23 are already connected internally. To connect different rows or across the center groove, jumpers are used, of different lengths, called breadboard wires.

The resistors, capacitors, and LED have long, bare wires. Don't let them touch each other; check each one before attaching the battery. You can cut them shorter if you wish. (You can buy wire cutters, but you can also just use household scissors although cutting wire may dull the scissors.)

The resistors and capacitors have no orientation so can go in any way. But the 555 chip does, it has a small circle or dot in one corner. Also, the LED has a flat side on its rim (hard to see but easy to feel) that tells you which way it goes.

If you bought the Radio Shack resistor assortment you may be wondering how you tell them apart! The answer is by the color of the bands on the cylinder. There is a chart on the back of the package, but to make it easy, the 1 KΩ resistor is brown-black-red-gold; the 2.2 KΩ resistor is red-red-red-gold; the 4.7 KΩ resistor is yellow-violet-red-gold; the 39 KΩ resistor is orange-white-orange-gold and the 270 KΩ resistors are red-violet-yellow-gold. All the resistors in the assortment end with a gold band, so when reading the colors, start at the non-gold end.

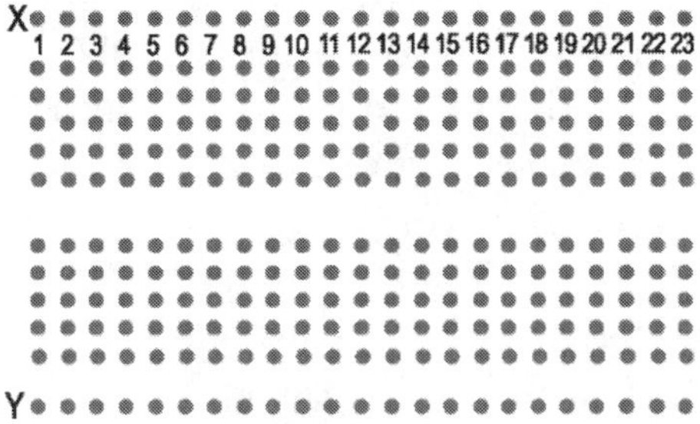

breadboard

The 555 timer chip is sensitive to static electricity. A good way to make sure you are not charged with static electricity is to touch a metal cold water pipe or faucet before handling the chip.

Although you are working with bare wires and electricity, there is little chance of harming yourself. During assembly the battery is not connected. Even while you are using the zapper, there are no voltages higher than the nine volts of the battery in this circuit. Still, take care not to come in contact with the components while the battery is connected in order not to make a spark or damage a component.

Plug in all the components as shown in the pictures.

Attach the battery last. Do this very carefully to avoid accidentally contacting its terminals backwards. Cover one battery terminal with tape first. Then snap in the free terminal. Remove tape and snap in the other terminal.

If you have a voltmeter and wish to check the output you will find it measures approximately 4.5 V. That is because the zapper is switching between nine volts and zero volts about 1000 times per second. The average of nine and zero is 4.5 V.

Step-by-Step Assembly

1. Examine the 555 timer chip. Find the dot or "cookie bite" at one end. This starts the numbering system for the legs, called "pins". The pin nearest to the dot is #1. Count them all. Find the 8th row on the breadboard and insert the chip across the "aisle" or groove as shown. Ease the chip in gently. If the pins refuse to go in evenly on both sides you may ease it out again with your fingernail and press the pins a bit closer together. The chip should lie flat against the breadboard when in place. Each pin connects to the row of 5 dots it is in. Identify the row of dots for each pin.

2. Insert the red wire of the battery snap connector. This will bring *Positive* (+) electricity to the whole row of 23 dots, called X, at the edge of the board.

3. Insert the black wire of the battery snap connector. This connects all the dots on the other edge, called Y, to the *Negative* (-) side of the battery. This is also called "ground". Do not attach the battery yet.

4. Insert the jumper (red) that will bring the (+) electricity to pin 8.

5. Insert the jumper that connects pin 1 to ground. Jiggle the jumpers till they go in smoothly or try a different one. Also try bending the wires slightly inward for easier fitting. You have now completed *Diagram A*.

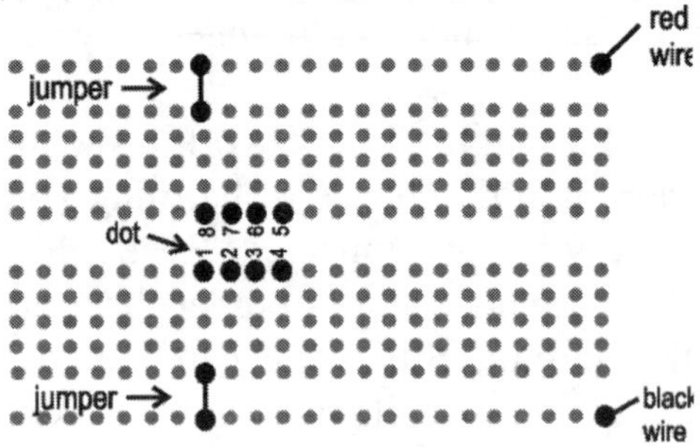

Diagram A

6. Connect pin 8 to pin 7 through a 1 KΩ resistor (brown-black-red-gold). Since this is a very short distance the ends of the resistor will seem too long. Bend one end over and down to make a "hairpin". Then cut both ends about ½ inch (1 cm) from the end of the resistor; then insert.

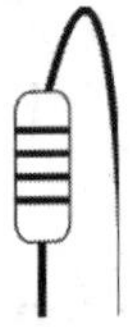

7. Connect the row of dots at pin 7 to pin 6

through a 270 KΩ resistor (red-violet-yellow-gold). Again, bend one end of the resistor in a hairpin; cut the other end off to make them even. Insert. Repeat with a second 270 KΩ resistor right beside it. This "parallel" configuration reduces the resistance to half, namely, 135 KΩ. This value is close enough to 144 KΩ as required on the parts list. This value works as well.

8. Next, you need to connect pin 2 on the 555 chip to pin 6. To do this, choose a jumper (green) that can take you away from the crowded conditions at pin 6, all the way to row 15 from row 10.

9. Then jump from here across the aisle (orange). From here jump to the row of dots at pin 2 (blue). Now pin 6 is connected to pin 2. You have completed *Diagram B*. (Some of your previous connections are omitted for clarity.)

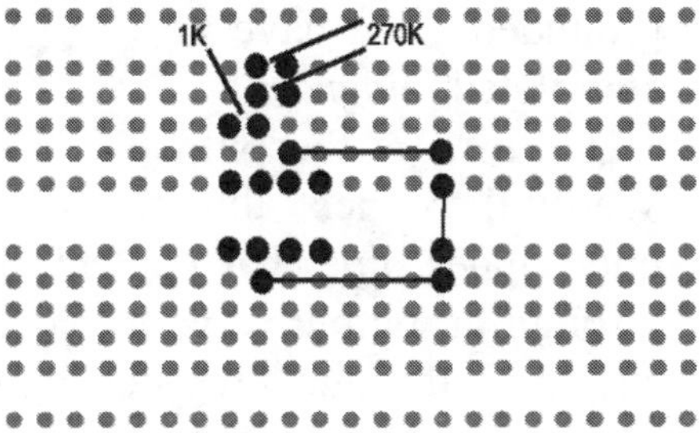

Diagram B

10. Connect pin 6 to another outlying row, such as row 17, through a capacitor, .0047 μF. Push the end at pin 6 in first; then bend the other end slightly inward to insert easily.

11. Insert the other capacitor, also .0047 μF, between pin 5 and the same row. After solid insertion straighten out the wires and make sure no wires are touching other wires inappropriately. If any insertion is especially difficult, use long nose pliers to grasp a wire near its end for firmer pushing.

12. Connect the outlying ends of the capacitors (row 17) to ground using a jumper that crosses the aisle (white).

13. Pin 4 also gets energized by the battery. Connect pin 4 to an outlying row (row 3) with a jumper (gray). Connect the

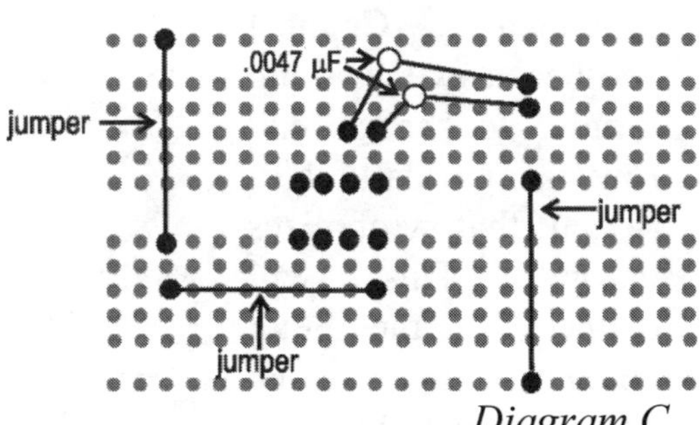

Diagram C

same row to the (+) side of the battery with a jumper. You have now completed *Diagram C*.

14. Now to connect the LED. Connect pin 3 to an unused row, such as 14, through a 2.2 KΩ resistor (red-red-red-gold). Find the flat side of the red dome on the LED. The flat side has the shorter wire.

15. Insert the longer wire of the LED at row 14, the shorter wire at ground. The flat side is grounded. You have now completed *Diagram D*.

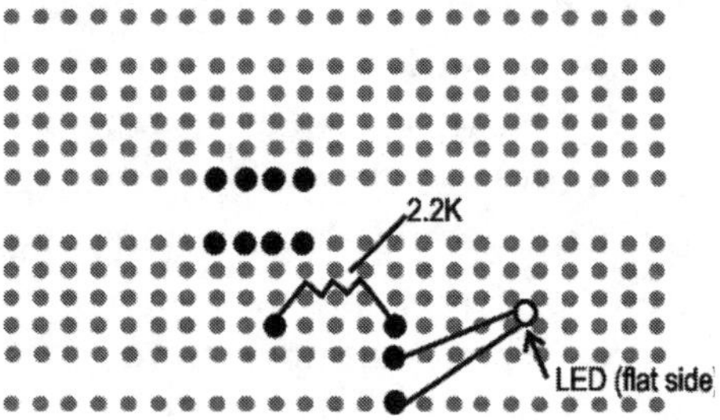

Diagram D

16. Pin 3 is the output. We will connect this to one copper pipe that contacts the body, but we will do this through an output resistor. Connect pin 3 to an outlying row, such as 2, through a resistor of 1000 Ω (brown-black-red-gold). This resistor protects the circuit if you accidentally short the two copper pipes as you hold them.

17. Connect an extra long jumper at row 2; it must reach to the outside of the box that will hold your zapper. Choose a light color that symbolizes the hot (+) wire. You have now completed *Diagram E*.

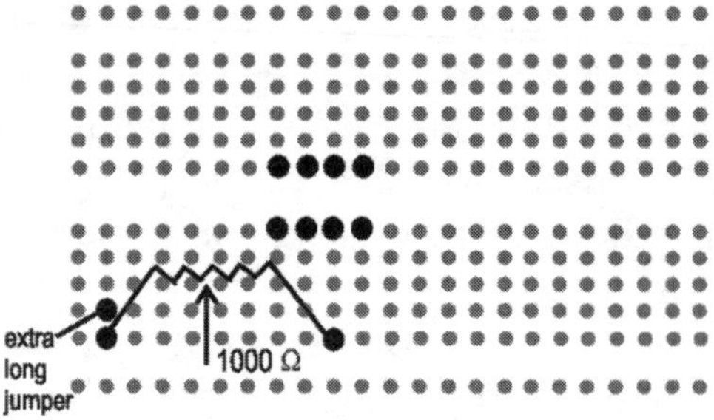

Diagram E

18. Pin 1 is already grounded. Connect another extra long jumper to the ground row, using a dark color (green) that symbolizes ground. This will connect to the other copper pipe that contacts the body.

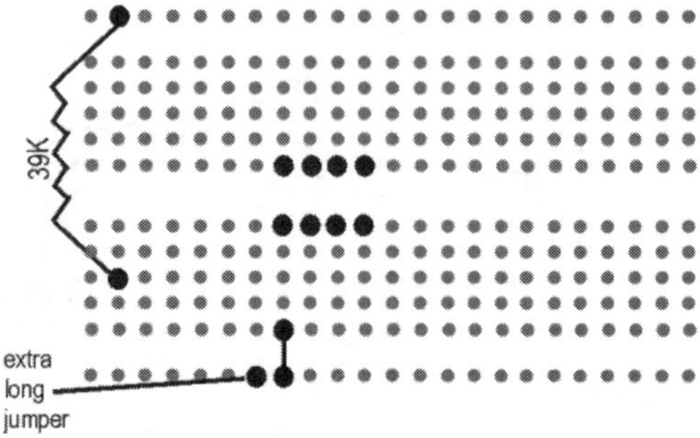

Diagram F

19. Now to add the offset resistor. Connect the 39 KΩ resistor between the battery and the output at row 2. This completes *Diagram F*.

20. To include a switch, pull out the red wire of the battery snap connector from its seat in the breadboard. Cut the red wire in half. Strip ½ inch of insulation from each newly cut end. Practice using the wire stripper on a different piece of wire first. Twist the bare ends into a tight form. Insert one end in the hole of one switch terminal. Make a tight connection. Connect the other bare end to the other switch terminal.

If possible, ask an electronics shop to solder these 2 connections for greater durability. Reinsert the red wire in the breadboard.

21. Connect the battery, but do this VERY CAREFULLY. Remember to cover one battery terminal with tape until the other terminal is safely seated in its holder. Then remove tape and seat the other terminal. You could destroy the chip if you touched the wrong terminals briefly.

22. The LED may now light. If it does not, throw the switch.

23. For protection you may place your zapper inside a plastic container with lid. Mount the switch and battery on the outside for convenience.

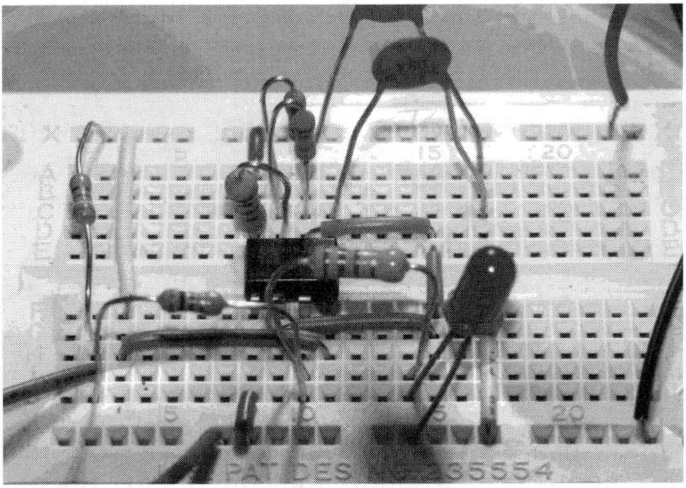

Fig. 124 Finished breadboard zapper (1 kHz) for zappicating foods

Troubleshooting

If the LED still doesn't light, it may be in backwards. Disconnect the battery, tape over one terminal, turn the LED around, and reconnect the battery. Being in backwards does not harm the LED. If it still does not light, or flickers, suspect the switch connections. Remove the switch or solder it.

If the battery gets hot, disconnect it immediately! Check that there are no bare wires touching each other. Double-check that your wiring matches the picture. You may have drained the battery a lot, so replace it with a new one.

If everything looks perfect, but the LED still doesn't light, you may have a defective component. That's why the Parts List advises getting a spare 555 timer chip. The 555 is the most likely component to fail. Disconnect the battery and try swapping chips (pay attention to which corner has the circle). None of the rest of the components are likely to fail, but you can try swapping them if you like.

Make sure your battery is fresh. Use a battery tester.

Seeing the Output

An oscilloscope shows you a high-speed picture of how the voltage changes. You can actually "see" the zapper go from zero to nine volts and back repeatedly. And you can calculate the frequency to make sure it is about 1000 hertz (low-frequency) or 30,000 hertz (regular zapper).

Oscilloscopes are expensive, so rather than buy one, it is better to ask your local television or VCR repair shop if they would use their oscilloscope to check your zapper. Here is how the zapper output typically looks. When your zapper is turned on, the bottom flat lines of each pulse should be ¼ volt above (more *Positive*) the zero line. To see the offset more clearly, change to .5 volts per division, see page 527.

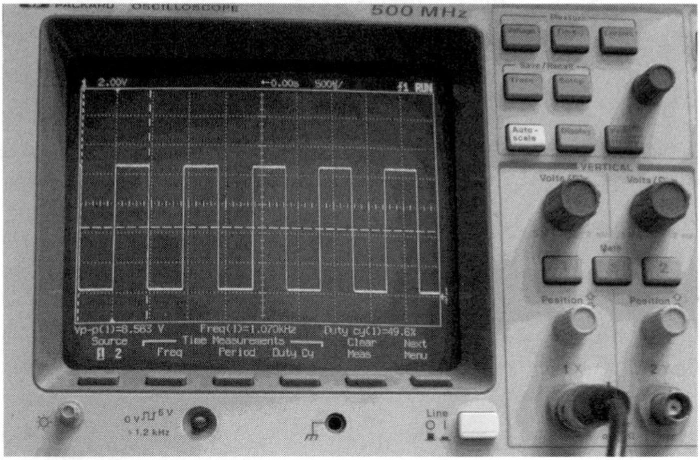

The *Positive* offset is visible just above the zero line.

Fig. 125 Output as seen at 2 volts per division range

Making the Zappicator Food Box

Get these supplies:

- zapper with a 1 kHz output, like you just made
- plastic carton, such as a cottage cheese or food container, or a plastic project box
- 4 ohm or 8 ohm loudspeaker, 2" or 2½" (5-7 cm) diameter, with a north pole face
- one alligator-to-banana clip lead (a piece of insulated wire with an alligator clip at one end and a banana clip at the other) to fit your zapper. Whatever fits is acceptable.
- compass
- roll of tape, sharp knife

Dropping the speaker or overheating it could change the polarity. Check yours before use with a compass once a week.

Many loudspeakers on the market are south pole. Be careful. Take your compass with you as you shop; the compass' north should be attracted to the face (see picture). A field strength of 10 to 20 gauss is preferred. This means the magnet on the speaker should be able to lift a loose chain of six paper clips. The current and watt ratings given for the speaker are not important. Some loudspeakers have "collars", or domes, or are encased, or shielded. Do not choose them. They do not work.

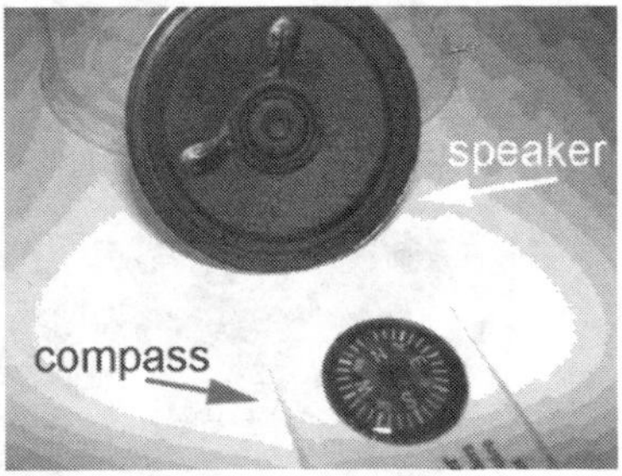

Fig. 126 Choose speaker with north pole face

The magnetic field is not necessarily stable either.

Assemble the zappicator food box parts.

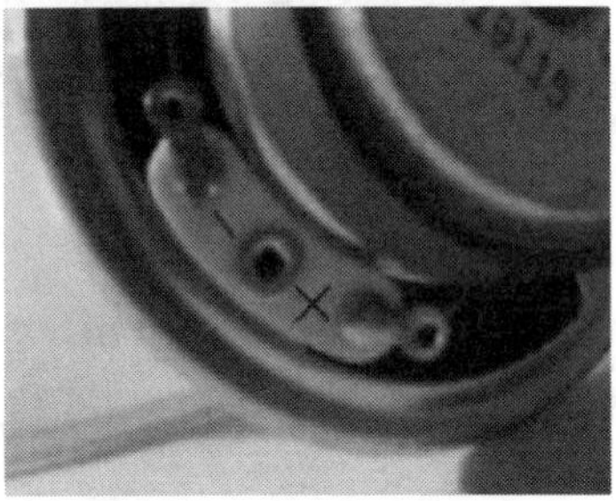

Fig. 127 Find the (+) sign on speaker

1. Find the (+) and (–) sign on the loudspeaker. You will be attaching a lead (wire) to the plus side.
2. Cut a hole, about ½ inch square in the side of the plastic carton for the lead to pass through.
3. Attach the loudspeaker to the bottom of the carton, inside, taping it down securely, or using hot glue around the edge of the cone.
4. Push the alligator clip lead through the hole and attach it securely to the (+) connection on the speaker. Attach nothing to the *Negative* terminal.
5. Find the (+) terminal of your 1 kHz zapper. You must be sure of this. If you did not build it and if it is not marked, take it to an electronics shop; the clerk can check this for you in a

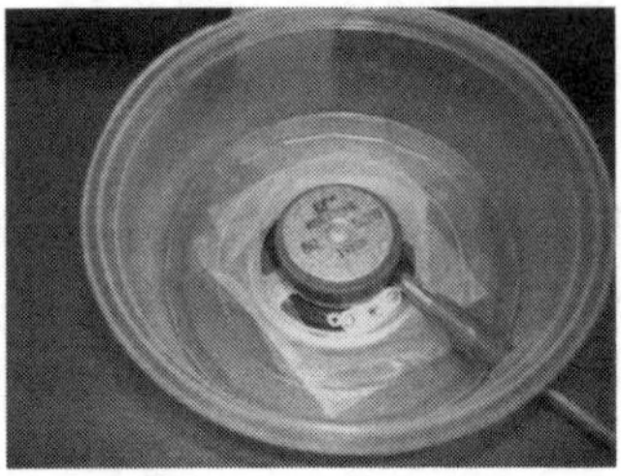

Fig. 128 Attach loudspeaker inside the carton

minute. Label it. Connect the free end of the clip lead to the (+) terminal of the zapper. If you need to use two leads to connect your speaker (+) terminal to your zapper (+) terminal, do so. Attach nothing to the *Negative* terminal.

6. Turn carton over to give you a flat surface for food placement. Place food, packaged food, beverage container, or filled plate on the top of the carton. It may hang over the edge. Turn zapper on for specified time.

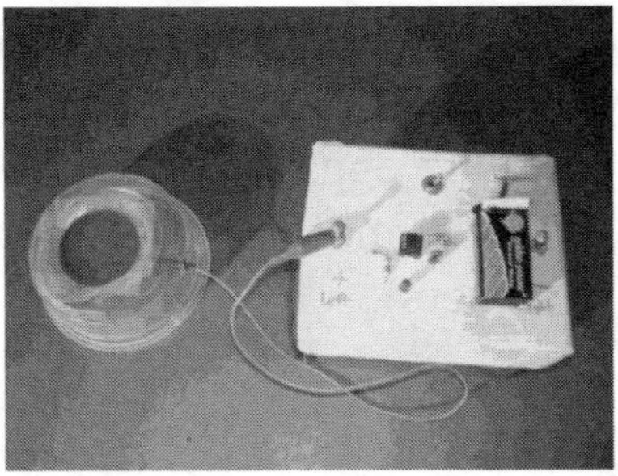

Fig. 129 Connect speaker to (+) output of zapper

Using the Zappicator Food Box

Metal objects, like cans, placed on the zappicator will become magnetized by zappicating, showing a south pole at the base and north pole at the top. Numerous poles are induced, not necessarily stable. The food inside the container shows the same polarity as the part of the container that is touching it (not opposite). For better quality food you should empty the can first and zappicate in a non-metal container. *All the canned food in the market place is half north and half south from the effect of the earth's magnetic field. This could be its worst feature.*

Glass jars should have their metal lids removed before zappicating. This gives all the food a north polarization like the polarity of the speaker. Otherwise the metal lid becomes polarized so that half the entire can becomes north and the other half south.

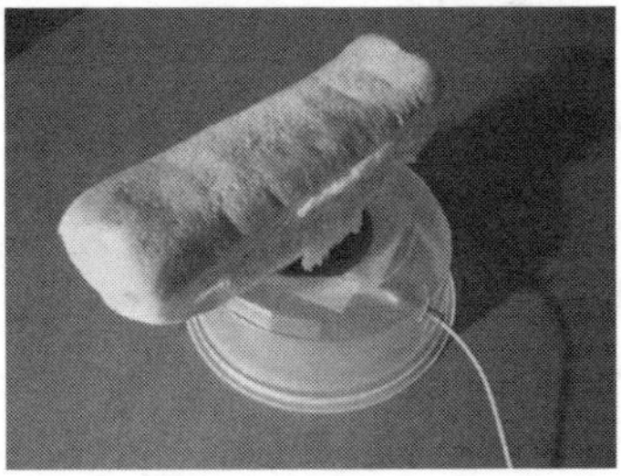

Fig. 130 Place food on top of carton

Foods and beverages become north polarized, although they may have started out south or without any polarization. This is because water is **diamagnetic** and takes on the same polarity as the field nearest to it instead of the opposite polarity as iron-like (tin can) metals do.

Changing your food to north polarized is an extra benefit of zappication. The other goals are to disable parasite eggs and other living things as well as changing harmful molecules, like food phenolics to harmless forms (isomers).

CHAPTER 22

RECIPES

For An Immune Depressed Society

Find old recipe books from before the time ingredients changed to packages and cans. Find new stainless steel blenders, juicers, choppers, that you have tested for chromium, nickel and vanadium releases. Home cooking without the taste of metal will bring flavor back…maybe even the children back…to the table. Children can often taste copper and chlorine in food. They feel tired and sleepy after eating malonic acid, nervous and hyper after eating chromium, especially after getting tooth fillings or sealant. When cooking from scratch you can hardly go wrong nutritionally.

The importance of this book is the emphasis on higher standards of food sanitation and safety. Sanitation from parasite eggs and bacteria or viruses; safety from the main immunity-destroyers: radioactivity, asbestos, benzene, PCBs, heavy metals, azo dyes, plus iron cyanides and polonium all from an inferior chlorination process.

To make food sanitary I have recommended several methods in earlier books. In this book I will emphasize deep freezing. Ozonating, sonicating, and washing in Lugol's water are still good choices for foods that should not be frozen.

Is all this necessary? It is years of using the Syncrometer® and listening to the sick that provides the answer.

Yes! It is necessary. It is long overdue. We have been wading in filth—our own, our animals', and others'—and unbeknown to us, in radioactivity. We are wading in toxins: metals, solvents, and dyes. But it “looks” clean and safe enough to us and we might think, “With a shiny floor and gleaming glasses on the table, what could go wrong? Surely it can’t be so significant.” Shine and spot-free gleam is quite deceptive. When cows were milked by hand, you could see any filth and remove it. When potatoes were peeled by hand you could see the fungus (Potato Ring Rot) and cut it away. Now milking machines cover up filth, traumatize the udder, and bring a higher incidence of Staph infected cows, all dealt with by increased antibiotic use.

Potato peeling machines care nothing about the fungus inside. And potatoes left unpeeled for “better nutrition” hide it all. Yet that has become the AIDS-fungus.

Food Sanitizers

The ancient ways were washing, cooking, baking, pickling, drying, frying! They made food more edible and quite sanitary in times when toxicity did not play a big role. Disease germs were not known although they might have been called “evil vapors” at that time. Yet, people certainly knew that filth was linked to illness.

Recently, we have begun grilling and microwaving. It is a huge experiment in overheating food. It should be watched closely. This denatures the food more than before so more minerals are oxidized to toxic metals. These metals feed our pathogens. It is happening on a global scale.

Neither of these methods is a solution for our immunodepressed society. We need food with undetectable Salmonella and E. coli by Syncrometer® standards (about 10^{-15}) compared to regular standards (about 10^{-8}).

Healthy people do not appear to get sick from regular standards, but very sick people get immediately better when using Syncrometer® standards. It suggests a subtle influence of plain filth on our immune status.

There are only a sprinkling of bacteria in your salt, flour, rice, sugar, beans, pills, peanut butter, ultra pasteurized milk, canned goods, baked goods, and manufactured supplements. There will be none detectable after using our special freezing method. Ultraviolet treatment also promises us total disinfection but has not been made safe enough for public use yet. Cancer patients benefit immediately from this level of sanitation and all their setbacks are due to accidentally eating a few filth bacteria, E. coli, again.

Super Freezing

With this method there is nothing to add or turn on. Just open the lid and put inside your bag of supplements or flour or beans. Leave it there for 24 hours or till no E. coli or Salmonella can be found by Syncrometer® testing. Ascaris eggs and tapeworm eggs will be destroyed. In 2 or 3 days your stomach will feel better than in a long time. You must have a **freezer thermometer** for this and it must go down to -20° F or colder! Keep it there without interruption for 24 hours, no less! **Freezing does nothing but KILL invaders, it does not detoxify.** Don't crowd or overfill the freezer. Buy a self-defrosting one or attach a timer to the electric cord, to defrost once a week.

Lugol's Rinse

Lugol's iodine has been used for decades by travelers to foreign lands to wash their fruit and vegetables. Whether cooking or eating you can sanitize fruit and vegetables in minutes.

- Lugol's iodine solution (see *Recipes*, page 584)
- water

Fill a sink or a bowl with a measured amount of water. Draw a line here, so future treatments do not require measuring again. **Add 1 to 3 drops Lugol's per quart (or liter) of water, or 5 to 6 drops diluted Lugol's, called Veggie Wash.** You should be able to see the color. Dip lettuce, spinach and any other produce in it so everything is well wetted for one minute or more. Rinsing is optional. (Eating traces of iodine is beneficial, not harmful). If you wash so many vegetables that you can no longer see the color of the iodine it has lost its effectiveness. Add a few more drops.

Keep Lugol's out of reach of children. Keep it in small (½ oz.) dropper bottles as further protection against accidental overdose. **Do not use Lugol's if you are allergic to iodine. Your doctor would know because it only happens after a special clinical procedure.**

Cautionary Note:

Lugol's iodine can "crawl" out of its bottle even when it is tightly closed! It can stain the sink and counter top. If this happens, use vitamin C immediately to make it colorless, then wipe away.

If your Lugol's was not made from scratch, it will probably have wood alcohol and isopropyl alcohol pollution. Be sure to order the dry compounds, not a ready made solution. You will only need diet scales, plastic spoon and cup besides a large HDPE bottle. Your local pharmacist would be glad to help.

Ozonation

Ozone can kill bacteria and viruses deep inside food and beverages with surprising speed. In less than 10 minutes all the food in your refrigerator could be sterilized. For food just purchased, simply place it all in a plastic bag so the ozone can build up a slight pressure. This pressure will push it to the bottom of a quart container, right through a stick of butter, and right through meat. Of course the containers or packaging should be open to allow the ozone to enter.

The advantage of ozone, besides speed, is that it turns into plain oxygen, leaving no toxicity behind.

Another advantage is that it can do oxidizing chemistry, although this takes more than 10 minutes. The Syncrometer®

shows that the estrogens in dairy products (estrone, estriole and estradiol) are destroyed in 15 minutes. Azo dyes sprayed on meats can be destroyed in 15 to 20 minutes, and many phenolic food substances can be destroyed in 15 minutes as well.

Ozone has great penetrating power, which Lugol's does not. Lugol's has great attaching ability so surfaces are immediately sterilized. Lugol's does not penetrate. Each property has special value.

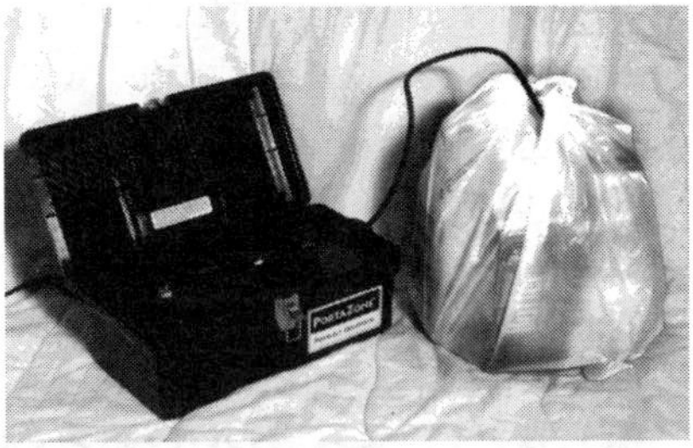

Plastic shopping bag holds groceries and ozonator hose. Ozonating semi-sterilizes and destroys many toxins.

Fig. 131 Ozonating food

Sanitizing with ozone only takes 7 minutes. Safety from dyes and other chemicals, including chlorine, takes 10 to 20 minutes. But metals cannot be destroyed. They will always be metals, even though they become oxidized metals. Can motor oil, wheel bearing grease, and PCBs be ozonated? This has not yet been tried.

Safety from heavy metals is not possible by ozonating them.

After turning off the ozonator, the packages and containers should be closed again. Ozonation continues, on its own, for about 10 more minutes, even while refrigerated.

Immunodepressed persons should ozonate all their food for its sanitizing effect. Excess ozone flavor can be blown away as the food is warmed later. Flavor changes can be compensated with spices. Do not ozonate supplements, medicines, or herbs to preserve their potency.

HCl Food Sanitizer (5% USP)

- 1 drop per cup water

Immerse produce. Agitate food well. Let stand several minutes. No need to rinse; this is edible (but don't put HCl directly in your mouth).

To kill most bacteria and parasite eggs, and to destroy traces of benzene and PCBs, add several drops directly to any food. Stir the food with a non-metal (hardened plastic) utensil while adding. Although 1 drop per cup is enough for clear liquids, three drops is safer when particles are present or the food is solid. Do not exceed 20 drops per meal, not counting food preparation.

What A Sonicator Can Do

Ultrasonic cleaners have been in use many decades. They are used to clean scientific instruments, even glassware, to a level not possible any other way. Sonicators can be bought in the form of jewelry cleaners. When jewelry is being cleaned, even the oily film of fingerprints comes off. We will use an ordinary jewelry cleaner, of a good size, but with water for the immersion fluid, not a solvent.

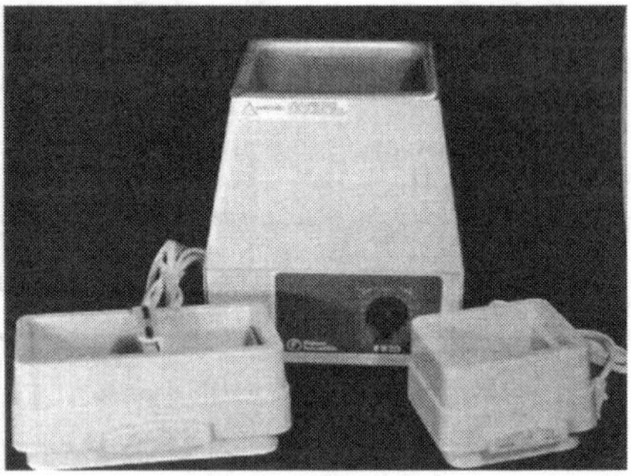

Fig. 132 Jewelry cleaners like these can remove PCBs

The food is placed in a plastic bag and lowered into the tank of water. The unit is turned on for five minutes.

But metals cannot be destroyed by sonication. They are elements; their form may be changed to an oxidized or hydrolyzed form, but this does not change the fact that a metal is present. Lanthanide metals are not destroyed either. Only hot water washes can remove these. Azo dyes as a group cannot be destroyed by sonication either. You must rely on ozonating and hot water washing for these ultra-important immune system toxins.

You can rely on sonication to destroy parasites, their stages, and bacteria even if they are deeply imbedded in meats, bones, or inside cans or packages. Viruses and prions will disappear, too, evidently disrupted by the same shaking action.

Molds on food, together with mycotoxins, are also shaken off and destroyed.

Tiny bits of pituitary gland and hypothalamus that float in eggs and dairy foods are destroyed in 10 minutes, slightly longer than bacteria.

Long sonication can destroy some food phenolics but cannot be relied on.

Large and small sonicators can be purchased from the Internet and from *Sources*. A five-minute built-in timer is also a great time saver. Avoid the variety that strictly forbids touching the bottom of the tank.

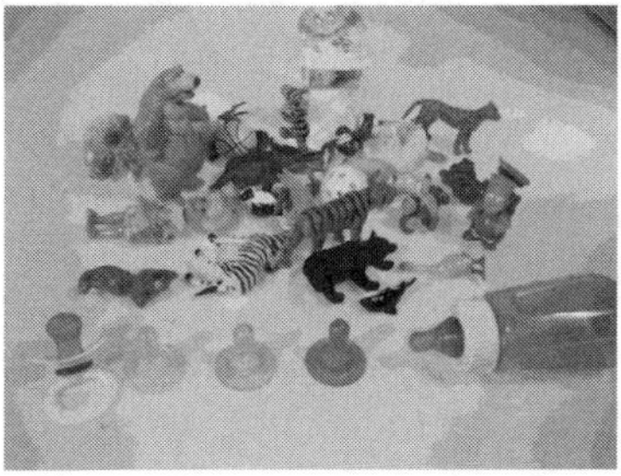

Clean PCBs off plastic toys and baby things.

Fig. 133 PCBs on plastic

Start with a general kitchen clean up as soon as you get your sonicator. Clean up baby things first; babies are the most vulnerable. Shake all the PCBs off baby toys, baby bottles and nipples, even though they have already been used and washed. PCBs don't "go away" by washing, they only spread. Sonicate baby medicine, swabs, band-aids, toys. Sonicate your kitchen sponges, your toothbrush and comb, your **dentures**, and everything else that goes in your mouth (yes, even cigarettes).

Hot Water Washes

All produce has been sprayed a number of times. More chlorox bleach with its polonium and immune destroyers gets stuck each time. Along with these come asbestos shreds from the conveyor belt, and a waxy coating dried onto the produce with hot air blasts. The result is a coating of PCBs, benzene, asbestos, azo dyes, heavy metals, malonic acid, motor oil, wheel bearing grease, and often water softener salts with uranium.

Run the hottest water you can from your faucet into a large stainless steel bowl used only for this purpose. Add all the produce so it is immersed. After 1 minute, dump it all, rinse everything and repeat. If the fruit has small milky-white patches on it, throw it away; it is pesticide residue.

This will not clean up waxed produce. Do not purchase such food. Certain foods show deep penetration of chemicals and should have 3 hot-washes with drying in between. Examples are potatoes, sweet potatoes, carrots, and tomatoes. They still need testing. Purchase from farmers' markets instead, if you can be assured it has not been sprayed against sprouting.

Dried produce needs 2 hot-washes as well, such as beans, rice, grains, lentils.

It is convenient to sanitize your produce right after hot-washing, using a few drops of Lugol's, hydrochloric acid, or by ozonating. Freezing is suitable for some.

No single method can do everything. Zappicating food has been added to reduce toxicity, and to improve its biological value. It is a magnetic treatment.

Magnetic Polarization Of Food

One of Nature's deepest mysteries is the influence of the earth's magnetic field on our bodies, on our health...perhaps on all living things. Fruit and vegetables, leaves and flowers, even nuts and grains are north polarized when they are freshly picked or purchased. Inside, where the seeds are, the polarization is southerly. But the soft parts begin to age and wilt and show deterioration within a week of being stored in the refrigerator. The northerly polarization is changing to southerly! It happens gradually. A large bunch of grapes will have some turned completely south in a few days, the wrinkled ones, while others are still completely north (the freshest looking ones). The seed does not change its polarization.

My conclusion is that we were meant to eat northerly polarized food, with just a little bit of southerly food in the form of seeds. Yet, most of the food we eat, even refrigerated food, has turned at least partly south. We are getting an overdose of south polarized food as well as water.

That is why I recommend zappicating our food, especially when we are sick.

Zappication

Water that is simply zapped gets electrical energy, just a voltage, impressed on it. We know, from bottle-copying, that water can hold very many frequencies of electrical energy. Food and our bodies are mainly water. Is it the same in food? Such research is badly needed.

Food that is simply put in a magnetic field has magnetic forces impressed on it. We can see that from making north and south polarized water (see page 242).

Electrical energy even generates magnetic energy and vice versa, so we always receive a dose of both even when only one kind is applied. This, too, needs much more research.

A third form of energy is physical, as our ears can sense when waves of air pressure reach them. Here we know that frequency is very important because it makes different sounds. Our ears can only hear sound when the frequency is under 20,000 Hz.

The zappicator combines all 3 kinds of energy and delivers them at the same frequency. The voltage from a zapper is brought to an electro magnet, which exudes its own magnetic field while pushing a diaphragm back and forth to create a physical effect at the same frequency. What does that do to food? A few things have been noticed, so far:

1. It changes the angle of light that is passing through each molecule of food further to the left if an amino acid is

zappicated. The d-amino acids are changed to l-amino acids this way. Remember, the body considers d-amino acids as allergens; it only uses l-forms itself. The food has been improved, to be less allergenic, before you eat it. Of course, changes can come after you eat it. It could change back to a d-form in a southerly zone, as happens to thyroxine (page 125).

2. It changes the polarization of the food to north, if the north side of the magnet faces the food. Food has been made "fresher".

3. Most bacteria, viruses and parasite eggs can't be detected afterwards. Were their growing points disabled by being turned northerly? This could be temporary, if it is reversible, but still useful.

4. Benzene gets oxidized to phenol, at least at trace levels. PCBs disappear, no doubt slightly changed, an important step toward detoxification.

5. Phenolic food antigens disappear if the correct frequency is used. Many are affected between 1000 and 1010 Hz. Perhaps they were oxidized further. The body could choose to reduce them again or make something equally toxic, but the ability to make food less allergenic beckons again.

6. A zappicator placed on plastic teeth in your mouth, instead of food, stops seeping of plastic, dyes, or malonic acid from them. Did it complete the polymerization process, or harden it all in some other way? Cerium is too dangerous to rely on this. Only cerium-free dental supplies should be used.

7. Placed on a cancerous lump on the skin, it seems to shrink in 24 hours. But much more improvement is needed in strength of magnet, and protection from stray south fields before you could experiment safely.

8. Finally, food seems to taste better. Maybe changing d- to l-amino acids or alpha to beta forms or l- to d-sugars can be tasted. These are all effects of zappication. Only more research can give us more advice.

Again, we must not demonize the opposite polarization. It is part of us, too, just as the seed belongs to the fruit. But much greater care is needed in handling south pole forces. Notice how Nature has its south pole seed securely encased. Don't do south polarization experiments till you have gained much experience with northerly ones.

Research on food and water, finding what is good for us and what is bad, has barely begun. Food is fascinating, all the more when we're hungry. As a species we are very hungry. Perhaps we would only need half as much food if it was correctly polarized for our bodies, and at the same time give us much more energy than we have now. With these purposes in mind, make yourself a zappicator (page 532) but don't throw away the Ancient Ways yet. **Don't depend on this to sterilize food.**

Zappicate food 10 minutes. Zappicate eggs and dairy foods 15 minutes or more. Check the polarity of your zappicator with a compass once a week. Some magnets can change their polarity by being heated, dropped, or wetted. Best of all, test the results in your food with a Syncrometer®.

Ultraviolet Disinfection

Ultraviolet includes the colors beyond violet. The wavelengths here are shorter than elsewhere. They are divided into A, B, and C, with C being the shortest at 254 nm. This short wavelength kills bacteria and viruses but you must be close enough to the bulb. Having 2 bulbs, each 20 watts, gives you 40 watts of power, enough to kill any bacteria quickly. But you must still find out for yourself, how high up or how far away the lamp can be and still be lethal in a convenient time.

Check if your vitamins are still there at the end. Do not take the disinfecting action for granted, you must find your distance from the lamp and time spent under it to be effective. The Salmonella and E. coli must be gone for proof of effectiveness at different settings. Be careful to obey the safety rules for all UV light, not to look at it directly, nor to allow children near the lamp. Make an enclosure for the lamp with lockable doors to guarantee safety. If you can't be in charge or children are about, it would be best to leave this one out. It is very convenient to dump all your groceries under the lamp for 15 minutes, then carry them all to the sink, or to set a plateful of food under the lamp for 10 minutes. But it does not penetrate dried foods or capsules of supplements.

Selecting Your Recipes

Get to know yourself. From your cancer location you can find your allergen. Then use the *Food Table* on page 97 to find foods that don't have this allergen. Notice, that overall there are about 50 times as many *N's* as *P's*. But, once you find your culprit food, you might realize you had been eating it much too often. Strengthen your resolve to get the nickel and radioactivity out of your body as soon as possible to stop all your allergies. Meanwhile find old cookbooks with recipes made from scratch.

A very good rule is not to eat the same food twice in a day or two days in a row. Have your refrigerator full of food, go shopping a lot, have help cooking; it is not a luxury when you have serious illness; it is necessary.

Kitchen Necessities

- a large set of stainless steel saucepans
- a blender, only if tested for seepage from blades (see *Sources*)
- an ozonator tested for nickel and rubber in the water.
- a bread-maker without Teflon coating (test basket for thallium, gold, and aluminum)
- stainless steel cutlery, utensils, bowls, meat platters, graters, funnels, strainers, choppers, all tested for nickel and chromium seepage
- food grinder (use for less than 4 seconds at a time to prevent nickel and chromium seepage)
- dishes, glasses and storage containers of HDPE or high impact plastic that you have tested for heavy metal seepage
- a conductivity indicator (see page 614)
- zippered plastic bags without chlorox bleach
- In previous books I recommended filter pitchers. I no longer do that because making it safe is too complicated. Errors

mean you will be drinking **ruthenium**. You can now purchase an automatic backwash filter with boiled coconut charcoal that removes ruthenium, iron cyanides, alkylating oils and dyes and radioactivity (please inquire to *Sources* shown).

- paper towels, napkins, scouring sponges, safe bleach, detergent, toilet paper without chlorox bleach
- a small low temperature chest freezer and thermometer that reaches -20° F as all purpose sterilizer and an automatic timer for the cord so it automatically defrosts

Test all items before purchasing them if possible.

To cook or fry, use stainless steel only, not aluminum or Teflon coated. To warm food, use a saucepan.

To store food, use HDPE and stainless steel containers. Make temporary bowls and place settings from water jugs until you are well.

> Be careful not to let the hydrochloric acid drip on your stainless steel sink or cookware, it will be stained. The Lugol's iodine should not be set on the kitchen counter or table; they will be stained.

Going Shopping

Shop for kosher foods whenever possible. Search for these symbols: K, U. Shop for Asian imports. This still does not guarantee their safety. Don't shop for anything in glass bottles unless you can test for thallium. That is a major seeped metal from both amber and clear glass, besides Teflon. If your legs ache be extra careful.

Organic produce has much less dye and pesticide pollution than regular produce, but buy it only if the local water, used to spray on the shelf for freshness, is not the chlorox bleach kind. Find a store with safe water by testing it for chlorox. Asbestos tufts adhering to the outside of foods is just as severe a problem with organic produce. When I tested some farmers' market produce, it was free of asbestos. Search for organic produce at farmers' markets. Potatoes and sweet potatoes, not sprayed against sprouting or greased against wilting, would be a rare find. The others have malonic acid deep inside. Next best might be a small corner grocery store. Ask which day their produce arrives to get it fresh.

No foods are safe, though, unless cleaned up with hot-washes and sterilized. Do not buy a spray that removes spray, either; the one I tested had more solvents than the original sprayed food. A UV lamp is the handiest for sterilizing fresh vegetables that have already been tested for chlorox and thallium.

RECIPES

Extremely advanced and abandoned cancer patients can still recover, but only if the diet chosen is correct. Choose your recipes carefully to comply with the program. Feel free to vary them.

Recently many new Asian and kosher foods have reached the marketplace, including bottled water. Choose kosher foods to avoid chlorination. Their heavy metals must still be tested, especially chromium. Make a list of safe foods for your area.

Rules For Making Recipes

1. Sterilize every item before or after preparation. It only needs to be done once.
2. Use stove top, not microwave to protect germanium and vitamin C.
3. All choices should comply with the *2-Week Program*.
4. c/s means "cut and sifted". Such herbs do not have heavy metals from grinding. Test for thallium and methylene blue.

Something Sweet

All granulated forms of all sugar varieties I purchased at USA grocery stores or health food stores had asbestos fibers and D-mannitol in them, not to mention chlorox.

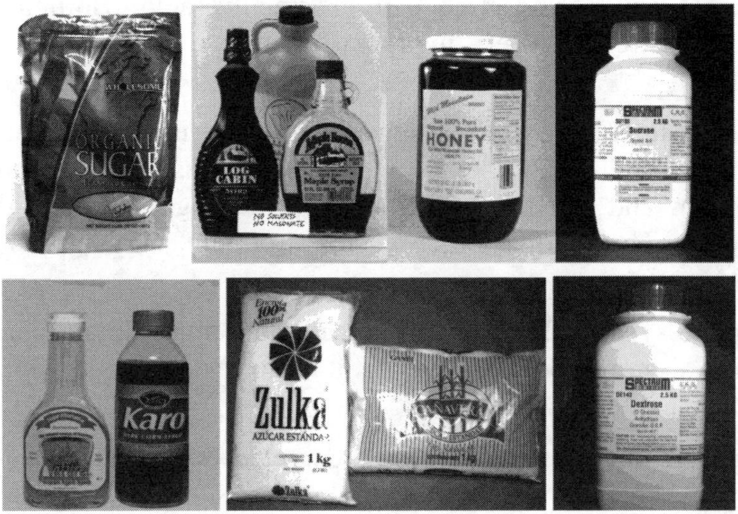

Organic sugar from Paraguay, maple syrup, locally produced honey, sucrose (crystal N.F. grade), agave syrup, dark Karo (corn) syrup, two Mexican sugars, and dextrose (made from corn).

Fig. 134 Safer sweetening

Organic sugar from Paraguay and Mexican sugars did not have asbestos.

Sucrose purchased from a chemical supply company did not have asbestos, nor D-mannitol or other pollutants.

Honey had asbestos fibers except when locally produced. Clover honey routinely had coumarin allergen. Orange blossom honey had many allergens.

All honey has fructose, normally a desirable form of sugar if not overdone. But fructose is the antigen for RBCs and should be *avoided in blood cancers, liver failure and malaria.*

Honey should be tested for gold and strontium, beryllium, vanadium and chromium, air pollutants that land on flowers.

Inositol is slightly sweet but the best choice of all. It is a much needed food factor. It does not feed yeast. Used daily it makes IP6 (inositol hexa phosphate) much more efficient at uranium removal.

Maple syrup very frequently has gallic acid. Boiling 1 minute destroys it. Very many varieties have ASA (aspirin); test first.

Dextrose is a "powdered sugar" variety. It is usually made from corn and carries CORN antigen as well as air pollutants, strontium and beryllium. Dextrose is the sugar used in IV solutions. They should be tested for strontium, beryllium and CORN antigen.

Agave syrup often has caffeic acid and cinnamic acid, but boiling destroys both. However, it also has fructose, which yields mannitol when boiled.

Plain fruit juices can be used as sweeteners. But when yeast is a problem even plain and natural sugars should be avoided. *Always avoid in breast, skin and brain cancers.*

The land of sweets is obviously strewn with land mines. If you are living dangerously, at least minimize each one by changing the variety at every meal.

Coconut Whipping Cream

- "meat" of 1 coconut with brown skin removed, frozen
- "milk" of 1 coconut, frozen

Place meat in blender for 4 seconds only. Then add ¼ cup "milk" and blend another 4 seconds. Continue adding bits of milk till consistency is perfect for you.

Something Sour

Use citric acid and vitamin C to give sour taste to foods. Safe vinegar (see *Sources*) is fine, but can't be used in colon and prostate cancer.

Citric Tangerine Dessert

- 2 tangerines
- 2 citric acid capsules or ¼ tsp.
- 1 tsp. safe sweetener

- heavy whipping cream without lactose (*optional*)

Hot wash tangerines and save peels in freezer. They have health value. Place tangerines in zippered plastic bag or non-seeping container (no need to disinfect). Add citric acid and sweetener. Mash and mix with stainless steel whip or roll over the bag with a glass jar. Top with cream. *Variations*: Boil tangerines with equal amount of water; add other ingredients. Serve on blended foods to provide flavor.

Lettuce A'la Crème – A TV Snack

- the greenest head lettuce you can find, with many loose outer leaves
- 2 citric acid capsules or ¼ tsp.
- ¼ cup heavy whipping cream, sterilized

Peel away many loose lettuce leaves to get away from adhering radon and sprays. Dip head in Lugol's water for 3 minutes. Add citric acid to whipping cream in a HDPE bowl. Tear pieces of lettuce off the head (don't cut) and dip into the sour cream. *Variations*: Use Romaine lettuce or Bok Choy. Add 1 Brazil nut or 4 Hazel nuts, ground.

Sour Cream - C

- 2 cups heavy whipping cream, already disinfected
- ¼ tsp. citric acid
- ¼ tsp. vitamin C powder
- pinch of pure salt

Stir until smooth. Refrigerate two hours before serving.

Coconut - Tangerine Juice (for organic germanium and selenium)

- one fresh coconut (keep the meat in freezer)
- 2 tangerines, hot washed
- milk of coconut

At a certain time of year the new coconut crop is in. The meat is soft and the "milk" plentiful. If someone would crack and clean it for you, you could consume one a week. Until you are no longer coughing, avoid coconut, though, because the natural oil somehow increases viruses. But after lungs improve you can get both organic germanium and selenium this delicious way. Pour the milk and a piece of "meat" into a blender. Add the whole tangerines, seeds and all. Blend 4 seconds only. Immediately strain through steel strainer. Do not store this; drink immediately.

Hydrangea Tea (for organic germanium)

- ½ cup hydrangea root, (c/s), organic, frozen
- 3 cups water
- stainless steel strainer

Soak the sterilized dried roots at least 4 hours to get the maximum goodness out of them later. Then simmer for ½ hour at low heat in a stainless steel pan. Let cool and strain into a HDPE container for storage. Several sips provide one dose of germanium for the 2-*Week Program*. Add sweetener to taste. Keep sterile by reheating daily.

Brazil Nut Split (for organic germanium and selenium)

- 1 whole nut in the shell
- sturdy nutcracker
- 1 frozen banana
- whipping cream, heavy, kosher, disinfected

Crack the nut when you are ready to use it. Choose a different nut if it is discolored or doesn't taste good after nibbling. Scrape away blemishes. Place frozen banana on stainless steel platter or HDPE dish. Dribble whipping cream over the banana. Before it freezes sprinkle ground Brazil nut over cream. Grind it by pounding in a plastic zippered bag or rolling it with a jar. All nuts have germanium and selenium, but eating more than one large nut a day challenges your digestion of linolenic acid too much so viruses can thrive. *Variations*: Add ground rose hips for organic vitamin C.

Rose Hips Tea (for organic vitamin C)

- 1 tsp. rose hips, coarse ground, with seeds, organic, frozen
- 1 cup water
- sweetener or heavy whipping cream, sterilized

Bring water to a boil in stainless steel saucepan. Add rose hips, cover, and then remove from heat. When cool pour into safe cup and drink right away. This can replace one dose of the capsules plus a vitamin C capsule in the program. You may add sweetener or whipping cream to taste.

Barley Water

This is an ancient "medicine". It has organic manganese.

- whole barley, frozen or ozonated to sterilize.

Test for bromine first; do not eat brominated grains. It cannot be removed. It sequesters polonium in you.

Add 4 times as much water as barley and let stand at least 4 hours. Then refrigerate. Decant and drink. Cooking changes some of it to plain manganese metal that feeds Shigella. Don't cook it if not necessary. It can be made into chewy, spicy, uncooked breakfast cereal. Vinegar kills Shigella, but can't be used in colon or prostate cancer. *Variation:* Any kind of safe rice can be made into a medicinal "rice water" that provides calories and B vitamins.

Barley Flakes, tested for bromine and chlorox

Add 1½ times as much water as flakes and let stand overnight in the refrigerator or 2 hours at room temperature. Serve with whipping cream and chopped fruit.

Tapioca - Barley Pudding

Put into a 2 quart pan.

- 1½ cups water
- $^1/_3$ cup small tapioca pearls (see *Sources*)
- 1½ teaspoons whole barley (grind first for 3 seconds)

Soak the above for one hour, then add:

- $1^1/_3$ cups water
- 2 cups heavy whipping cream
- ½ to $^2/_3$ cup safe sweetener (*optional)*
- ¼ to $^1/_3$ cup pure maple syrup (*optional*)

Bring to a boil and let boil for only one minute, stirring constantly with a stainless steel spoon. *Optional*: Add contents of two nutmeg capsules and a tsp. of the spice mix below. Serve warm or cold. Makes approximately eight 4 oz. servings. *NOTE*: For thinner consistency use ½ cup more water.

Spice Mix

- 1 tsp. coriander seeds, frozen
- 1 tsp. cardamom seeds, frozen
- 1 tsp. anise seeds, frozen

Grind 3 seconds; then let grinder blades cool and grind another 3 seconds. Store in freezer to keep potency.

Spice Mix TV Snack

These spices (above) can be chewed whole; no grinding needed if your teeth are up to it. Adding sweetener or whipping cream makes it a dessert to be nibbled on for hours. A few detox symptoms next day will be a real reward. Make sure it all got sterilized at some point.

Burdock Tea

This is called an herb, but it is too delicious and flavorful for this simple label.

- 2 Tbsp. burdock root, organic, (c/s)
- 1¼ cups water

Bring water to boil in stainless steel saucepan. Add burdock and turn down heat to simmer, covered. Simmer for about 20 min. Cool. While it is cooling, it will turn sweetish, and the grounds will settle. Then you can pour it off without a strainer. It is so good straight, nothing needs to be added. Even the "grounds" are good, spooned up with cream or sweetening. Do not make herb teas in the microwave. Some organic germanium would get destroyed and phenolics that should be destroyed would escape. Burdock fights E. coli and more. Sterilize first.

Eucalyptus Tea

This tea is too flavorful to be considered an herbal tea, more so if you can pick it off the tree! Best of all is to find it cures your flu's, Salmonella attacks and even malaria. Most important…it does not need to be tested for thallium or other pesticide. There are several varieties. Gather:

- 5 long leaves or 10 short-variety leaves
- 2 inches of twig (that holds the leaves)
- a marble size piece of bark, if available

Rinse under faucet and place in stainless steel pan. Add 2¼ cups water. Bring to a boil, covered. Then turn down heat to simmer for 10 minutes. Cool. Notice the beautiful red color it develops and delicious aroma. You may add whipping cream. During a cold or cough, sip it throughout the day for 2 days (if it lasts that long). It is the only herb, besides oregano (oil) that I have found can kill Clostridium bacteria. Be sure to sterilize every bit.

There are many other herbs used to improve health, discussed in this book. Make these as teas if you have chills or sore throat, adding whatever makes them enjoyable. Do not combine them with other herbs unless they are traditionally combined. They could destroy each other. You need the extra liquid, besides, to stimulate more urine flow.

Although I advised sterilizing them I have never found Salmonella or E. coli bacteria on growing leaves, even if there is dust and the branches hang over streets.

About Eggs

In earlier books I gave egg recipes, knowing they had malvin and gallic acid allergens, and knowing they had hypothalamus and pituitary cells afloat in them. I thought they could be made safe with special treatments. But since then I have found the MYC virus, the SV40 virus and sometimes even OPT itself in eggs. It makes no sense to eat them anymore. Not all eggs have all of these. It probably depends on the animal waste and preservatives in their feed. Free-range chickens could present a different picture. But without testing by Syncrometer®, it seems to me to be quite unwise to eat either chickens or eggs.

About Milk

When cows were free and roamed in meadows of grass and flowers, they produced a moderate amount of milk, a moderate amount of manure and money and a large amount of health in growing children. Allergies and disorders were not so rampant.

But now cows are fed quite unnatural food (soybeans, yeast culture, carbohydrates) to increase milk production. These processed concentrates and even the water in their trough now give her daily doses of chlorox bleach. In fact, dairymen are encouraged to pour extra bleach into their water trough, and no mention is made of the NSF kind or that 2 kinds exist. Nor does the Dept. of Agriculture. Now cows are becoming immunodepressed, like humans, getting recurrent mastitis and necessitating lots of antibiotics. They, too, develop increased parasitism. We would expect many "Flu" attacks as a cow's body manages to kill its own flukes. Cows also get more than their share of digestion problems from their unnatural food, so that phenolic allergens would be expected. She could be expected to get prion protein attacks from so many free hypothalamus cells and not enough pepsin to digest them. Periods of dizziness, loss of appetite and staggering would result, which could explain BSE. Lowered productivity as a goal(!) for cows seems like an intelligent solution, so all these trends can be reversed while it is still possible. If we lose the milk industry to prion increase we will lose the beef industry, too. Dairy and beef producers should take a preventive approach, not adversarial.

With a heavily parasitized cow we would expect to see Bacillus cereus and tyramine in her milk. And we always do, even in cheese and all other dairy products. In fact tyramine is considered to be a headache-causer in allergy textbooks. (Nutmeg kills these bacteria.)

Switching to goat milk by sick people is another intelligent solution, to reduce allergens obtained from cow's milk.

Even goat milk provides more lactose than can be quickly digested. We use only Mexican heavy whipping cream, without lactose, and only for recovering patients. After you are well, goat milk, frozen to disinfect, then boiled 10 min. to denature allergens, would be a great help for your nutrition.

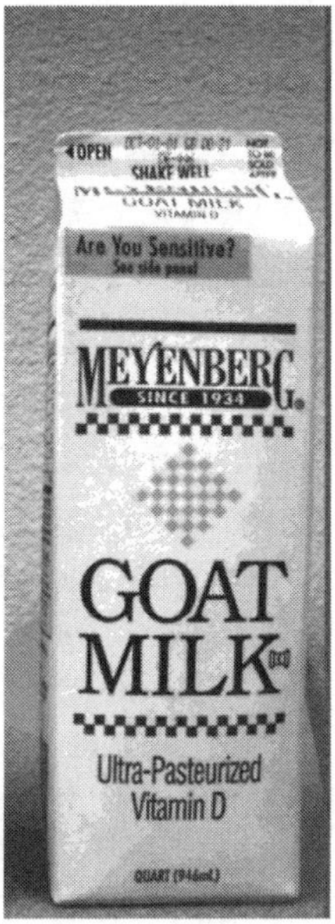

Fig. 135 Popular variety of goat milk

Plain Goat Milk

There is no way of knowing whether a dairy is using chlorox bleach to sanitize equipment or NSF bleach, or steam, or old fashioned Lugol's iodine. For this reason you should send a sample to a Syncrometer® tester before becoming a milk consumer.

Raw goat milk has not been studied for its medicinal value although it has been used for such purposes from antiquity. Now that sterilization can be done by freezing or ozonation, it should be reevaluated, (as should raw cows' milk).

C – Milk

- milk
- nutmeg
- vitamin C powder

Cold milk can absorb a lot of vitamin C without curdling or affecting the flavor. Try ½ tsp. vitamin C and a pinch of nutmeg in a HDPE "glass" of ice cold goat milk. Start with small amounts.

Buttermilk - C

Mix equal amounts of heavy whipping cream and ultra pasteurized goat milk, first frozen, then boiled when cold. Stir in 1½ tsp. vitamin C powder per 8 oz. glass. Add ⅛ capsule of nutmeg powder, zappicate. If it does not form flakes readily, add ¼ tsp. citric acid per glass.

Raw Certified Milk

Undoubtedly, fresh goat milk is the most nutritious food in existence for a young, sickly or allergic child. But don't use it unless you can find which disinfectant is being used at the farm. Have your milk streamed straight into a HDPE water jug. Cut away the part across from the handle of a gallon bottle to make this easy for the milker. Or purchase a milking bucket designated only for your child—test it yourself for seeping metal or use a large plastic zippered bag as a liner. Supply the strainer and strainer holder yourself, too, selected for no conductivity of their soak-waters. Do not use cloth or paper strainers of a single-use kind; use a stainless steel kind.

Or make your own strainer from boiled cheesecloth (see *Sources*). Then dip in Lugol's water before placing in stainless steel strainer or funnel.

After straining into a fresh jug add 1 drop Lugol's to each cup (without measuring) while stirring. The Lugol's should be made from scratch, not bought ready made.

Except for this special circumstance Lugol's should not be added directly to food.

5-Minute Raspberry Ice Cream

Why buy ready made ice cream when homemade is twice as delicious?

- 1 pint heavy whipping cream previously treated with ¼ capsule lactase enzyme for several hours and then ozonated
- 1 carton raspberries from a farmers' market, disinfected by deep freezing after rinsing. Test for thallium if imported.
- wheat germ (freshly opened, nitrogen packed, frozen)
- ½ cup safe sweetener
- nuts (optional)

Dump frozen raspberries into blender. Pour whipping cream and sweetener over them. Blend for 4 seconds (only). Pour it all into a stainless steel bowl, already chilled in freezer. Don't clean the blades. Quickly sprinkle wheat germ or ground nuts over the top. Cover with close fitting zippered bag and place in freezer. Prepare it a day ahead. Try using other frozen fruit like blueberries, peaches, but not strawberries. Strawberries are very heavily fertilized now with very radioactive fertilizer. In fact, when you dry strawberries (or oranges or purple grapes) they can be tested with a handheld inexpensive Geiger Mueller counter and found to be 10% or more radioactive than the background level. Raspberries have a special anti-cancer factor, **ellagic** acid, as do Brazil nuts. Freeze many pints.

Pear Slush

- 1 large pear
- ⅛ tsp. citric acid
- 1 Tbsp. safe sweetener
- 1 Tbsp. water

Sterilize in Lugol's water or ozonate. Peel and cut away the stem and flower end, leaving no blemishes. Place in blender with sweetener, water, citric acid, seeds and all (pear seeds are powerful virus killers). Blend 4 seconds (only). Scoop into chilled stainless steel sherbet servers and freeze inside a zippered bag. Serve frozen. *Variations*: Add topping of pounded or rolled nuts and whipping cream. *NOTE*: Use any other raw fruit desired, but always add the citric acid.

Complete Meal Drinks

When a meal is missed weight is lost and the body is stressed. During dental work, especially, weight is easily lost that cannot be regained. Every effort should be made to keep up the usual calorie intake. You can make a drinkable "meal" that needs no preparation, and provides the fat, protein, and carbohydrate essential for life. The principles are:

(1) no vegetable oil to avoid triggering viruses
(2) no eggs or milk

- ½ cup heavy whipping cream
- ½ cup water or barley water
- 1 Tbsp. safe sweetener
- 5 capsules mixed amino acids This is the protein source. (Read label for phenylalanine or tryptophane presence in case you must avoid these). *Variations*: ½ capsule nutmeg, a pinch of cloves or any other spice, ground nuts.

Stir all together. The whipping cream should already have been treated (overnight) with ¼ capsule lactase per pint, then ozonated. Take lipase-containing digestive enzymes with this. Change the spice and sweetener at each meal. CALORIES: 477

Blender Meals (to prevent weight loss)

You won't lose weight during dental work with these recipes, even if you don't know what you're drinking. For emaciated patients, add 1 Tbsp. safe butter to each recipe.

Blended Turkey

- cooked rice, 1 serving
- cooked turkey, 1 serving
- water, about 1 cup
- pure salt
- avocado, ripe but without mold spots inside

Place rice, turkey, water, salt in blender and blend 4 seconds at a time till drinkable. Add chunks of avocado later, to provide something solid.

Blended Stew

- any cooked meat or fish dish
- any vegetable dish
- anything raw and green or yellow
- water, about 1 cup
- pure salt
- an herb, like oregano leaf, thyme leaf, cilantro, disinfected

Put a serving of each in the blender along with water, salt to suit taste and herbs. Blend 4 seconds at a time, adding more water till drinkable. *Variations*: Use less water to keep it thick and spoonable. Adjust salt to needs as seen on blood test if it was already added earlier.

Salt

Plain Salt

Use pure salt only (see *Sources*), like for laboratory use. Grocery store salt and sea salt as well as other kinds of salt have processing contaminants, not to mention aluminum additives, and often have Ascaris eggs and mold. Sterilize.

B - C Salt

This is the easy way to get vitamin B_2 and vitamin C into all your food:

- ½ cup pure salt
- 1 capsule vitamin B_2
- ½ tsp. vitamin C (ascorbic acid) powder (also try 1 tsp.)

Shake together in HDPE bottle or non-seeping jar. Zappicate. When using this salt in cooking, wait until the end to add it, to preserve its vitamin power.

Regarding potassium salt, some varieties of potassium-containing salt and supplements were seen to be radioactive, using a Geiger Mueller counter, so are no longer listed. Those mentioned in this book were tested.

Spreads

Real Butter

Use butter for baking and all other purposes, not oil. Find undyed, organic, kosher butter. Ozonate or sonicate the whole pound for 10 minutes after opening each quarter; then plop it into a bowl of cold water for 5 minutes to draw out metals. Turn after 5 minutes for another treatment, since it floats.

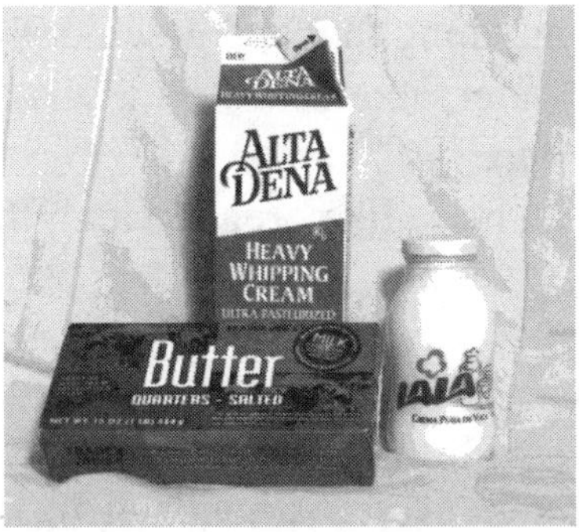

No wrong bleach in this food. Lala is a Mexican brand of heavy whipping cream. The glass bottle does not seep, either! Sanitize by deep freezing or ozonating.

Fig. 136 Safe butter & cream

Lala is a Mexican brand of heavy whipping cream without lactose. The glass bottle does not seep, either! Sanitize by deep freezing or ozonating. Never eat fake butter, as in margarine. Nickel is used as a catalyst to make it!

Don't use special grease-sprays, they contain silicones, which accumulate in tumors.

Emergency Disinfection

If you are stuck with the food on an airplane or while stranded, put a tiny drop of Lugol's on your butter, mix it well. Put another tiny drop on each other food you are served, as well as in the water. This is the second exception when you may put Lugol's in a food. You may request kosher food on an airplane now, but it still needs Lugol's treatment. It will have no chlorine disinfectant. Tiny drops are made by merely touching the food to leave a dot of color.

Preserves

- 1 cup fruit
- 1 Tbsp. water
- ¼ tsp. citric acid
- sweetening

Only use fruit that tests *Negative* for chlorox bleach. Send several varieties to a Syncrometer® tester and stick to them. Peel if possible. Cut into cubes keeping seeds with the fruit. Heat to boiling in water, stirring with stainless steel spoon. When done, add citric acid and half as much sweetening as there is fruit. Bring to a boil again. Cool. Zappicate.

Fruit is often unevenly ripened. This changes its nature. I suspect this is the reason that bad chemicals like phloridzin and chlorogenic acid appear in them. Save such fruit for cooking, as in jams or jellies because this destroys these phenolics.

Dressings

Queen of Hearts Dressing (hides all supplements)

Fruit juices are easily made into dressings for many purposes, over vegetables, over rice, and even over a pile of vitamins dumped from their capsules.

- 1 cup fruit juice
- ½ tsp. (or more) citric acid powder
- 1 Tbsp. sweetening
- 2 Tbsp. thickener (rose hips, hydrangea powder, vitamins)
- extra spice (thyme, turmeric, fennel, nutmeg, cardamom, coriander, ginger); choose to suit the meal

Avoid fruit juice in brain cancer.

Boil fruit juice. Add to thickener slowly, while stirring to make a paste first. Add sweetening, spice, and citric acid.

The thickener can be any assortment of dry supplements that needs to "go down" at that meal. By keeping the fruit juice and citric acid mixture always handy and varied, any pile of vitamin powders can be consumed the easy way: on top of a lettuce salad. Rotate spices.

Tomato Sauce

Choose perfect cherry or Roma tomatoes because they do not produce malvin and are often unsprayed. Test for malonic acid, though. Sterilize with Lugol's water or ozonation or freezing.

- 2 cups whole tomatoes
- ½ cup water¼ tsp. sodium chloride (pure) salt
- 1 tsp. oregano or thyme leaves, organic, or fresh (garden)

Purchased oregano needs testing for thallium besides chlorox. Bring all ingredients to a hard boil for 2 or 3 minutes in a stainless steel saucepan. Empty this into a polyethylene container as soon as cool enough. Keep refrigerated or frozen. Keep oregano frozen, too. You can use a manual "food mill" to separate peels, seeds, etc. (see *Sources*). Eat the peel if there is no danger of sprays. *Variations*: Use fresh basil, if unsprayed, as seasoning.

Baked Goods

Bake cookies, cakes and pies from scratch, using unprocessed ingredients. Do not use paper cupcake cups, the wax coating has benzene. Do not use aluminum baking pans, bowls, measuring spoons, or foil wrapping. Do not use stretchable plastic film. Do not use plastic or wood utensils; use stainless steel. Plasticware can be hardened in boiling water for 30 minutes. Use aluminum-free baking powder, pure salt, and butter instead of oils.

Use flour that is not brominated; bromine attracts polonium to be stored in the spleen.

Cereals

Barley is the best choice, because it does not have the menadione phenolic allergen, even when stale. Other cereal grains should be nitrogen packed to avoid developing menadione. Store in freezer after opening. Do not ozonate, to avoid oxidation. Test for bromine.

Choose only the coarse varieties, not finely ground or very thin flakes to avoid nickel and chromium contamination from the blades. Don't risk this with breast cancer, which develops pain so easily.

Corn is a poor choice because it picks up air pollutants like strontium, beryllium, vanadium, chromium, each of which feeds an important pathogen.

Rice is second best, with least antigens.

Maria's Best Pancakes

- 32 ounces of Bob's Red Mill rice flour
- 1 stick of butter (Trader Joe's salted, turquoise package)
- 2/3 to ¾ cup of heavy cream (Lala crema Pura de Vaca brand in Mexico)
- 24½ oz. water (depending on consistency)
- raisins (Fairfield, Sun Maid) or currents (Sun Maid)
- 1 Tbsp. baking soda
- 1 tsp. salt
- ½ Tbsp. vitamin C
- 2 eggs (Mexican, unbleached)

Disinfect all ingredients. Combine all, except water, in large bowl. Mix together then add water slowly to desired consistency. Fry in butter.

Chewy Barley Pearls

- ¼ cup pearled barley (unbrominated)
- water to cover
- sweetening
- spice

Place sanitized barley and water in HDPE bowl and cover. Next morning drain liquid. Add sweetener. Eat straight. Save liquid to drink with spice.

Fish and Seafood Recipes

Since all varieties of fish and seafood had Fast Garnet dye and "shrimp" antigen (*the cause of lymphomas and lymph node metastases*) these recipes have been omitted. But you may fish it yourself and eat it within 6 hours. Don't use "household" chlorox bleach to clean up, nor buy fish at a fish market. Unpolluted fish is available in Mexico in several supermarkets.

Beans, Dried Peas, Lentils, and Garbanzos

In the uncooked state, these have no ONION chemicals. But if they are cooked at too high a temperature many ONION sulfides are made. They must not be heated higher than boiling water. This excludes frying, pressure cooking, and microwaving. When they are warmed up later, they must again not be heated higher than boiling water. Valuable, nutritionally, as they are, I consider them too hazardous for cancer patients because they form the alkylating agents along with onions, garlic and mustard that make part of the cancer-complex.

Meats

Sanitation of meats is quick and easy now that freezing and ozonation are available to penetrate deep into the interior. Safety from chlorox bleach treatment can be found by testing with a Syncrometer®. But the extra dyes used everywhere now and unsaturated oils dispersed in the meat create almost unsolvable problems. USA animals have been fed unsaturated oils, gallate-sprayed grains and given chlorox-bleached water to drink, like their owners.

Heightened parasitism is seen in chickens and beef. The animals seem sickly, judging by frequent antibiotic use (read the ads in animal feed stores), and not fit for consumption even by a healthy person. Four kinds of free-range raised (vegetarian) animals did not show these weaknesses:

(1) free-range, organic turkey
(2) free-range lamb
(3) free-range beef (test for Macracanthorhynchus, prions and gold)
(4) buffalo

Bone Marrow - Beef Broth

Buying long bones cut into short pieces where the bone marrow can be gotten out brings you **lactoferrin**, much needed in anemia and bone marrow disease (blood cancers). It is one of the few "meats" that is not dyed in the USA. Test for prions.

Part of the fat in the bone marrow of regular beef will be the unsaturated oils, linoleic and linolenic acid. You should avoid these if you have respiratory diseases because they are the triggers for most of these viruses. Stick to the free-range varieties or wait till your coughing is gone.

- 3 or 4 beef bones, cut to expose the bone marrow
- vegetable soup already made
- 1 bay leaf, tested
- sodium chloride salt (to taste)

Treat bones in original package in sonicator, or ozonate for 10 minutes or freeze at -20° F. In my tests only sonication destroyed prions. Place soup in large stainless steel pan. Bring to boil. Remove and discard foam that develops at first during cooking, using stainless steel spoon.

Add bones and cook five minutes more. Cool. Eat some bone marrow as soon as cool enough. (If it is absolutely delectable, due to a craving, eat the whole thing and make more in a few days.) Pour off the broth into HDPE container. Add 5 drops HCl. Drink one cup a day. Refrigerate. If fat solidifies at the top, do not throw this away. It belongs with the broth. Reheat it daily so it can be mixed. *Variations*: Make a cream soup out of leftovers: choose a vegetable and seasoning herb, like thyme, and lastly add cream.

Vegetables And Fruits

Most are sprayed with combinations of wax, dye, pesticide (thallium!), antisprouter, antimold, etc. Azo dyes (Fast Green and Fast Garnet) are present in most sprays, as are heavy metals and malonic acid. They penetrate the food deeply. But double soaking in hot water for one minute each time removes it. Even organic pears, plums and oranges must be double soaked this way. Peeling is not sufficient. Potatoes and yams will not come clean, though. Thallium pesticide and malonic acid penetrate too deeply to come out. If you have leg pain (caused by thallium), or effusions, shop only at a farmers' market and test even these.

If the food has chlorox bleach, implying polonium, cerium and ferrocyanide, do not try to salvage any part of it.

Ozonate produce to destroy leftover traces of dyes.

Parasite-Killer Recipes

Detox-Tea

Prion protein is present in all of us, repeatedly, as our hypothalamus gland becomes inflamed and releases free cells in the blood and lymph. If there is not enough pepsin to digest them, the remains turn into prions. These results are tentative. The true source is not yet certain. Our WBCs eat prions promptly. But if our WBCs do not have enough germanium, selenite, and vitamin C, the prions are not killed but escape and enter the brain and nerves. Light headedness and disorientation is felt. That contributes to detox-illness. You can kill them in hours with:

- 1 tsp. fennel seed (freshly ground), use capsules
- 1 tsp. sage, organic, (freshly ground)
- 3 heaping tsp. birch bark
- 1 Tbsp. sweetener
- 3 cups water

All herbs should be tested for thallium besides chlorox bleach because most are imported.

Birch bark is the strongest prion killer and could be used alone. Make birch bark tea by adding to boiling water and then simmering for 5 minutes. Add other ingredients to the birch bark tea. Set to cool. Drink 1 to 3 cups a day till symptoms stop. *Variation*: Reishi mushroom, unboiled, instead of birch bark. Make fennel-sage tea. Let cool; add 1 tsp. Reishi, also called Ganoderma.

Buski Tea

- 1 tsp. anise seeds
- 1 tsp. coriander seeds
- 1 tsp. fennel seeds
- 2 cups water
- ½ tsp. whole cloves
- 4 capsules nutmeg

2 cups barley water sweetener

Make barley water recipe first (page 563) and refrigerate. Add seeds to water and simmer 10 minutes (longer times cause lost activity). Add cloves and remove from heat. When cool, add cold barley water, nutmeg and sweetener. Refrigerate. Strain 1 cup to drink and put back solids. Next day, repeat. On 3rd and 4th day, eat the solids, with extra sweetener if desired. This tea reaches leftover Fasciolopsis in "unreachable" places like eye muscles, jawbone, spine, so expect minor pain here and <u>protect yourself from detox-illness</u>. If no detox is felt, take the 4 cups closer together until you can feel the effects.

Be sure all spices are tested; store them in freezer.

Pomegranate Seed

- 1 pomegranate, tested for chlorox, and refrigerated

Sanitize with Lugol's water. Cut in quarters. Then peel. Place seeds in blender. Blend 10 seconds at a time if fruit is cold, till seeds are fine enough to drink (about 8 sessions). Refrigerated fruit keeps blades cooler. The peel is also medicinal. It eliminates E. recurvatum.

Six Fresh Seeds

- 6 large apricots OR 6 peaches OR nectarines (in order of effectiveness). They do not need to be tested for chlorox since it does not penetrate the pit.

Let them completely ripen if you have time and chlorox is *Negative*.

Remove the pits. To crack open pits: find a rock or piece of cement brick. Slide it into a zippered plastic bag. Position it in your sink over the drain. Or, if you are near a cement sidewalk, slip the 6 pits into a double zippered plastic bag for cracking. Procure a heavy hammer. After cracking the pits, remove the seeds and place in grinder. If you are very sick choose the larger seeds, at least the size of your thumbnail. Adding the following is optional:

- ¼ tsp. nutmeg
- ¼ tsp. ground barley (raw)
- 3 tsp. shredded coconut or flakes

Grind 1 Tbsp. whole barley first for 4 seconds (only) in coffee grinder and store in freezer. Grind all ingredients together for 3 seconds only. Eat it all within one hour. The raw barley provides the drying effect that keeps fresh seeds from clogging the grinder and also brings organic manganese.

It may be thought that amygdalin or "laetrile" is the active ingredient of the 6 seeds, but there is no evidence for this. Clinical trials got stalled decades ago after finding it promising against cancer. Amygdalin keeps its potency but the active ingredients in this recipe do not.

Apricot kernels in health food stores have lost their potency, in spite of refrigeration, so you must prepare your own. Do not crack these pits ahead of time nor store seeds, although you may store pits. The Syncrometer® finds that the active ingredient is already a part of our metabolism, somewhat like a vitamin, and in similarly small amounts. It is not yet identified, chemically. Sick organs have none. The correct amount is essential for us but large amounts are toxic, somewhat like trace elements and hormones. I have not seen any side-effects. Nevertheless, do not take more. Six Fresh Seeds can single handedly kill SV40, Fasciolopsis buski, the tumor nucleus, and prions, as well as destroy many phenolics.

The dose is one set of 6 kernels daily for 3 days, using half of them in a suppository and the other half by mouth at the same time. Then take 1 or 2 days off and repeat till you are much better. You may grind by pounding seeds with a hammer.

NOTE: Apricot seeds have had this warning label to let you know they were once deemed toxic (LOW QUANTITIES MAY CAUSE REACTION. NOT SUITABLE FOR FOOD USE WITHOUT FURTHER PROCESSING-SECTION 10786 TITLE 17, CALIFORNIA ADMIN. CODE). Six fresh seeds has not resulted in stomach aches, headaches, diarrhea, or even fatigue. Their cancer-curing magic is easy to monitor by Syncrometer®. Read more on Internet.

Green Black Walnut Hull Tincture

- your largest stainless steel (not aluminum, ceramic, plastic, glass, enamel, or Teflon) cooking pot
- Black Walnuts, in the hull, each one still at least 50% green, enough to fill the pot to the top
- grain alcohol, about 50% strength, enough to cover the walnuts
- unfiltered, unchlorinated water, tested with a Total Chlorine test strip (see *Sources*), or kosher bottled water.
- vitamin C powder (capsules are fine).
- 1 or 2 ounce amber glass bottles and HDPE bottles without rubber droppers
- 1 gal. HDPE jugs as used for vinegar or water, with screw on lid

The Black Walnut tree produces large green balls in fall. The walnut is inside, but we will use the whole ball, uncracked, since the active ingredient is in the green outer hull.

Wash the walnuts carefully with water that does not have chlorox bleach disinfectant. Put them in the pot and cover completely with the alcohol. Sprinkle 1 tsp. vitamin C over them. Cover with lid. Let set for three days. Add another tsp. vitamin C. Pour into HDPE gallon jugs, using stainless steel funnel or homemade HDPE funnel. Discard walnuts. The vitamin C helps to keep the color green, as does the non-chlorinated, unfiltered water. Potency is strong for several years if unopened, even if it darkens slightly. Pour as soon as possible into 1 or 2 oz. amber glass or HDPE bottles. Freeze these after opening, to preserve green color.

When preparing the walnuts, wash only with cold tap water. Rinse with unfiltered, unchlorinated or kosher water to remove all chlorine. Distillers have filters attached. Beware of this problem or you will destroy your entire crop. You may need to use a brush on areas with dirt. If you are not going to use all of them in this batch, you may freeze them in a zippered plastic bag. Simply refrigerating them does not keep them from turning black and useless. The pot of soaking walnuts should not be refrigerated. Nor does the final tincture need refrigeration. But freezing it before opening protects it from turning dark.

Exposure to air causes the tincture to darken and lose potency very quickly. To reduce air exposure, fill the pot as much as possible while still keeping a snug fitting lid. Even more importantly, the HDPE jars or bottles you use to store your tincture should have as little air space as possible and should not be repeatedly opened before use. A large jar should be divided into the 1 or 2 oz. size bottles all at one time. Quality is better if poured originally into 1-serving containers.

There are several ways to make a 50% grain alcohol solution. Some states have Everclear™, 95% alcohol. Mix this half and half with unfiltered, unchlorinated, or bottled kosher water. Other states have Everclear™, which is 76.5% alcohol. Mix this two parts Everclear™, to one part water. Do not use vodka or the flask-size Everclear™; it must be 750 ml or 1-liter. Smaller bottles have wood alcohol or isopropyl alcohol pollution.

This is the second time that purchased water is allowed in this very important recipe. A half-million lives of cancer patients could be saved in a year. There is a lot at stake. You may buy bottled water in 1-gallon jugs if it passes these tests:

- Syncrometer® testing for chlorox bleach, ferricyanide, ferrocyanide, polonium, methylene blue should be *Negative.*
- Heavy metals and sodium hypochlorite should be *Negative.* Any variety of chlorine bleach has hypochlorite.
- Thulium and gold should be *Negative.*
- Isopropyl alcohol should be *Negative.*
- Malonic acid should be *Negative.*
- Radon and alpha, beta, gamma radiation *Negative.*

Any brand of bottled water will not be the same in different sizes and in different parts of the country. Be sure to use only the size and source you have tested. You may also use rainwater stored in HDPE water jugs and only filtered through washed cheesecloth, see page 202.

Lugol's Iodine Solution

It is too dangerous to buy a commercially prepared solution for your internal use. It is certain to be polluted with isopropyl alcohol or wood alcohol. Make it yourself or ask your pharmacist to help you. You must see the stock bottles, not trust the pharmacist. The recipe to make 1 liter (quart) is:

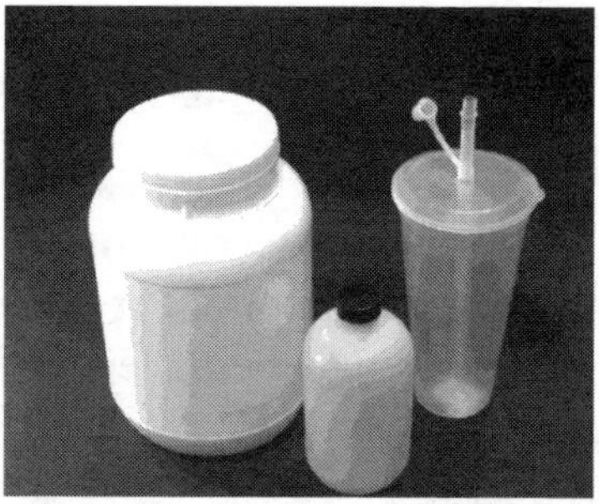

Suitable high density polyethylene containers can be found on the Internet.

Fig. 137 Containers that do not seep

- 44 gm (1½ ounces) iodine, granular, USP
- 88 gm (3 ounces) potassium iodide, granular, USP
- diet scales and plastic cup and spoon
- large HDPE bottle with screw cap (see *Sources*)

Dissolve the potassium iodide completely in about a cup of water in a HDPE container. Then add the iodine crystals and wait till they are all dissolved. This could take ½ hour with frequent shaking. Then fill to the liter mark (quart) with pure water. (Draw a permanent line here.) Be careful to avoid chlorox bleach water for preparation or you would pollute it yourself. Use kosher water if unsure. Place a plastic zippered bag, not kitchen wrap, over the top; then close tightly before storing. Keep out of sight and reach of children.

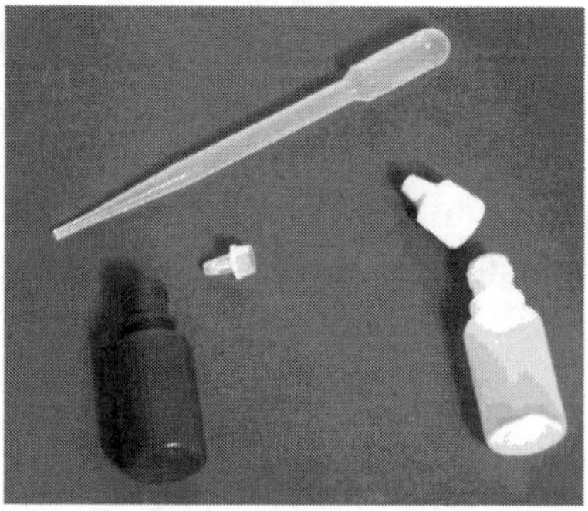

Fig. 138 Drop dispensers

Do everything inside the kitchen sink. Wipe stains up promptly with vitamin C powder. The dropper bottle for dispensing should be made of polyethylene with built in drop dispenser or a separate pipette free of chlorox.

Lugol's Iodine Drops

- 6 drops Lugol's iodine solution
- ½ cup water

This specifically kills Salmonella bacteria in your body. It can be taken at any time. If taken at end of meals, it helps to sterilize the food just eaten so gives you double benefit. Do not use if allergic to iodine (see page 548). Do not add it to other beverages. Do not take together with vitamins since these will become over oxidized. If the problem has not cleared up in two days, do the Lugol's-turmeric enema for several days (see page 469. Lugol's gives the fastest relief for most food-related stomach distress; it takes about one hour. The turmeric kills E. coli.

White Iodine

- 88 gm (3 ounces) potassium iodide, granular, USP

Add potassium iodide to one quart/liter cold water. Potassium iodide dissolves well in water and stays clear; for this reason it is called "white iodine". Label clearly and keep out of reach of children. Do not use if allergic to iodine. It is useful for disinfecting the mouth and helpful to the dentist but it is not as strong as Lugol's.

Benzoquinone (BQ) (for clinical use only)

- 500 mg. benzoquinone powder (not hydroquinone). (One size 00 capsule filled with powder, by hand.)
- 1000 ml (1 liter/qt.) pure water. The variety "for injection" often has chlorox bleach contamination. Distilled water that shows no conductivity nor chlorination or kosher water is much safer.

This should be made and supervised by a physician. Prepare 2 non-seeping HDPE bowls by cutting off the bottom ends of 2 water jugs of 1 gallon size. Pour 1 pint of water into each bowl. Empty the BQ capsule into one bowl, stirring with a non-seeping plastic spoon until completely dissolved (about one minute). Further dilute this as follows: ½ ml BQ solution, as prepared above, is added to a second pint of water in the second bowl. It may be drawn up with a HDPE pipette tested for chlorox. All quantities can be approximated, since the final concentration should be one part per million but need not be exact. After the second dilution, the BQ solution must be used within 20 minutes. If there is further delay, the solution must be made up from the powder again. The containers should be emptied but not rinsed. A dose of one cc (2 cc for persons over 100 lb.) is given in the muscle (IM) in the hip after cleaning skin with ethyl alcohol. This is 1 mcg. Give the shot slowly to reduce burning. Patients may exclaim over their improvement by the time the needle is out.

The BQ solution is thrown out when it is 20 minutes old. All containers are used only for this purpose. Before first use, they are rinsed with pure water to remove any adhering antiseptic. It is only rinsed and drained after that—never chemically cleaned or brushed.

ORGAN IMPROVEMENT RECIPES

The Bowel Program

Bacteria are always at the root of bowel problems, such as pain, bloating and gassiness. They cannot be completely killed by zapping, because the high frequency current does not penetrate the bowel contents.

The worst bowel bacteria are the Salmonellas, Shigellas, and E. coli because they have the ability to grow in the rest of your body. One reason bowel bacteria are so hard to eradicate is that we are constantly reinfecting ourselves by keeping a supply on our hands and under our fingernails. The second reason is that the bacteria are themselves infected by oncoviruses and carry radioactive particles that give them protection from your WBCs.

1. The first thing to do is improve sanitation. Use 70% (approx.) grain alcohol in a spray bottle at the bathroom sink.

Or Lugol's iodine, one drop per cup water. Sterilize your hands after bathroom use and before meals by spraying or dipping them.

2. Second, take Lugol's solution, six drops in ½ cup water 4 to 6 times daily. This is specifically for Salmonella, which is responsible for at least half of all bowel distress. If your Lugol's solution is only 2% iodine, as in Veggie Wash, use 10 drops.

3. Third, use turmeric (6 capsules, 3 times daily). This is the common spice, which I find helps against Shigella, as well as E. coli. Expect orange colored stool.

4. Fourth, use fennel (6 capsules, 3 times daily). Take turmeric and fennel, one after the other and 5 minutes after Lugol's for fastest relief.

5. Fifth, take four digestive enzyme capsules all together, any variety.

6. Sixth, take 1 tsp. tincture or 2 capsules freeze-dried Black Walnut Hull, preferably at bedtime.

7. Seventh, do a Lugol's-turmeric enema or a Lugol's-turmeric-fennel enema once a day. Do them one right after the other using a Fleet bottle and 2 capsules of each herb. Use 10 drops Lugol's first (see page 589).

8. Eighth, <u>if you are constipated</u>, take Cascara Sagrada, an herb. Start with one capsule a day, use up to maximum on label. Take extra magnesium (300 mg. magnesium oxide powder, two or three a day), and drink a cup of hot water (flavored is fine) upon rising in the morning. This will begin to regulate your elimination. Constipation is usually caused by *Clostridium botulinum*, which makes its own chemicals in your colon to inhibit the neurotransmitters there. These are the normal driving force for intestinal movement. Use betaine hydrochloride capsules, three with each meal, to keep Clostridium out of your colon. Constipation can also be caused by other bowel bacteria. Certain drugs, such as morphine or similar painkillers produce constipation as a side-effect. You must work hard to be sure you expel bowel contents at least once a day...if necessary, with an enema.

There are more ways to empty the bowels. For some people, senna tea works well. For others ½ cup prune juice works fine. For still others, milk of magnesia or Epsom salts work well. Finally, for immediate action, a glycerine suppository works in 15 minutes. These are available at all pharmacies. Be sure all items are sterilized.

With this powerful approach, even a bad bacterial problem should clear up in two days. If it doesn't, you are feeding them their special requirements. They all require special heavy metals (see page 328). This is like fanning flames. Test all your dishes and cookware for seeping heavy metals with a conductivity indicator. Throw out all stored food in your refrigerator. It may have bacteria. Eat only ozonated, frozen or sonicated food. Keep your own hands sanitary. Keep fingernails short. Do not put fingers in mouth. Your tummy can feel flat, without gurgling, and your mood can be good. Remember, cancer is not the cause of your bowel problems. You ate polluted food and nurtured the bacteria.

It may take all the remedies listed. Afterwards, sanitize all your food, put hydrochloric acid drops in all your food, and eat out of non-seeping dishes. Test all supplements and drops for Salmonella and E. coli.

Moose Elm Drink-also known as-Slippery Elm

For sensitive stomachs when nothing wants to stay down, and for obstructions:

- 1 Tbsp. moose elm (also called slippery elm) herb
- 1 cup cold water
- sweetener (*optional*)

Start by making a paste of the powder and a bit of water as if it were cocoa. Gradually add more water to consistency desired. Sweeten. Zappicate. This can be drunk hot or cold. Sip one cup a day. You may use heavy whipping cream, diluted with water or other beverage. Test the herb first for pollution.

Alginate/Intestinal Healer

For intestines or stomach that are sore from surgery or cancer.

- 1 tsp. sodium alginate powder
- 1 cup water

Soak alginate in water about 4 hours or overnight until completely dissolved and pourable (instead of boiling, as in old recipes). Add to soup, stew, moose elm drink, pudding or pie filling. Alginate is not digested—it merely forms a long ribbon of soothing gel that coats trouble spots and finds its way through the narrowest passageway to keep it open. Use 1 cup a day. It is quite tasty combined with Moose Elm. Add more water or more alginate to suit consistency desired.

Lugol's Enema (not if allergic to iodine)

Add ¼ tsp. (25 drops) of Lugol's iodine to 1 pint of very warm water; pour into Fleet™ bottles (giving yourself several doses), or enema apparatus (see *Sources*). Administer enema slowly and hold internally as long as possible. Cold water will cause spasms and inability to hold it. Prepare only a cup, with 12 drops Lugol's or 20 drops diluted Lugol's, the first time; do not force yourself to hold more than is comfortable.

Lugol's-Turmeric-Fennel Enema

This is a "super" enema that can improve your sick-feeling immediately. Timing is important for this since Lugol's can kill bacteria, but not the oncoviruses sheltered inside the bacteria.

After the Lugol's enema, do a second one right away, within minutes after emptying the bowel from Lugol's treatment. Prepare it ahead of time.

Have ready 6 capsules turmeric already emptied in the bucket; close valve and add 1 cup very warm water. Run it in <u>slowly</u> to avoid expelling it. None of this super enema is to be expelled <u>at all</u>. That is why so little water is used. Do not pull out the tube yet. Sit on it or lean back to reduce pressure. After

20 to 30 minutes empty 6 fennel capsules in the bucket, add ½ to 1 cup water and run it in very slowly. Do not pull out the tube yet. After another 20 minutes, open 2 coenzyme Q10 capsules into hot water, they will cool en route. Keep these in for 15 minutes. Then add a final ½ tsp. of Lugol's to top of tube. After running each one in, lie down, read or watch entertainment till all urgency to expel is gone. Leaning back helps, too.

If you did need to expel, reduce the water volume next time.

This "super" enema, given correctly, has the most powerful effect on how sick you feel. Even if you feel immediately better though, these bacteria and viruses will all come back unless you complete the whole program. Do not premix Lugol's or other items with each other. Wash the bottle, nozzle, bucket and hose using Lugol's in water until color is visible, it kills everything it contacts. For more help, read earlier books by this author.

Black Walnut Hull Enema

Add 1 tsp. of Black Walnut Hull Extra-Strength, or homemade, to 1 pint of very warm water. Repeat as for Lugol's enema.

Apricot Suppository

Crush 6 apricot seeds in a zippered plastic bag using a hammer or rock inside a zippered bag. Mix half of them with some soft butter so you can roll it up in a piece of plastic, into a pencil shape, about 1" long.

Put in freezer or refrigerator for 5 minutes just to get hard. Soon it will be hard enough to insert as a suppository.

Shove it as far as you can reach with your middle finger. Wear a single finger cut from a plastic glove to cover yours.

Buy apricot pits and crack them only an hour before using the seeds. Do not buy seeds – they have no potency. Pits do not need testing; chlorox does not penetrate. Do not refrigerate or freeze pits or seeds to store them.

Go to bed with it in. Do not expel.

Chew the other 3 seeds after the suppository is in.

Take 9 wormwood and 9 cloves before or after apricots.

Giving Yourself the Perfect Enema

Any drop you spill and everything you use to do the enema will somehow contaminate your bathroom. Yet you must leave it all perfectly sanitary for your own protection. So follow these instructions carefully.

Spread out a large plastic trash bag on top of paper towels on the bathroom floor. Place a plastic zippered bag beside it. Set a chair nearby, too. The trash bag is for you to lie on. Lie on your back if you have nobody to help you.

The enema apparatus shown is best for larger volumes. It is easy to see through every part, to know what is happening (see *Sources*).

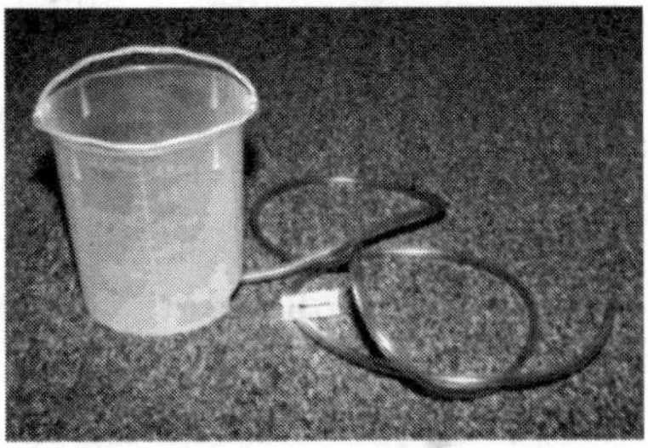

Fig. 139 Enema container, tube, pinchcock

Test the apparatus first, in the bathroom sink to see how it works. Wipe away the grease that comes with it on the applicator; it is sure to be a petroleum product and be tainted with benzene.

Place a dab of butter onto the zippered bag for the lubricant. Or place a wet bar of homemade soap on it. Also alcohol and paper towels.

Do a practice session first.

After filling the container with the enema solution, run some through the tubing until the air is out of it and close the pinchcock. Place it on the trash bag.

Insert the applicator tube as far as you comfortably can. Then lift the container with one hand while opening the valve with the other. The higher you lift it, the faster it runs. Take as much time as you need to run it in. You may wish to set the container on the chair. Very warm liquid is easier to hold. Don't force yourself to hold it all. At any time you may close the valve, withdraw the applicator, and place it on the paper towel.

If you cannot insert the tube, you will need to do a pre enema with just a Fleet bottle of warm water first. Use only the bottle, not the purchased contents.

Cleaning up the apparatus, the bathroom, and yourself: This topic is seldom discussed, but very important. Notice that some bowel contents have entered the container by reflux action, which is unavoidable. Consider the whole apparatus contaminated. For this reason you must never, never use anybody else's apparatus, no matter how clean it looks.

First, wipe the applicator tube with toilet paper. Then fill the container with hot water and run it through the hose into the toilet. Repeat until it appears clean; this is appearance only; you must now sterilize it. Fill it with hot tap water and add Lugol's iodine (not your pure variety!) or povidone iodine (from a pharmacy) until intensely red in color. Place the tube to soak, rinsing the whole length of it with the iodine water. Empty both tube and container; then wipe the outside of the tube with paper. Do not dry the container. Store it all in a fresh plastic shopping bag. Throw away the bags and soap. Clean the sink with chlorine bleach (NSF variety, 5 or 6%). Then wash your hands with Lugol's water for several minutes.

Kidney Cleanse

- ½ cup dried hydrangea root, organic, (c/s)
- ½ cup gravel root, organic, (c/s)
- ½ cup marshmallow root, organic, (c/s)
- 4 bunches of fresh parsley, frozen
- ginger capsules
- Uva Ursi capsules

- Black Cherry Concentrate, 8 oz., tested
- vitamin B_6, 250 mg.
- magnesium oxide, 300 mg. in powder form

All herbs should be tested for thallium and chlorox bleach pollution. Organic varieties are less likely to have these. Do not ozonate them nor UV them. Deep freezing is the best disinfectant.

Measure ¼ cup of each root (this is half your supply) and set them to soak, together, in 10 cups of water, using a stainless steel saucepan tested for seeping. After four hours or overnight, add 8 oz. black cherry concentrate, heat to boiling and simmer for 20 minutes. Drink ¼ cup as soon as it is cool enough. Pour the rest through a stainless steel strainer into a HDPE container. Refrigerate.

Find fresh parsley at a small neighborhood grocery store where the water has the correct disinfectant bleach. Give it 2 very hot washes. Boil the fresh parsley in 1 quart of water, or as much as needed to cover it, for five minutes (rolling boil). Drink ¼ cup when cool enough. Freeze 1 pint and refrigerate the rest. Throw away the parsley. Alternatively, you may crush the frozen parsley and eat 1 Tbsp. daily, straight or mixed with food.

Dose: Each morning, pour together ¾ cup of the root mixture and ½ cup parsley water, into a safe cup. Drink this mixture in divided doses throughout the day. Refrigerate. Do not drink it all at once or you will get a stomachache and feel pressure in your bladder. If your stomach is very sensitive, start on half this dose. But if your problem is very severe, such as ascites, increase to a double dose by the 3rd day and keep this up till the ascites is reduced.

Save the roots after the first boiling, storing them in the freezer. After 13 days when your supply runs low, boil the same roots a second time, but add only six cups water and simmer only 10 minutes. This will last another eight days, for a total of three weeks.

After three weeks, repeat with fresh herbs. You need to do the *Kidney Cleanse* for six weeks to get good results, longer for severe problems.

Also take:

- ginger capsules: 2 with each meal (6 a day) for 1 week only
- Uva Ursi capsules: 2 with each meal (6 a day) for 1 week only
- vitamin B_6 (250 mg.): one a day
- magnesium oxide (300 mg.): one a day 10 minutes before a meal

Ginger and Uva Ursi remove methyl malonate from the kidneys, which clogs them. It is also the cause of kidney failure and cystic kidneys (see page 459). Take these supplements 5 to 10 minutes before your meal to avoid burping. If you are already taking these supplements, omit them here. The parsley combines with each one of the 5 malonic acid members that I call the M Family, and removes them.

Some notes on this recipe: this herbal tea, as well as the parsley, can easily spoil. Heat it to boiling every third day if it is being stored in the refrigerator to reduce bacteria. After this you may take it to work without refrigerating it (use a HDPE container or a zippered plastic bag inside a jar). Fold the bag over the edge to drink it.

When you order your herbs, be careful! Herb companies are not the same! These roots should have a strong fragrance. If the ones you buy are barely fragrant, they have lost their active ingredients; switch to a different supplier.

Liver Cleanse

This is particularly important in any disease-prevention program. Cleansing the liver of gallstones dramatically improves digestion, which is the basis of your whole health. You can expect your allergies to disappear, too, more with each cleanse you do! Incredibly, it also eliminates shoulder, upper arm, and upper back pain. You have more energy and increased sense of well being.

It is the job of the liver to make bile, 1 to 1½ quarts in a day! The liver is full of tubes (*biliary tubing*) that deliver the bile to one large tube (the *common bile duct*). The gallbladder is attached to the common bile duct and acts as a storage reservoir (see page 178). Eating fat, protein, or citric acid triggers the gallbladder to squeeze itself empty after about 20 minutes, so the stored bile finishes its trip down the common bile duct to the intestine.

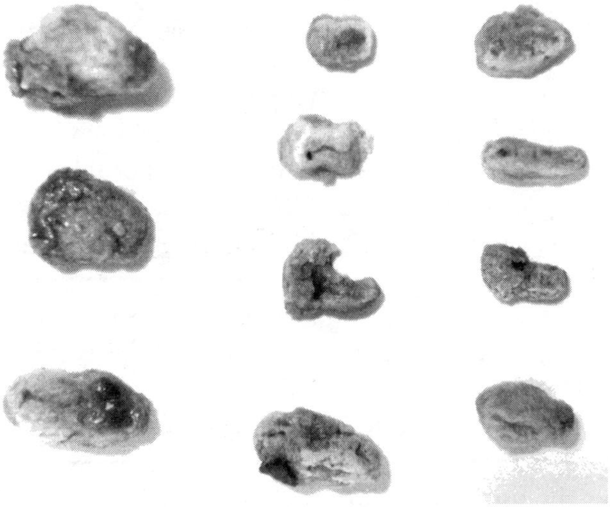

Fig. 140 These are gallstones

For many persons, including children, the biliary tubing is choked with gallstones. Some develop allergies or hives but some have no symptoms. When the gallbladder is scanned or x-rayed nothing is seen. Typically, they are not in the gallbladder. Not only that, most are too small and not calcified, a prerequisite for visibility on x-ray. There are over half a dozen varieties of gallstones, most of which have cholesterol crystals in them. They can be black, red, white, green or tan colored. The black ones are full of wheel bearing grease and motor oil, which turns to liquid in a warm place. The green ones get their color from being coated with bile. Notice in the picture how many have imbedded unidentified objects. Are they fluke remains? Notice how many are shaped like corks with longitudinal grooves below the tops. We can visualize the blocked bile ducts from such shapes. The ducts have been too weak to open for a long time. Weakness comes from interrupting the nerve impulses with the insulator-like automotive greases. Other stones are composites—made of many smaller ones—showing that they regrouped in the bile ducts some time after the last cleanse.

At the very center of each stone is found a clump of bacteria, according to scientists, suggesting a dead bit of parasite might have started the stone forming.

As the stones grow and become more numerous the backpressure on the liver causes it to make less bile. It is also thought to slow the flow of lymphatic fluid. Imagine the situation if your garden hose had marbles in it. Much less water would flow, which in turn would decrease the ability of the hose to squirt out the marbles. With gallstones, much less cholesterol leaves the body, and cholesterol levels may rise.

> Emptying the liver bile ducts is the most powerful procedure that you can do to improve your body's health.
> But it should not be done before the parasite program, and for best results should follow the kidney cleanse.

Gallstones, being sticky, can pick up all the bacteria, viruses and parasite eggs that are passing through the liver. In this way "nests" of infection are formed, forever supplying the body with fresh parasite eggs and bacteria. No stomach infection such as ulcers or intestinal bloating can be cured permanently without removing these gallstones from the liver.

Cleanse your liver twice a year.

Preparation:

You can't clean a liver with living parasites in it. You won't get many stones, and you will feel quite sick. Zap daily the week before, or get through three weeks of parasite-killing before attempting a liver cleanse. If you are on *Maintenance Parasite Program*, you are always ready to do the cleanse.

Completing the kidney cleanse before cleansing the liver is also highly recommended. You want your kidneys, bladder and urinary tract in top working condition so they can efficiently remove any undesirable substances incidentally absorbed from the intestine as the bile is being excreted.

Choose a day like Saturday for the cleanse, since you will be able to rest the next day.

Take no pills or vitamins that you can do without; they could prevent success. Stop the *Parasite Program* and *Kidney Cleanse*, too, the day before. Even stop zapping and taking drops.

Ingredients	
Epsom salts	4 tablespoons
Olive oil	½ cup *(light olive oil is easier to get down)*
Fresh pink grapefruit (*for brain and spinal cord cancer use apple juice, with citric acid, see page 600*)	1 large or 2 small, enough to squeeze ½ cup juice *(you may substitute a lemon, adding water or sweetener to make ½ cup liquid)*
Ornithine	4 to 8, to be sure you can sleep. Don't skip this or you may have the worst night of your life!
Pint jar with lid	
Black Walnut Hull tincture, any strength	10 to 20 drops, to kill parasites coming from the liver.

Double hot wash the grapefruit. Zappicate the oil to destroy traces of benzene and PCBs or add a few drops of hydrochloric acid to the bottle and shake.

Eat a no-fat breakfast and lunch such as cooked cereal, fruit, fruit juice, bread and preserves or sweetening (no butter or milk). This allows the bile to build up and develop pressure in the liver. Higher pressure pushes out more stones. Limit the amount you eat to the minimum you can get by on. You will get more stones. The earlier you stop eating the better your results will be, too. In fact, stopping fat and protein the night before gets even better results. Finish eating by 12 noon with only sips later.

2:00 P.M. Do not eat or drink after 2 o'clock. If you break this rule you could feel quite ill later.

Get your Epsom salts ready. Mix 4 Tbsp. in three cups water and pour this into a safe jar. This makes four servings, ¾ cup each. Set the jar in the refrigerator to get ice cold (this is for convenience and taste only).

6:00 PM. Drink one serving (¾ cup) of the ice-cold Epsom salts. If you did not prepare this ahead of time, mix 1 Tbsp. in ¾ cup water now. You may rinse your mouth, but spit out the water.

Get the olive oil and grapefruit out to warm up.

8:00 P.M. Repeat by drinking another ¾ cup of Epsom salts.

You haven't eaten since two o'clock, but you won't feel hungry. Get your bedtime chores done. The timing is critical for success.

9:45 P.M. Pour ½ cup (measured) olive oil into the pint jar. Squeeze the grapefruit by hand into the measuring cup. Remove pulp with fork. You should have at least ½ cup. You may use lemonade. Add this to the olive oil. Also, add Black Walnut Hull Tincture. If you haven't gotten stones out in the last few cleanses, add citric acid to bring success. Also, using 2/3 cup water for Epsom salts instead of ¾ can bring success. Close the jar tightly and shake hard until watery (only fresh citrus juice does this).

Now visit the bathroom one or more times, even if it makes you late for your ten o'clock drink. Don't be more than 15 minutes late. You will get fewer stones.

10:00 P.M. Drink the potion you have mixed. Take 4 ornithine capsules with the first sips to make sure you will sleep through the night. Take eight if you already suffer from insomnia. Drinking through a large plastic straw helps it go down easier. You may use salad dressing, syrup, or straight sweetener to chase it down between sips. Take it to your bedside if you wish. Get it down within five minutes (15 minutes for very elderly or weak persons). If you had difficulty getting stones out in the past add ½ tsp. citric acid to the potion. You may put it in capsules.

Lie down immediately. You might fail to get stones out if you don't. The sooner you lie down the more stones you will get out. Be ready for bed ahead of time. Don't clean up the kitchen. As soon as the drink is down walk to your bed and lie down flat on your back with your head up high on the pillow. Try to think about what is happening in the liver. Try to keep perfectly still for at least 20 minutes. You may feel a train of stones traveling along the bile ducts like marbles. There is no pain because the bile duct valves are open (thank you Epsom salts!). **Go to sleep**, you may fail to get stones out if you don't.

Next morning. Upon awakening take your third dose of Epsom salts. If you have indigestion or nausea wait until it is gone before drinking the Epsom salts. You may go back to bed. Don't take this potion before 6:00 am.

2 Hours Later. Take your fourth (the last) dose of Epsom salts. You may go back to bed again.

After 2 More Hours you may eat. Start with fruit juice. You may add another ½ tsp. citric acid to it (or capsules) and get even more stones. Half an hour later eat fruit. One hour later you may eat regular food but keep it light. During the day take the parasite-killing herbs and zap. By supper you should feel recovered.

Alternative Schedule 1: Omit the first Epsom salts dose at 6 p.m. Take only one dose, waiting till 8 p.m. Change nothing else. Many people still get stones with one less dose. If you do not, do the full course next time.

Alternative Schedule 2: Add ½ tsp. citric acid to the oil-grapefruit mixture. Stir till dissolved. Next morning, add ½ tsp.

citric acid again to the first fruit juice you drink when done with Epsom salts.

Alternative Schedule 3: For brain and spinal cord cancers, caffeic acid is the antigen to be avoided. This includes grapefruit. Blend whole apples instead, Red or Golden Delicious. Strain to get ½ cup juice. Add ½ tsp. citric acid to oil-juice mixture.

If you don't get stones…

- Use slightly less than ¾ cup water for each Epsom salts dose, such as 5/8 or 2/3 cup.

CONGRATULATIONS!

You have taken out your gallstones without surgery! I like to think I have perfected this recipe, but I certainly cannot take credit for its origin. It was invented hundreds, if not thousands, of years ago, THANK YOU, HERBALISTS!

How well did you do? Expect diarrhea in the morning. This is desirable. Use a flashlight to look for gallstones in the toilet with the bowel movement. Look for the green kind since this is proof that they are genuine gallstones, not food residue. Only bile from the liver is pea green. The bowel movement sinks but gallstones float because of the cholesterol and automotive grease inside. Count them all roughly, whether tan or green. You will need to total 2000 stones before the liver is clean enough to rid you of allergies or bursitis or upper back pains permanently. The first cleanse may rid you of them for a few days, but as the stones from the rear travel forward, they give you the same symptoms again. You may repeat cleanses at two-week intervals. Never cleanse when you are ill.

Sometimes the bile ducts are full of cholesterol crystals that did not form into round stones. They appear as "chaff" floating on top of the toilet bowl water. It may be tan colored, harboring millions of tiny white crystals. Cleansing this chaff is just as important as purging stones.

At the first diarrhea, search for parasites, using the photos in this book to help find them. Use the Gary Technique (page 184) if possible to keep them in good shape till you can identify them or photograph them. Save a dozen shallow plastic bowls to keep the varieties separate for easier identification.

How safe is the liver cleanse? It is very safe. My opinion is based on over 500 cases, including many persons in their seventies and eighties. None went to the hospital; none even reported pain. However it can make you feel quite ill for one or two days afterwards, although in every one of these cases the *Maintenance Parasite Program* had been neglected. This is why the instructions direct you to complete the parasite and *Kidney Cleanse* programs first.

Warning: If you do change these recipes in your own way you might expect problems. The liver is quite sensitive to details. It is recommended to seek the help of a therapist.

This procedure contradicts many modern medical viewpoints. Gallstones are thought to be formed in the gallbladder, not the liver. They are thought to be few, not thousands. They are not thought to be linked to pains other than gallbladder attacks. It is easy to understand why this is thought: by the time you have acute pain attacks, some stones are in the gallbladder, are big enough and sufficiently calcified to see on x-ray, and have caused inflammation there. When the gallbladder is removed the acute attacks are gone, but the bursitis and other pains and digestive problems remain.

The truth is self-evident. People who have had their gallbladder surgically removed still get plenty of green, bile-coated stones, and anyone who cares to dissect their stones can see that the concentric circles and crystals of cholesterol match textbook pictures of "gallstones" exactly.

Dental Recipes

Hardening Dentures

Various kinds of dentures, including colored, can be hardened using this recipe. This means they will not seep acrylic acid, urethane, bisphenol-A, phthalates, metals, or dyes, to a detectable level. But it will not stop polonium or uranium radiations. The hardening was tested with a Syncrometer® by soaking dentures of various kinds and colors in water for many hours and sampling the soak-water. If you will not be able to test, repeat this 3 times:

- Place dentures in a saucepan and cover with tap water. Heat till it is steaming but not boiling. Turn off heat. Cover. Let stand ½ hour. Remove and rinse. Repeat twice with fresh water.

Your mouth should have no reaction, no redness, no burning, and no odd symptoms from wearing your dentures. If symptoms occur, repeat the hardening recipe. Also repeat after every visit to the dentist even for the most minor adjustments.

Dental Bleach

This recipe is easier to make than ever before. This is because NSF bleach is now available in 5 to 6% strength like regular bleach. Find the varieties listed in *Sources*.

This is for use during dental work and for occasional denture cleaning. Do not use it as a regular mouthwash or as a daily denture soak. You would get too much chlorine.

The chemical name for bleach is **hypochlorite**. There are different grades. The grade used only for laundry is not acceptable.

Bleach is very caustic. It must be diluted before you can use it without harm. Please follow these directions carefully.

- 1 tsp. (5 ml) bleach, USP (NSF) grade, 5-6% hypochlorite

- 1 pint water (500 ml) from your outside faucet. Remove garden hose first. If this is not NSF quality use rainwater or kosher water, see *Sources*.

Use a HDPE pint bottle (see *Sources*). Fill with water. Add bleach (1 teaspoon). Use a plastic teaspoon to measure and mix. The result is .05% hypochlorite. This is only a quarter as strong as the .2% solution recommended by Bunyan* for oral surgery, but is strong enough for *Dental Bleach*.

Keep out of reach of children. If any kind of bleach is accidentally swallowed, give milk to drink and see a doctor at once.

Hardening Toothbrushes and Other Small Plastic Things

Buy a new toothbrush of the straight-stick variety. Many new styles and brightly colored brushes have come into the market place. They seep large amounts of plasticizer and dyes! They are especially dangerous to children and sick persons. Harden them by placing them in a saucepan and covering with tap water. Heat slowly till steaming. Then turn heat off and let stand for 30 minutes, covered. Drain. Wash the brush in fresh water and repeat twice.

Only the straight-stick kind of toothbrush can be hardened this way. Buy them by the dozen (see *Sources*). The sculptured kinds with fat portions of plastic cannot be hardened at all. BEWARE!

---

* Bunyan [in The Use of Hypochlorite For The Control of Bleeding, Oral Surgery, v. 13, 1960, pp. 1026-1032] reported that rinsing with 0.2% hypochlorite solution stops postoperative bleeding within 1 minute after a tooth extraction or other oral operation. The hypochlorite solution functions also to contract and harden the blood clots and make them more resistant to infection. In addition to the effective hemostasis and the change in the character of the clot, the author reported a reduction of swelling of traumatized gingival tissues and diminution of the postoperative pain.

Oregano Oil Toothpowder

- 10 tsp. baking soda, disinfected by freezing
- 10 drops oregano oil, disinfected by freezing

Be sure these ingredients are chlorox-free (ask for test results).

Place ingredients in zippered plastic bag. Squish the mixture in the bag till well mixed. Store in HDPE closed jar or keep in original bag. Freeze again to sanitize later. This is about a 2-month supply. Brushing daily will keep Clostridium bacteria at undetectable levels. Dip dry toothbrush in powder. But be careful, oregano oil straight in your mouth could make you jump with burning sensation although it does not harm you. If you accidentally get too much, chew bread and keep your tongue at the roof of your mouth.

Immediately after dental work your mouth is too sore to brush your teeth. In fact, it is unwise to use a brush at this time. Simply **rub** your teeth after flossing. Wind a strip of paper towel around your finger. Dampen with a few drops of water and dip into the powder. *Variations*: Essential oils are too strong to be used daily, unless they are of the culinary variety. You may use 1 drop clove, ginger, basil, cardamom, peppermint, fennel, sage oil, but only once a day to avoid allergy.

Straight Dental Bleach is 4 times stronger than the mouthwash variety. It is .2% sodium hypochlorite. Use it to sterilize your dentures overnight.

Denture Cleaner

To keep your denture free of bacteria, disinfect it every night, rotating the disinfectant.

- Dentures that acquire gray or fine-lined discoloration are growing Clostridium bacteria! Kill them by brushing with *straight Dental Bleach* (see *Sources*). Let denture stand without rinsing until the discoloration is gone. Rinse with vitamin C water (add ½ capsule vitamin C to ½ cup water). Rotate the following treatments:

- Soak in *straight Dental Bleach* overnight once a week. This is 0.2% sodium hypochlorite (NSF grade). Rinse with vitamin C water. If you use it more often you could get allergic to chlorine! BEWARE.
- Sonicate once a week in a small jewelry cleaner.
- Ozonate twice a week.
- Soak in salt water, ¼ tsp. pure salt to ¼ cup water three times a week.

Alcohol, Lugol's and weak salt solution are not strong enough. Commercial solutions have dyes, sweetener and must be tested.

Don't keep partials or dentures in your mouth at night. Your mouth should <u>always</u> smell sweet.

Denture Adhesive

- 1 rounded tsp. sodium alginate
- 1 cup water
- 2 tsp. grain alcohol (Everclear only), tested for chlorox bleach, isopropyl alcohol, and wood alcohol. This is only for preservation, not essential.

Let mixture stand in water 4 or more hours till completely dissolved. To make it stronger, add more alginate and wait longer. Keep notes on your favorite concentration. Don't use commercial sources that are colored blue or green. The coloring is due to methylene blue dye or a cobalt compound.

This powder can be used straight, dusted lightly on denture after wetting denture surface. Use slim plastic salt shaker.

Soap and Shampoo

For Dishes

Take care of your cleaning and personal needs using <u>only homemade recipes</u>. There are many more in earlier books.

Use borax for all cleaning purposes except for dishes in the sink. For laundry see instructions on box; for dishes use in granular form to scour; for dishwasher, 2 tsp. plus 1½ tsp. citric acid as the rinse. (It takes 3 dishwasher loads to remove old scum and give you gleaming glasses. You only need to do this once). Also use borax to shampoo and for personal soap. It inhibits bacteria, leaving a residue that deters them. For the shower keep it in a vitamin bottle. Open and stick in 2 fingers to pick up enough for special places. Then wash each hand. Soapless showers are easy to get used to.

Borax Liquid Soap

- 8 heaping Tbsp. borax powder
- 1 gallon plastic jug
- funnel

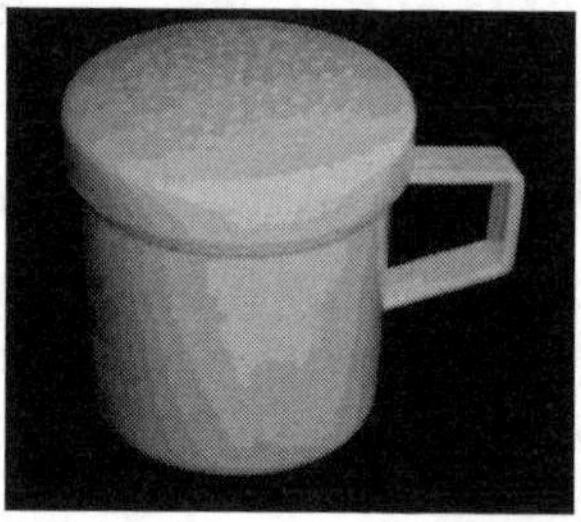

Fig. 141 Salt shaker makes nice dispenser for powders

Pour the borax into the jug, fill with the hottest tap water you can get. Shake a few times. Let settle. There should be no crumbs. Add hot water if there are. Pour into dispenser bottles. It will not suds or bubble much, but it should feel slippery between your fingers. The most common mistakes are not using hot enough water and pouring crumbs into your dispenser bottles.

For dishes in the sink, add as much homemade liquid soap as you have liquid borax. For really greasy dishes use homemade lye soap straight. This is much too strong for regular use on your skin, though. Find gentler recipes in earlier books. For ungreasy dishes use no soap at all, simply wash by hand under hot faucet.

Shampoo

- 1 heaping Tbsp. borax
- 2 cups very hot water.

Pour a heaping Tbsp. borax into a plastic container and enough very hot water to dissolve. There should be no crumbs left at the bottom. If there are, add more hot water. Scoop it up over your hair by hand. Rub it in lightly. By the time all your hair is wetted, it will already be squeaky clean. Massage scalp, too. Borax removes dandruff bacteria. To rinse, use citric acid (see *Sources*). Remove traces of benzene from citric acid by microwaving the entire bottle for 1 or 2 minutes first. Ascorbic acid, lemon juice or vinegar are not strong enough to rinse out borax. Put 1 or 2 teaspoons citric acid in a plastic container like a cottage cheese carton. Add about 1 cup of your shower water when you are ready for it, otherwise it will be cold. Leave rinse in hair for one whole minute while showering your body; then rinse out lightly. After rinsing, your hair should already feel silky. If it does not, make more rinse while you are still in the shower and leave it on longer.

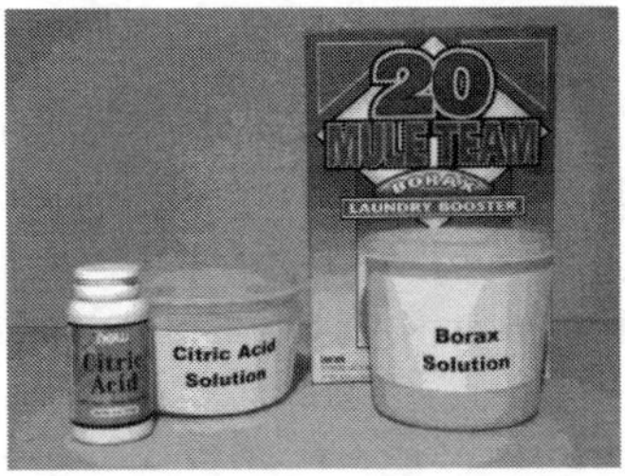

Make a bottle of borax liquid to fill your soap dispensers and shampoo bottle. Use citric acid to rinse and condition hair.

Fig. 142 Borax & citric acid for the shampoo

For Dyed Hair: Add 2 tsp. citric acid to the borax solution when shampooing. Be sure it is dissolved. It will preserve more dye. A cancer patient should use no commercial dye.

Baking Soda Shampoo

- 2 Tbsps. baking soda (remove traces of benzene by microwaving the whole box for two minutes first)
- 2 cups very hot water

Place both in a plastic container and stir with your fingers until dissolved. This is the soap. To shampoo scoop it up over your hair by hand; if you pour it, too much runs off. This time rinsing with ascorbic acid (1 tsp. to 1 cup water) or vinegar (equal parts vinegar and water) works well. Leave rinse in hair one minute. To add sheen to hair, wash a whole lemon twice in hot water; then press lemon against hair.

Baking Soda Shampoo II

Place baking soda box within reach while you are in the

shower. Prepare the conditioner and set nearby. After wetting your hair, take a handful of baking soda straight from the box. Spread it through your hair, rubbing gently. Condition with lemon juice, vinegar, or citric acid.

DO'S and DON'TS for hair

- Never put alcohol on your scalp, it will kill hair follicles.
- Never let very hot water reach your scalp, it will kill your hair follicles.
- Your hair should always have a final acid rinse (vinegar, lemon juice, or citric acid). It combats bacteria.
- All these hair shampoos do wash some color out of dyed hair. Nothing is known yet to prevent this. But adding citric acid to the shampoo reduces it.

Hair Dye

BEWARE: Recently some black henna varieties were found to have chromium metal contamination. Test yours. This could add to the pain already present for many sick persons. A cancer patient should use no commercial hair dye.

Light Golden Blonde

...for totally gray hair. This recipe is enough for short hair. Double everything exactly for medium long hair. It has not been tried for middle age hair, but it is so easy and quick, it's worth a try. You won't need any help.

- 1¼ cup cold water
- ½ cup white vinegar
- 2/3 cup Black Walnut Hull powder (see *Sources*)
- 1 qt. saucepan
- Optional for darker color: 1 heaping tsp. Pure Red Henna from Nour (see *Sources*)

Heat water to near boiling. Turn down heat to steaming. Add vinegar. Dip out 2 Tbsp. for later use. Measure Black Walnut powder into cup carefully—over the sink. Add to liquid and stir till smooth with fork. It should still be steaming. Cover to prevent spattering the stove. Let stand for 20 min. at low stove setting, not boiling, for dye to be extracted. Add the extra water 1 tsp. at a time if consistency needs adjusting. If too thin, heat longer. It should be like medium gravy.

No mess. Prepare the bathroom. Lay 4 to 6 paper towels in shower or bathtub for instant clean up. This dye did not stain my tile or shower.

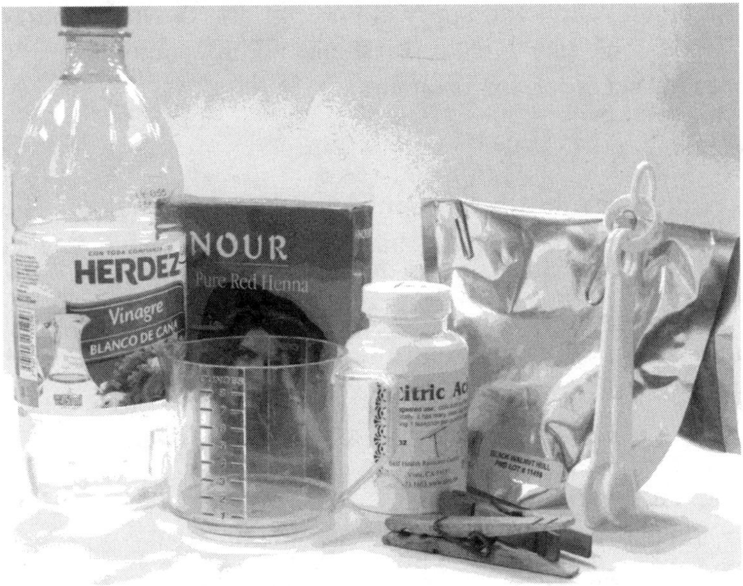

Set nearby: a shower cap or plastic grocery shopping bag; 2 or 3 clothespins; 1 strip of paper towels (2 sheets long, folded twice down the middle, lengthwise, to get a long neckband); 2 single sheets of paper. Turn bathroom rugs upside down, although black drips will wash out in regular laundry.

Before applying stir one more time and adjust consistency.

Apply to dry hair when just cool enough. You can stick your head in the shower for this, without undressing. Set the saucepan on a plastic chair. Pick up handfuls of dye (do not pour) and place directly on top of hair. Mix thoroughly with hair by hand. If consistency is too thick it will spatter; if it is too thin it will run off the hair. Remedy both immediately with

1 tsp. hot water or 1 level Tbsp. powder at a time. Keep notes for next time.

If your mixing-hand turns brownish, you know the dye is taking to your hair, too. When done, tie the long paper band around your neck very loosely. Use a clothespin to help. Tie a second one around your neck, too.

To cover hair with plastic shopping bag, cover head first, then bring handles forward and up to forehead. Twist handles round and round and apply clothespin. Pat down the puffy bag till you look like a baker or sheik, adding a clothespin where needed. Set clock for 1½ hours.

To Wash Out…

…Prepare the bathroom again giving yourself several choices of shampoo and conditioner until you have reached the best recipe for yourself.

Make egg shampoo with 2 raw eggs in a bowl. Beat with fork about 50 times. You might never go back to your old shampoo after this!

OR – Prepare Low pH Shampoo to keep dye in

- 2 cups very hot water
- 1 Tbsp. borax
- ½ Tbsp. citric acid

Stir all together till dissolved. Set near shower. The acidity should be about pH 6, using litmus paper.

Wash away dye without very hot water, till all particles are out. Then shampoo. The more alkaline your shampoo is, the more dye you will lose. You may add citric acid to any shampoo to make it less alkaline, but these are experiments for you. Condition hair with citric acid, after washing out shampoo (3 tsp. to 1 cup water) for one full minute. Another choice is straight vinegar. Let hair soak in vinegar for 2 to 3 minutes. Meanwhile finish your shower. Rinse hair lightly.

Comb first, dry later, for curly or wavy hair. Dry with single sweeps from front to back, not back and forth motion. Dry in the sun for glossy hair, or wash a lemon in hot water and press on hair in single strokes at a later time. To keep hair glossy and wavy, do not use a hair blower; keep hair still till completely dry. This is a failsafe and forgiving recipe with very little work or clean up.

Deodorant

Sweating removes toxins from the body especially the iron cyanides and MUSTARD oils. By taking enough MSM as a supplement the odor of it disappears. A cancer patient should use no chemicals to retard sweating. Sweating in the armpits undoubtedly protects the breast. Of course, you will ruin your clothing, though! Try 1/8 tsp. baking soda as an absorbent in each armpit. Wash this out of shirts and blouses by hand in cold water to prevent staining before laundering or dry cleaning. After you are well, you could use straight alcohol (Everclear only) on clothing as well as yourself. Oregano tooth powder works well as deodorant, too. Essential oils must be tested for chlorox, namely polonium, first.

Laundry Recipes

Borax is not strong enough to remove chlorox from clothing.

The following recipes remove wheel bearing grease, polonium, iron cyanides and alkylating agents (mustard oil) from clothing in one wash cycle. You will not need borax or NSF bleach in addition to the recipe.

Choose any dry uncolored detergent marked kosher, or tested for chlorox and methylene blue dye. Your choice may not be strong enough to remove cyanide and polonium. For this reason, use extremely hot water and double the alcohol in the recipe given.

You have a choice of dry detergents. In Mexico choose:

1.) Bold, con aloe vera   2.) Dona Blanca

In the USA choose:

1.) Cheer, free & gentle   2.) Gain, island fresh

Instructions

- Use hottest water possible (barely able to hold hand in it).

- 2 cups dry detergent
- 2 cups alcohol (Mexican Las Canitas) (USA Everclear 95%; use more alcohol if it is a lower percentage, page 582).

Wipe the washing machine first with a paper towel and detergent if it is shared by others.

Put ingredients in the machine, then add clothes, then turn on water. DO NOT switch these around. One cycle is enough to remove the cancer-complex from laundry. After this, use borax as usual for cancer patients.

NOTE: Do not use Mexican alcohol for any other purpose. It has not been tested for metals or solvents.

Skin Lotion

After finding major air pollutants in all corn products, it seems wiser to switch to a different starch. Beryllium, strontium, vanadium, and chromium are now present in large amounts, causing multiple chemical sensitivities. Even one capsule using cornstarch can start an allergic reaction later.

- 3 tsp. pure arrowroot starch (see *Sources*)
- 1 cup water

Test starch for chlorox bleach. Boil starch and water until clear, about one minute. Cool. Pour into dispenser bottle. Keep refrigerated. **For Rashes And Chafe** use arrowroot starch dry on rashes, fungus, moist or irritated areas and to prevent chafe. Adding magnesium oxide or zinc oxide makes it even drier.

Lipstick

A stick of raw red beet cut like a "French fry" is more convenient and useful than any recipe. Store in plastic bag in refrigerator. Use also on cheeks for rosier complexion.

Eyeliner

Use washed and tested charcoal.

CHAPTER 23

SAMPLING AND TESTING

How To Test Your Water

Only water that is disinfected with chlorox bleaches have oil and grease in them, and the correlation is 100%. The difference between these kinds of waters is easy to see with the naked eye if they are carefully prepared. I will describe 3 ways to find which water has chlorox bleach disinfectant.

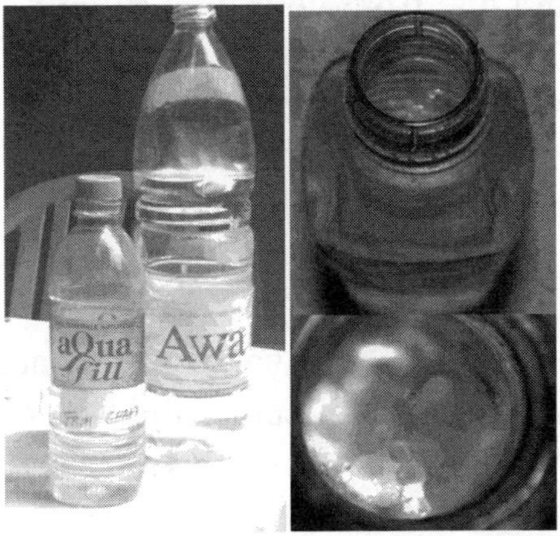

Unopened water bottles from Africa develop oil slicks at the surface in 3 to 6 weeks, if left undisturbed.

Fig. 143 African bottled water

The Theory

The principle underlying these methods is that oil rises in water. The top portion of the water will then have more oil and grease than the bottom. The top portion will have less electrical conductivity because electricity travels less well through oil than water. A conductivity meter or a handmade device could be used to compare the conductivity at the top and bottom of a water sample. On the other hand, oil detection paper could be dipped into the surface. Only very oily water could be detected this way, though, such as water from Africa. Thirdly, a flashlight could detect oil if there is a film on the surface and if the beam makes the correct angle to see it. These methods do not identify the oils chemically, but they are more reliable than laboratory methods, for simply finding them present.

There are no quantitative aspects to consider. If any oil is seen in a water sample it has chlorox bleach in it. And you can infer the presence of PCBs, benzene, polonium, ferrocyanide and the other toxins.

Making A Water Sample To Test

Now that it is easy to test by Syncrometer® which bleach has been used in your water, it is not necessary to make many samples. One sample from an outside faucet and one from your kitchen cold faucet is all that is needed. Bottles used to sample should be rinsed 3 times in the water you are sampling.

Wash your hands, without soap, between different samples or you will cross-contaminate them.

The Conductivity Way

There are a variety of conductivity indicators on the market. By collecting the water in a large container with a spigot at the bottom you can compare top with bottom water more easily.

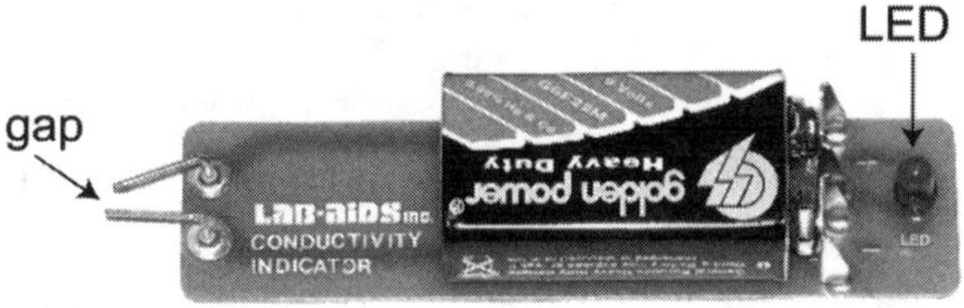

Fig. 144 Conductivity indicator

An inexpensive device is available that has a very short gap (.5 to 1 mm) between two wires that connect to a battery and tiny LED light. When current is flowing the LED lights up. When the two wires are stuck into clean tap water, considerable electricity will flow. You can adjust the gap to be more or less sensitive. Water with oil in it is less conductive, so the light will be dimmer. Compare the top and bottom layers of water that has stood over a month. Draw it from the bottom to compare with the top. Water that is flowing cannot show you the conductivity differences.

How to Use the Conductivity Indicator

1. Use a fresh 9-volt battery, not rechargeable variety. Keep it in a separate bag. It will last a long time.
2. Handle the tester with great care. Everything depends on the gap at the tips of the wires.
3. Buy distilled water, more than one kind. You need to find a variety that shows <u>no</u> conductivity.
4. Attach battery to tester. Fit one side of battery first. Then swing battery into the other side of connector. This prevents accidental damage.
5. The tester light should not be on. If it is, separate the tips of the wires with a piece of paper. Bend them apart very gently till no light comes on when the paper is removed.
6. Turn off all room lights. It should be dark.
7. Open water jug, stick tester into distilled water, not above the wires. Light should not go on.
8. If the light goes on it is not suitable water. Try a different distilled water. When you have a distilled water that does not turn on the light you are ready to start.
9. Pour distilled water into the containers you want to test for metal seepage. Allow a suitable time, like 2, 12 or 24 hr.
10. Rinse the device before each test, in the distilled water, giving it a shake to dry it. Do not use anything to dry it except a very <u>soft tissue</u>. Use a <u>very soft touch</u>. If you do not dry it before you lay it down it could short later and turn the light on by itself. That would drain the battery.
11. Now dip the device in each water container, not above the wires. Keep it in about 20 seconds, moving it around. Cup your hands around it to make it darker so you can see better. There should be no light, not even the faintest glimmer. That is a

good container, such as bowl, saucepan, dishes. Even the faintest glow is too much; discard the container.

12. After each test, wash the electrodes in the distilled water as in #10.

13. Well water, chlorinated water and rainwater all have considerable conductivity. Only distilled water may not.

14. This does not test for malonic acid or solvents or dyes. It is not as sensitive as a Syncrometer®. A conductivity meter is better in some ways. But it does not detect the weaker metals such as germanium or thallium.

The Centrifuge Way

The method: Purchase an inexpensive table centrifuge, with centrifuge tubes for holding liquids and a small brush (similar to a bottle brush) for cleaning them. Caps are not needed. You need not wait for oil and grease to rise with this method. The centrifuge speeds it up.

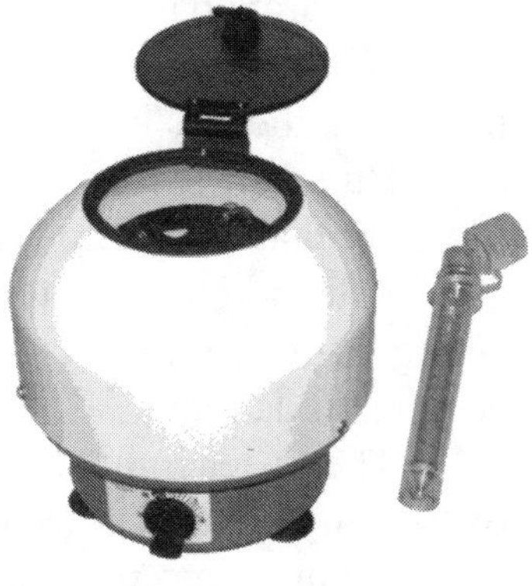

Fig. 145 Centrifuge & tube

Pour water to fill 2 centrifuge tubes nearly to the top. Label them and arrange them across from each other in the centrifuge, leaving the other holes empty. Or use other holes to test other kinds of water, including clean water. Arrange them all symmetrically. This keeps the centrifuge from wobbling. After centrifuging at least 30 minutes at the highest speed it is capable of, set the tubes upright in a drinking glass to store till you can test for grease at your convenience.

Then choose one of these test methods:

1. Dip your conductivity indicator into the surface and note light intensity or other kind of evidence of the conductivity. Compare this with the conductivity of this same water that has not been centrifuged.

2. Wait till an oil film appears at the surface. It may take the form of grease "particles" instead of a flat film at the surface. It may come in patches or swirls. It could take a week.

How To Make Saliva Test Samples

Homeographic Saliva Sample

Being able to capture the frequency pattern of a saliva sample in pure water is important to be able to transport it safely and to be able to store it for an indefinite time. You can capture it in a small bottle of water (Method 1 M) or in a zippered plastic bag of water (Method 2 M).You will need:

Method 1 M

This method has been modified to leave out the added water in earlier recipes. This will reduce the possible errors that stem from using impure water.

- a small bottle that fits snugly in your hand so there is maximum surface contact between hand and bottle. A ½ oz. amber bottle of glass or plastic, with non-metal cap, is fine.
- paper, such as kitchen towel, unfragranced, uncolored, tested for chlorox. Cut or tear a 3" x 3" piece (8 cm x 8 cm).
- zippered plastic bags, tested for chlorox, about 6" x 6", not stretchable.
- rainwater, stored in HDPE container, untreated.

A sample of the paper should be made as "control". Place in separate zippered bag. Label it CONTROL.

Stuff the square of paper in your mouth, dry, and chew till wet but not dripping. Spit it into a zippered plastic bag without touching it with your hands. Zip shut. Set aside.

Next, prepare the water sample that will receive the frequency pattern.

Put 2 tsp. water, up to the shoulder, but not measured, in the ½ oz. bottle. This leaves room for shaking. Close.

Holding the bag with saliva sample in your hand, place the bottle of water on top of it (the bag). The bottle should be positioned above the paper wad. Grip both tightly. If you used too big a bag this will not be possible. Shake 130 times vigorously (20 shakes per 5 seconds; practice this beforehand). Label the bottle "Saliva #1, Manual".

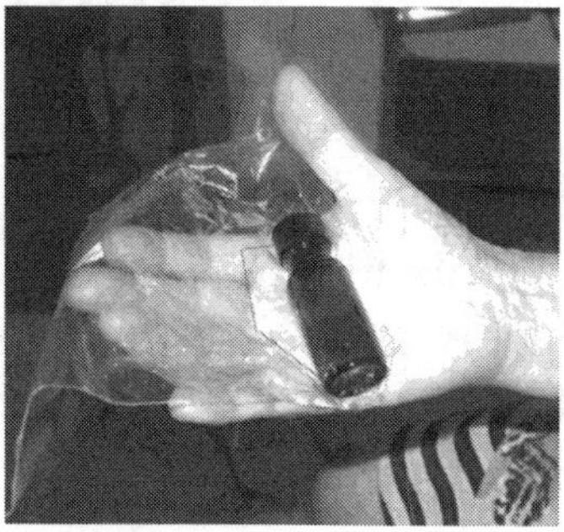

Chewed paper wad is in bag under bottle.

Fig. 146 Homeographic saliva sample

Explanation: Saliva, as you produce it, is given the number "1". After adding water, it is called #2; its electronic properties are changed. The copy of #2 is called #3; if copied by hand it is called "Manual". If it is copied on copy maker, it is called "electronic".

Protect your copy of saliva from direct sunlight and magnetic fields. That is why the amber color and plastic lid were chosen. Wrap the bottle in layers of packaging material, or "bubble wrap" to keep it safe from magnets while traveling. Always ship in baggage compartment. No refrigeration needed.

Evidently, your body is supplying the high frequency energy needed to "carry" (modulate) the pattern from the saliva sample through the glass or plastic into the water. The action may be similar to homeographic copy-making (see page 198).

After shipping the bottle should be tested for "shipping damage" (see page 200).

Method 2 M

This method has been modified, too, omitting the water added to the saliva sample.

You will need only the paper, water and zippered plastic bags. First we will make the saliva sample; then we will copy it into some clean water in a second bag.

Cut or tear a piece of paper towel without fragrance or a printed pattern. The size should be about 3 inches square. Stick it all in your mouth and chew it till it is quite damp. Spit it into a zippered plastic bag of sandwich size, about 6 inches square (not bigger) without touching it with fingers. This is called a #1 sample because it has had nothing added. Close the bag securely. Set aside.

Put about 1 Tbsp. of rainwater into a second zippered bag.

We will copy the frequency pattern of the saliva sample into this water sample.

Check each bag for leaks, expelling some air so the bags will lie flat on each other.

Place the saliva sample bag in your strongest hand so the corner with the sample is in your palm. Place the water sample on top of it, also in your palm. Fold the empty portions of the bags inward so you are holding all of it in your hand. If you chose large bags this will not be possible. Gripping it tightly, shake it 150 times, as fast as you can. Aim for 4 shakes per second. You may take rests. You may switch hands without starting the count over. It is better to change hands to rest than to slow down. Stop the count while you rest.

Even if the bags loosened and got misaligned, and a few drops escaped, the frequency will probably transfer. If water escaped, close the bags again very tightly. Rinse them with rainwater and dry each side carefully. Finish shaking. Then throw away the bag with saliva sample. For shipping, place the newly made water sample in a second zippered bag and both of these in a plastic bottle (used vitamin bottle). Put bottle in a third zippered bag.

During shipment all the seals will open! Each sample needs its own 3 bags. Label it Homeographic Saliva Sample #1 copy.

It is safe and can be shipped without special precautions.

How To Stop Your Pitcher Filter From Seeping

Take out the filter unit. Bring tap water to a near-boil and pour it into the pitcher. Fill the pitcher to the top. Cover and let stand for ½ hour. If the plastic is very flexible, you should do this twice, because there may be a lot of DAP in it. (DAP is a known carcinogen.)

Next we will stop the metal seepage from the filter unit. If you are not very handy, draw it first, so you can put it back together correctly.

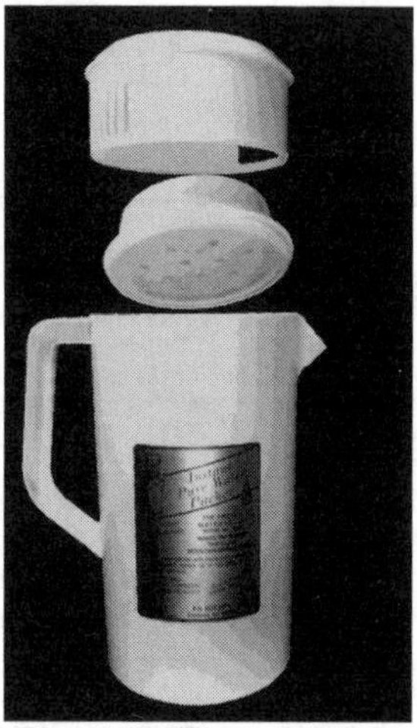

Fig. 147 Water pitcher with filter

Take it apart. Pour the charcoal into a steel saucepan and set aside. Put the white fiber or other cushioning into its own saucepan and set aside. Place the plastic parts into a third saucepan. Cover them with tap water. Bring to a near-boil. When steaming, turn heat off. Cover and let stand for ½ hour. Drain and rinse twice with tap water.

Cover the fiber with near-boiling water. Let stand 5 minutes and drain. Repeat 2 more times. Rinse with tap water.

Cover the charcoal with a huge excess of tap water (nearly a quart). Bring to a boil and boil 5 minutes. Drain carefully so charcoal stays in pan. Add a bit more tap water and drain a second time. If you used distilled water you will recontaminate the charcoal. Spoon the charcoal back onto its padding and reassemble the filter unit. Pour your distilled water into the filter pitcher. DO NOT FILL IT SO FULL IT TOUCHES THE FILTER. Leave 1 inch (2½ cm) of space. Pour through the filter into a non-seeping glass or a zippered bag. Test with conductivity indicator.

You could, of course, test each part separately before reassembling it. Clean your charcoal by boiling it 5 minutes every 2 weeks. Other parts do not need reheating.

Trouble Shooting the Filter

You can't assume the filter is doing its job even if you put it all together correctly. Test the water by Syncrometer® for ruthenium, strontium, aluminum, beryllium, rubidium, and rhodium, even if the conductivity indicator detects nothing. You may make the tester more sensitive by making the gap smaller. Be sure to rinse and dry very gently after each test now to avoid accidental "shorting". Keep the test water covered to reduce carbon dioxide absorption from the air, which raises conductivity.

If the water shows you some conductivity, don't drink it. Study your filter. The fit of the filter unit may be so loose that the distilled water is bypassing the filter. In this case test the filtered water by Syncrometer® for malonic acid, DAP, thallium (which is not very conductive), and traces of strontium, beryllium, aluminum, ruthenium, and rubidium. The ruthenium comes from the charcoal itself and from the distilled water, even if properly disinfected. That is why the boiling is done in tap water.

How To Clean Activated Charcoal For Filter Pitcher

Dump new or used NSF grade charcoal, wet or dry, into a stainless steel pan. There will be 3 or 4 Tbsp.

Cover with about 3 cups tap water (NSF bleach disinfected). Boil charcoal 5 minutes. Drain. Add another ½ cup tap water and drain again. (If you accidentally rinse with distilled water you will reload the filter with ruthenium.) Finally, spoon the charcoal back into its padding.

This does not clear chlorox bleach from charcoal.

Filter Padding

Save the fiber padding from old filters to use in homemade ones. They are easily cleaned, just under the hot faucet. When padding is not available, a piece of nylon hose tested for chlorox bleach works well, too. Boil the whole hose 5 minutes first and rinse under faucet. When dry cut a 5 or 6 inch length, tying a knot at one end. Spoon in the clean charcoal and tie other end. This can be made to lay flat in the pitcher filter or HDPE gallon filter (here it is tucked into the funnel).

CHAPTER 24

SOURCES

Many sources for herbs, vitamins and minerals have used the name Clark to promote their products and to help you identify products that I recommend.

Please be careful in your choices. This whole book is about products that contain polonium, uranium, and other unthinkable toxins that cause cancer. Yet there is no way for YOU to distinguish these from others in the market. I am well aware of the dilemma it creates for you.

The customary logo that has always identified products that I have tested by Syncrometer® is an outstretched hand with a sine wave held in it. This signifies that the frequency is an important part of its action and unless it has been very carefully crafted and tested by Syncrometer® it could not be relied on.

And there is no way for the manufacturer to distinguish between ingredients that contain chlorox and those that do not. Hopefully, testers will soon be available for this most important of jobs. At present, about 80% of all edible things and 90% of all objects that touch you (like toothbrushes, floss, toothpaste, lotions) have chlorox bleach disinfectant, with its traces of polonium.

Brands can be quite deceptive, copying portions of other logos, or using similar colors. Beware. Brands can break even the ground rules of construction of a sensitive device. Imagine a watchmaker using polished nickel instead of silver inside, but neglecting to check how well it keeps time.

If you are a manufacturer but cannot test, you must be doubly careful to follow instructions, exactly. All the homemade zapper builders, for instance, did so successfully, showing you it can be done by anyone.

If you, the consumer, detect any substitution in a recipe or device, buy elsewhere. Raising our standards of performance will benefit us all.

The logo to identify devices that have been tested by me is still in production. Hopefully the self-imposed standard that is implied in the stamp will yield big dividends in health.

This list was accurate as this book went to press. Only the supplement sources listed here were found to be pollution-free. Only the herb sources listed here were found to be potent and chlorox-free. There are, of course, many sources worldwide that could not be tested. Hopefully, this new technology will soon be automated so that all manufacturers and vendors can take leadership again in providing quality products.

The author has no financial interest in any company listed.

Note to readers outside the USA:

Most sources listed are companies in the United States because they are the ones I am most familiar with. You may be tempted to try a more convenient manufacturer in your own country and hope for the best. I must advise against this! In my experience, an uninformed manufacturer most likely has a polluted product! Your health is worth the extra effort to obtain the products that make you well. One bad product can keep you from reaching that goal. Best of all is to learn Syncrometer® testing yourself. Nearly all the caregivers and about 1/3 of the patients learned while they were at the clinic.

When contacting these sources, ask first for their **retail department**. They may wish to direct you to a nearby distributor. Be patient. **When ordering chemicals for internal use, always ask for the food grade variety.**

Item	Source
Activated carbon	See charcoal
Amber glass or polyethylene bottles, ½ ounce	Continental Packaging Solutions (large quantities); Self Health Resource Center; Drug store
Amino acid mixture, liquid for IV use and other IV liquids in glass bottles	Abbott Laboratories; Mexican pharmacy
Amino acids, dry	Spectrum Chemical Co.; Seltzer Chemicals, Inc., Self Health Resource Center
Anatomy set	See microscope slides
Anesthetic (topical, for dentistry)	Blistex Inc. a) Kanka gel; b) Kanka Blistex (with benzoina)
Anise Oil	Nature's Alchemy; San Francisco Herb & Natural Food Co. , Self Health Resource Center
Arrowroot starch, #P170	San Francisco Herb & Natural Food Co.
Aspartic acid	Spectrum Chemical Co.
Baking soda (sodium bicarbonate)	Karlin Foods Corp.; Spectrum Chemical Co. , Self Health Resource Center
Basil Oil	Nature's Alchemy; San Francisco Herb & Natural Food Co.
Beeswax	Brushy Bee
Benadorm	Mexican pharmacy
Benzocaine (20%)	Pharmacy
Betaine hydrochloride	Seltzer Chemicals, Inc.
Birch bark tea	San Francisco Herb & Natural Food Co.
Black cherry concentrate	Bernard Jensen Products; health food store
Black Walnut Hull powder	See hair dye
Black Walnut Hull tincture	See Green Black Walnut Hull
Bleach, USP ((NSF) also see Dental Bleach	Smart and Final; Wal-Mart; Target and others; Colgate Palmolive; Arctic White; Hilex, Javex
Blender	Proctor-Silex; Wal-Mart; Target and others
Boneset	San Francisco Herb & Natural Food Co. , Self Health Resource Center
Bottled water (kosher)	Acadia (distributed by Foodhold USA);

Item	Source
	Niagara Bottling LLC; Whistler Water Co.
Bottle-copies	See homeographic copies
Bottles	See HDPE bottles
Bottle-copy shields (electrical conduit pipe, 1 inch diameter, 2¾" long and 2 ¼" long	Hardware and plumbing stores; Testers, place the shorter ones over bottles when testing (amplifies about 2X).
Borax	Grocery store
Boric acid	Spectrum Chemical Co.; health food store; pharmacy; animal feed store
Bread maker (no Teflon)	Breadman (Ultimate Plus), available – Target; Wal-Mart
Bromelain	San Francisco Herb & Natural Food Co.
Burdock	San Francisco Herb & Natural Food Co.
Cactus, Prickly Pear, tablets (Nopales)	Plantas M. Anahuac, C.A. de C.V. Raw is available seasonally. , Self Health Resource Center
Cardamom oil	Nature's Herb Co. (kosher and parve); San Francisco Herb & Natural Food Co. Self Health Resource Center
Cascara Sagrada	San Francisco Herb & Natural Food Co.; Self Health Resource Center
Catnip	San Francisco Herb & Natural Food Co.
Charcoal (NSF chlorinated)	Self Health Resource Center
Cheesecloth	Protec (Mexico pharmacy)
Chlorination supplies	Pool and spa store (Desert Star, Sani Clor, Water Guard); (also see Bleach, USP)
Chlorine test (Total-Chlorine, Free Chlorine) test strips	Industrial Test Systems, Inc. (sensitivity at least 0.05 mg/L [.05 ppm]). Use for testing wells, filters; Pet stores; Self Health Resource Center
Cholecalciferol	See vitamin D_3
Chrysanthemum	San Francisco Herb & Natural Food Co.
Cigarettes (polonium-free) Djarum Black	Kretek International, Inc.
Cilantro	San Francisco Herb & Natural Food Co.
Citric acid	Univar
Cleaning sponges	Scotch-Brite (Heavy-Duty 3M); U.F.O., Inc.; grocery store
Cleavers	San Francisco Herb & Natural Food Co.
cloves	San Francisco Herb & Natural Food Co.

Item	Source
	(Ask for fresh); Starwest Botanicals, Inc. Self Health Resource Center
Coenzyme Q10	Self Health Resource Center; Seltzer Chemicals Inc.
Coffee mill (hand grinder)	Lehman's
Colloidal silver maker	CTS Originals
Compass	Camping store; science store
Conductivity indicator	Lab-Aids, Inc., Self Health Resource Center
Coriander oil	Nature's Herb Co. (kosher and parve); San Francisco Herb & Natural Food Co.
Cosmetics	New Ways, Self Health Resource Center
Cumin	San Francisco Herb & Natural Food Co.
Currants	Sun-Maid
Decaris (levamisole)	Not available in USA, but it is non-toxic and very helpful in amounts recommended, visit another country for it.
Dental Bleach (NSF)	Self Health Resource Center
Denture Bleach (sterilizing)	Self Health Resource Center
Dental chemicals	I have not found dental chemical supply companies to be reliably pure. Order your dental chemicals from regular chemical companies like Spectrum Chemical Co. and others.
Dental help in Europe	Naturheilverein
Dental impression compounds	Bosworth Company (Plasto-paste Base-White and Accelerator-Brown; also Superpaste, Base-White and Accelerator Green); GC America, Inc.; DENTSPLY (Jeltrate regular); Kerr Corporation Company; Patterson's Dental Supply, Inc.
Denture material	Fricke Dental International, Inc.; other acrylics
Denture powder (adhesive)	Self Health Resource Center; Super Corega (Mexico pharmacy)
Dental probe	Make your own
Dental supplies Anesthetics – Scandonest (brown ring) 2% vial adrenaline 18 mg.; 30/0 (green ring)	Net 32; or check individually on Internet;

Item	Source
vial without adrenaline Anesthetic, local: Mepivicaine with adrenalin, in brown ring vial; Anesthetic by injection – Mepiseal Fillings Crowns Sutures – Ethicon 3-0; silk, black braided CE; silk, black braided 3-0; Ethicon 5-0; black silk; white braided mersilene, polyester Teeth – artificial	 Laboratorios Pisa S.A. de C.V. Point 4 by Kerr; TPH by DENTSPLY; FILTEK Z250 by 3M Targis Newtek; Co-oral-ite
Detergent- dry, no chlorine	Cheer (free & gentle); Gain (island fresh); Ultra Tide 2X; Bold- con aloe vera (Mexico); Dona Blanca (Mexico)- should have no blue or green granules or powder
Detergent- dishes	Colgate Palmolive (green bottle)
Detergent- dishwasher, liquid, no chlorine	Cascade
Digestive enzyme mixture	Self Health Resource Center
Drop cloths (Trimaco) plastic and paper	Self Health Resource Center; hardware store
Earplugs (Mack's Ultra Soft Foam Earplugs)	McKeon Products, Inc.
EDTA (calcium disodium), chelating agent	Arizona Natural Products, Inc. Self Health Resource Center
Elecampane	San Francisco Herb & Natural Food Co. , Self Health Resource Center
Electronic parts	Radio Shack; Mouser
Empty gelatin capsules, size 00	Self Health Resource Center; Health food store
Enema equipment	Medical Devices International; Source of Health, Inc.; "Fleet" bottle is available at pharmacies; Drug store
Epazote	San Francisco Herb & Natural Food Co. , Self Health Resource Center
Epoxy coating for copper pipes	ACE DuraFlo; American Pipelining; Cura Flo

Item	Source
Eucalyptus leaf, organic	San Francisco Herb & Natural Food Co.
Fat emulsion for IV use	Abbott Laboratories; Mexican pharmacy
Fennel	San Francisco Herb & Natural Food Co. , Self Health Resource Center
Filters, backwash, Clark	Self Health Resource Center
Filters, coconut charcoal	Pure Water Products (pitchers); Self Health Resource Center (faucet, shower, whole house)
Folic acid	Spectrum Chemical Co. , Self Health Resource Center
Food mill	See coffee mill
Freezer (FrigidAire)	Sears - Commercial -20C Type: CF07
Geiger Mueller counter	Less EMF Inc.; the INSPECTOR model has automatic counting & timing, not intended for liquids
Germanium, organic	Hydrangea, coconut or other nuts
Ginger capsules	San Francisco Herb & Natural Food Co. (bulk) , Self Health Resource Center
Ginkgo leaf	San Francisco Herb & Natural Food Co. , Self Health Resource Center
Glutathione	Seltzer Chemicals, Inc. , Self Health Resource Center
Goat milk	Meyenberg Dairy; health food store
Goldenrod tincture	Blessed Herbs; Self Health Resource Center
Good food (free of chlorine bleach)	Summer Kitchen (flour, tapioca perles, tapioca starch, currants, Demerara sugar, noodles [white & organic whole wheat], potato starch, arrowroot flour, raw pumpkin seeds, barley flakes, Red Star yeast)
Good water in Europe	see listings on page 642
Good grains	Bob's Red Mill (test to be sure)
Grain alcohol (ethyl alcohol)	Liquor store; search for the ¾ liter or 1 liter size of Everclear.
Grain alcohol	Alcoholes de Guadalajara (Etílico alcohol - Mexican)
Gravel root (herb)	San Francisco Herb & Natural Food Co.; Starwest Botanicals, Inc. , Self Health Resource Center
Green Black Walnut Hull freeze-dried capsules	Consumer Health Organization; New Action Products; Self Health Resource Center

Item	Source
Green Black Walnut Hull tincture	New Action Products; Self Health Resource Center
Hair Dye, Black Walnut Hull (powder), Light Golden Blonde Medium Brown	San Francisco Herb & Natural Food Co. (Item #P246) Light Mountain Natural
hair dye (NOUR), pure black, Henna red	Karabetian Import; San Francisco Herb & Natural Food Co; Self Health Resource Center
Herbs, in bulk	San Francisco Herb & Natural Food Co.
HCl	See hydrochloric acid
HDPE (high density polyethylene) bottles	Spectrum Chemical Co. (lids of different plastic need to be hardened) , Self Health Resource Center
Homeographic copies	The Natural Health Choice, Ltd.
Hydrangea (herb)	San Francisco Herb & Natural Food Co.
Hydrochloric acid, USP	Spectrum Chemical Co. (You must dilute the 10% solution purchased (#HY105) to a 5% solution by adding an equal volume of water. For internal use, must be made by pharmacist.)
Hydrogen peroxide 17½ % (food grade)	Univar; Do not use straight. You must dilute with an equal volume of water. , Self Health Resource Center
Inositol	Self Health Resource Center
Insulation, house	Bonded Logic, Inc.
Intravenous saline & 5% dextrose solutions in 500ml glass bottles	Pisa Farmaceutica Mexicana
Iodine, USP	Spectrum Chemical Co.
Juniper Berry Oil	Nature's Herb Co. (kosher and parve)
Kosher meat	S'Better Farms
Lactase enzymes	Mother Nature Advanced Enzyme System (Rainbow Light)
Pancreatin-lipase enzyme mixture	See individual ingredients
l-glutamic acid powder (this is not glutamine.)	Spectrum Chemical Co.
Lipase	Spectrum Chemical Co
l-lysine powder	Spectrum Chemical Co.
Lugol's iodine	For slide staining (*not internal use*) from Spectrum Chemical Co.; or farm animal supply store. For internal use must be

Item	Source
	made from scratch. (For disinfecting food, *Veggie Wash* 2% iodine from Source of Health; New Action Products).
Magnesium oxide	Spectrum Chemical Co. , Self Health Resource Center
Magnopatch, only North side touches skin	The Cutting Edge; craft store, Cut a 1 inch square from a magnetic sheet. Glue on 1/3 inch round magnet in the center, south side up. Round bottom magnet .312 x .125
Maple syrup	US Foods
Marshmallow root (herb)	San Francisco Herb & Natural Food Co.; Starwest Botanicals, Inc. , Self Health Resource Center
Melatonin	Self Health Resource Center; Benadorm (Mexico) , Self Health Resource Center
Microscope slides	Carolina Biological Supply Co.; Ward's Natural Science, Inc.; Southern Biological Supply Co.
Milk thistle seed	San Francisco Herb & Natural Food Co. , Self Health Resource Center
Mullein leaf	San Francisco Herb & Natural Food Co. , Self Health Resource Center
Niacinamide	Spectrum Chemical Co. , Self Health Resource Center
Nutmeg	San Francisco Herb & Natural Food Co. , Self Health Resource Center
Oil detection test paper	The Science Source, Self Health Resource Center
Olive leaf powder	San Francisco Herb & Natural Food Co.
Olive Oil	Bertolli Classico; Bertolli Extra Light; Self Health Resource Center
Oregano oil	Starwest Botanicals, Inc.; North American Herb & Spice Co. , Self Health Resource Center
Oregon grape root	San Francisco Herb & Natural Food Co.
Organ samples preserved on microscope slides	See microscope slides
Ornithine	Spectrum Chemical Co.; Seltzer Chemicals, Inc. , Self Health Resource Center
Ortho-phospho-tyrosine	Use homeographic copies

Item	Source
Oscillococcinum, homeopathic for flu	Boiron Borneman; Self Health Resource Center; health food store; drug store
Ozonator	Superior Health Products (ask for non-black tubing - test for nickel in ozone)
P24 antigen sample	Use homeographic copies
Painkiller, narcotic, free of chlorine	TYLEXCD, by prescription only in Mexico
Painkiller, OC (free of chlorine)	Advil; Tylenol Extra Strength and others; Dorixina Forte (Mexico)
Pantothenic acid	San Francisco Herb & Natural Food Co.
Paper towels	Kleenex Jumbo; Marathon; Max Soft (Mexico)
Parasites, bacteria, viruses preserved on microscope slides	See microscope slides
Pancreatin	Spectrum Chemical Co, Self Health Resource Center
Pau D'Arco	Starwest Botanicals, Inc.
Peanut butter	Laura Scudder's; Wild Oats, others
Peppermint leaf	San Francisco Herb & Natural Food Co.
Peppermint oil	Starwest Botanicals, Inc. , Self Health Resource Center
Periwinkle	San Francisco Herb & Natural Food Co.
Peroxy(17% H_2O_2)	See hydrogen peroxide
pH strips	Self Health Resource Center; Pharmacies; drug store
Plastic-coated water pipes	See epoxy coating
Plastic sheet	See drop cloths
Polyethylene dropper bottles (1/2 oz., 1 oz. amber & opaque)	Self Health Resource Center: Spectrum
Pomegranate seeds, fresh (grind in your own blender); pomegranate peel capsules	San Francisco Herb & Natural Food Co. (for peel); Self Health Resource Center
Potassium chloride	Spectrum Chemical Co. , Self Health Resource Center
Potassium iodide	Spectrum Chemical Co.
Pump, water lubricated	F.E. Myers
Pump, well water, hand operated (*harden internal plastic impellers*)	GROCO
Q-Tips (Limpiecitos	Desechables Quirurgicos e Industriales

Item	Source
aplicadores) Mexico	
Reishi mushroom	San Francisco Herb & Natural Food Co. , Self Health Resource Center
Rose hips	San Francisco Herb & Natural Food Co. , Self Health Resource Center
Salt (sodium chloride)	Spectrum Chemical Co. , Self Health Resource Center
Salt (sodium-potassium)	Self Health Resource Center, Self Health Resource Center
Shampoo	Self Health Resource Center
Sheep sorrel	San Francisco Herb & Natural Food Co.
Shields	See Bottle-copy shields
Shopping bags (plastic, no chlorine)	Grupo AEEG S.A. De C.V.
Slides	See microscope slides
Soap, homemade	See *Recipes*; Self Health Resource Center; see individual ingredients
Sodium alginate	Self Health Resource Center; Spectrum Chemical Co.; health food store
Sodium hypochlorite, NSF	See Chlorination supplies; Bleach
Sonicator	Any ultrasonic jewelry cleaner, use water
Sonicator (fits eyeglasses)	Self Health Resource Center
Stainless steel cookware	Restaurant supply stores, department stores – 18/10 quality (still must test)
Stainless steel platters	Tableware International Inc.
Stevia powder, extract	Self Health Resource Center
Strainer, stainless steel	San Francisco Herb & Natural Food Co.; Self Health Resource Center
Sucrose	Spectrum Chemical Co. (#SU103, Crystal, N.F.)
Syncrometer® diploma	International Syncrometer® Educational Science Center (ISC)
Syncrometer® video/ DVD	New Century Press
Tapioca pearls	See Good food
Tea ball, stainless steel	San Francisco Herb & Natural Food Co.; Self Health Resource Center
Teeth, artificial	Newtek, Co-oral-ite; see Dental supplies
Thioctic acid	Self Health Resource Center
Thyme leaf	San Francisco Herb & Natural Food Co.
Thyroid pill, 1 grain	By prescription only
Timer, automatic	Appliance or electrical store
Toilet paper	Kirkland (Costco brand)
Toothbrush, slender style	Nutramax Products, Inc.; Drug and

Item	Source
	grocery store
Tubes, shielding	see Bottle-copy shields
Turmeric	San Francisco Herb & Natural Food Co. , Self Health Resource Center
Unchlorinated bottled water	Buhl; kosher (*This is not an endorsement of bottled waters)*
Uva Ursi, herb	San Francisco Herb & Natural Food Co. , Self Health Resource Center
Vermiculite insulation	See insulation
Vinegar (rice)	Mitsukan Rice Vinegar (no need to freeze; it has no bacteria); white vinegar for hair and cleaning – Herdez (Mexico)
Vitamin A (acetate)	Spectrum Chemical Co.
Vitamin B_1	Spectrum Chemical Co. , Self Health Resource Center
Vitamin B_{12}	Spectrum Chemical Co. , Self Health Resource Center
Vitamin B_2	Spectrum Chemical Co.; Seltzer Chemicals, Inc. , Self Health Resource Center
Vitamin B_6	Spectrum Chemical Co.; Seltzer Chemicals, Inc. , Self Health Resource Center
Vitamin C (ascorbic acid), synthetic; chlorine-free	Self Health Resource Center, , Self Health Resource Center
Vitamin C, organic (Rose hips)	San Francisco Herb & Natural Food Co.
Vitamin D_3	Spectrum Chemical Co. , Self Health Resource Center
Vitamin E	Bronson Laboratories, Self Health Resource Center
Watercress, tablets (Berro)	Plantas M. Anahuac, C.A. de C.V. , Self Health Resource Center
Water filter pitchers	See filters
Water-lubricated pump	See pump
Wild lettuce	San Francisco Herb & Natural Food Co.;
wormwood capsules, mixture	New Action Products; San Francisco Herb & Natural Food Co.; Self Health Resource Center
wormwood seed	R.H. Shumway
Yeast for bread making	Self Health Resource Center; Industria Mexicana de Alimentos S.A. de C.V.
Yunnan Paiyao	China Healthways Institute; health food

Item	Source
	store; the Internet
Zinc gluconate	Self Health Resource Center
Zinc oxide	Spectrum Chemical Co. , Self Health Resource Center

3M
www.mmm.com

Abbott Laboratories
100 Abbott Park Rd.
Abbott Park, IL 60064
(847) 937-6100
www.abbott.com

Acadia Natural Spring Water
(see Foodhold USA)

ACE DuraFlo
USA & Canada
(888) 775-0220
Fax (714) 854-1833
www.aceduraflo.com

Alcoholes de Guadalajara
Av. Not 4618 Craftsmen Col.
Craftsmen 45590
Guadalajara, Jal. Mexico
(33) 3606-1002
Fax (33) 3606-1571
www.alcoholesgdl.com

American Pipelining
PO Box 5045
El Dorado Hills, CA 95762
(916) 933-4199
www.americanpipelining.com

Arizona Natural Products, Inc.
9849 N. 19th Dr., #3
Phoenix, AZ 85021
(800) 255-2823
www.arizonanatural.com

Bernard Jensen Products
535 Stevens Ave.
Solana Beach, CA 92075
(800) 755-4027
www.bernardjensen.org

Bertolli
www.bertolli.com

Blessed Herbs
109 Barre Plaines Rd.
Oakham, MA 01068
(508) 882-3839
(800) 489-4372
www.blessedherbs.com

Blistex Inc.
1800 Swift Dr.
Oak Brook, IL 60523-1574
(800) 837-1800
www.firstaidsuppliesonline.com
www.suncareking.com

Bob's Red Mill
5209 SE International Way
Milwaukie, OR 97222
(800) 349-2173
Fax (503) 653-1339
www.bobsredmill.com

Boiron Borneman
6 Campus Blvd.
Newtown Square, PA 19073
(800) 258-8823
(610) 325-7464
www.boiron.com

Bonded Logic, Inc.
411 East Ray Rd.
Chandler, AZ 85225
(480) 812-9114
www.bondedlogic.com

Bosworth Company
7227 N. Hamlin Ave.
Skokie, IL 60076
(800) 323-4352
www.bosworth.com

Bronson Laboratories
350 South 400 West, Ste. 102
Lindon, UT 84042
(800) 235-3200 retail
(800) 610-4848 wholesale
www.bronsonlabs.com

Brushy Mountain Bee Farm
(800) 233-7929
www.beeequipment.com

Buhl Water Co.
(218) 258-3258
www.buhl-water.com

Carolina Biological Supply Co.
PO Box 6010
Burlington, NC 27216-6010
(800) 334-5551
(336) 584-0381
www.carolina.com

Century Nutrition of Mexico
S. de R.L. de C.V. Mexico
Fax 52-664-683-4454

China Healthways Institute
100 Avenida Pico
San Clemente, CA 92672
(949) 361-3976
(800) 743-5608
www.chinahealthways.com

Co-oral-ite
www.pearsonlab.com

Consumer Health Organization of Canada
1220 Sheppard Ave. E,
Ste. 412
Toronto, Ontario M2K 2S5
Canada
(416) 490-0986
www.consumerhealth.org

Continental Packaging Solutions
230 West Monroe St.,
Ste. 2400
Chicago, IL 60606
(312) 666-2050
www.cgppkg.com

CTS Originals
PO Box 64
Lemon Grove, CA 91946
Fax (619) 644-8635

Cura Flo
1265 North Manassero St.,
Ste. 305
Anaheim, CA 92807
(800) 620-5325
Fax (714) 970-2105
www.curaflo.com

DENTSPLY
www.dentsply.com

East Coast Olive Oil Corp.
75 Wurz Ave.
Utica, NY 13502
(351)797-7070
Fax (315) 797-6981
www.gem-ecoo.com

Ecolab
(651) 293-2233
www.ecolab.com

F.E. Myers
1101 Myers Parkway
Ashland, OH 44805
www.globalspec.com

Foodhold USA
Landover, MD 20785
(877) 846-9949

Fricke Dental International, Inc.
165 Roma Jean Pkwy.
Streamwood, IL 60107
(800) 537-4253
(630) 540-1900
Fax (630) 540-1916
www.frickedental.com

GC America, Inc.
3737 W. 127th St.
Alsip, IL 60803
www.gcamerica.com

GROCO
7240 Standard Dr.
Hanover, MD 21076
(410) 712-4242
www.groco.net

Grupo AEEG S.A. De C.V.
Blvd. Sanchez Taboada 110
Local 22 Tijuana, Mexico
22320
(664) 684-1899

Henry's Market place
www.wildoats.com

Industria Mexicana de Alimentos S.A. de C.V.
Km. 70.5 Carretera Federal
Mexico – Puebla, San Martin,
Texmelucan, Puebla
52 (5) 541 9602
Fax 52 (5) 541 9675

Industrial Test Systems, Inc.
1875 Langston St.
Rock Hill, SC 29730
(800) 861-9712
(803) 329-9712
Fax (803) 329-9743
www.sensafe.com

International Syncrometer® Educational Science Center (ISC)
757 Emory St., PMB #398
Imperial Beach, CA 91932

Karabetian Import
2450 Crystal St.
Los Angeles, CA 90039
(323) 664-8956
Fax (323) 664-8958

Karlin Foods Corp.
1845 Oak St., Ste. 19
Winnetka, IL
(847) 441-8330
www.karlinfoods.com

Kerr Corporation Co.
1717 West Collins
Orange, CA 92867
(800) 537-7123
Fax (800) 537-7345
www.kerrdental.com

Kretek International, Inc.
Moorpark, CA USA
www.rokokzone.com

Lab-Aids, Inc.
17 Colt Ct.
Ronkonkoma, NY 11779
(800) 381-8003
Fax (631) 737-1286
www.lab-aids.com

Laboratorios Pisa S.A. de C.V.
International private company
Avda Espana 1840, Colonia Moderna, Guadalajara, Mexico
52 33 3678 1600
Fax 52 33 3810 1609
www.pisa.com.mx

Lehman's
(888) 438-5346
www.lehmans.com

Less EMF Inc.
(518) 432-1550
www.lessemf.com

Light Mountain Natural
(800) 742-5841
www.bytheplanet.com

McKeon Products, Inc.
25460 Guenther
Warren, MI 48091
(586) 427-7560
www.macksearplugs.com

Medical Devices International
512 Lehmberg Rd.
Columbus, MS 39702
(800) 438-7634
www.cprmicroshield.com

Mitsukan
www.mizkan.com

Mother Nature
322 7th Ave., 3rd Floor
New York, NY 10001
(800) 439-5506
Fax (212) 279-4290
www.mothernature.com

Mouser
1000 North Main St.
Mansfield, TX 76063-1514
(800) 346-6873
www.mouser.com

Nature's Alchemy
c/o Natural Products Shopping
PO Box 489
Twin Lakes, WI 53181
(800) 905-6887
Int.Toll Free (262) 889-8591
www.naturesalchemy.com

Nature's Herb Co.
410 Washington St.
Salisbury, MD 21804
www.herbalhut.com

Naturheilverein "Hilfe zur Selbsthilfe"
e.V. Postfach 1238
D-65302 Bad Schwalbach
Germany
49-06128-41097
www.drclark-verein.de

Net 32
(800) 517-1997
www.net32.com

New Action Products (USA)
PO Box 540
Orchard Park, NY 14127
(800) 455-6459 (USA only)
(716) 662-8000
New Action Products (CANADA)
PO Box 141
Grimsby, Ontario
(800) 541-3799
(716) 873-3738
www.newactionproducts.com

New Century Press LLC.
(Book Publisher)
1055 Bay Blvd., Ste. C
Chula Vista, CA 91911
(800) 519-2465
www.newcenturypress.com

Newtek
www.dentodental.com

Niagara Bottling, LLC
Irvine, CA 92614
(877) 487-7873
www.niagarawater.com

North American Herb & Spice Co.
PO Box 4885
Buffalo Grove, IL 60089
(800) 243-5242
www.internatural-alternative-health.com

Patterson Dental Supply, Inc.
1031 Mendota Heights Rd.
Saint Paul, MN 55120
(651) 686-1600
(800) 328-5536
www.pattersondental.com

Plantas M. Anahuac, S.A. de C.V.
Oriente 255 no 57 col.
Agricola
Oriental CP 08500 Mexico D.F.
52-557-63-75-20
Anahuac (U.S. office)
7522 Scout Ave.
Bell Gardens, CA 90201
562-927-6414

Pisa Farmaceutica Mexicana
Av. Spain 1840
Modern 44190
Guadalajara, Jalisco
Mexico
(33) 36781600
www.pisa.com.mx

Pure Water Products, LLC
10332 Park View Ave.
Westminster, CA 92683
(800) 478-7987
Box 2783
Denton, TX 76202
(940) 382-3814

R.H. Shumway
PO Box 1
Graniteville, SC 29829
(803) 663-9771
www.rhshumway.com

San Francisco Herb & Natural Food Co.
47444 Kato Rd.
Fremont, CA 94538
(800) 227-2830 wholesale
(510) 770-1215 retail
www.herbspicetea.com

S'Better Farms
www.sbetterfarms.com

Scotch-Brite
3M Home Care Division
PO Box 33068
St. Paul, MN 55133

Seagull Distribution Co.
3670 Clairemont Dr.
San Diego, CA 92117
(858) 270-7532
www.seagulldistribution.com

Self Heath Resource Center & Source of Health, Inc.
1055 Bay Blvd. Suite A
Chula Vista, CA 91911
(800) 873-1663
(619) 409-9500
www.drclarkstore.com

Seltzer Chemicals, Inc.
5927 Geiger Ct.
Carlsbad, CA 92008-7305
(800) 735-8137
(760) 438-0089
Fax (760) 438-0336
www.nutritionaloutlook.com

Southern Biological Supply Co.
PO Box 368
McKenzie, TN 38201
(800) 748-8735
(901) 352-3337

Spectrum Chemical Co.
14422 South San Pedro St.
Gardena, CA 90248
(800) 791-3210
(310) 516-8000
www.spectrumchemical.com

Starwest Botanicals, Inc.
11253 Trade Center Dr.
Rancho Cordova, CA 95742
(800) 273-4372
(916) 638-8100
www.starwestherb.com

Summer Kitchen
13110 Emerson Rd.
PO Box 221
Kidron, Ohio 44636
(866) 748-8500
Fax (330) 698-0413
www.summerkitchenonline.com

Sun-Maid
www.sunmaid.com

Superior Health Products, LLC
13808 Ventura Blvd.
Sherman Oaks, CA 91403
(800) 700-1543
(818) 986-9456
www.superiorhealthproducts.com

Tableware International Inc.
770 12th Ave.
San Diego, CA 92101
(619) 236-0210
Fax (619) 236-0130
Tableware@pacbell.net

The Cutting Edge
P.O. Box 4158
Santa Fe, NM 87502
(800) 497-9516
Fax (505) 982-3194
www.cutcat.com

Trimaco
www.trimaco.com

The Natural Health Choice, Ltd.
44 292 055 4943
Fax 44 292 055 3779
www.the-natural-choice.co.uk

The Science Source
PO Box 727
Waldoboro, ME 04572
(207) 832-6344
info@thesciencesource.com
"What's in the Water 1500 Kit"

Univar (wholesale only)
2100 Hafley Ave.
National City, CA 91950
(800) 888-4897
(619) 262-0711

U.F.O., Inc.
2110 Belgrave Ave.
Huntington Park, CA 90255-2713
(323) 588-6696
Fax (323) 588-6780
www.ufobrand.com

US Foods
www.usfoodservice.com

Ward's Natural Science, Inc.
5100 West Henrietta Rd.
Rochester, NY 14692
(800) 962-2660
(716) 359-2502
www.wardsci.com

Whistler Water, Inc.
(604) 606-1903
www.whistlerwater.com

GOOD WATER IN EUROPE

By Karl Nussbaum – Fax: 0049/2234/273963

***NOTE**: Some of these listings date back to 2002. They were found Negative for chlorox bleach...please send any information on other good water sites to the author. It will be greatly appreciated.*

GERMANY

Marpingen (Saarland) - 100 meters west of the Forest Chapel in the Hārtelwald. Marpingen is a little village 5 km west of St. Wendel and 40 km north of Saarbrűcken. The spring in the forest is an underground pipe, newly constructed.

Heroldsbach - A small village 6 km southwest of Forchheim and 25 km south of Bamberg. Spring water is in the middle of the sanctuary in the southeast of the village Heroldsbach. A fresh fountain.

Sievernich - 47 km southwest of Cologne. Autobahn A1 until "Euskirchen" road Nr. 56a direction Zűlpich/Vettweib to the little village of Sievernich. Tap water in the village without chlorox near the church "St. Johann Baptist" and in the future in the Garden of the Vicarage as a fountain (in construction).

Kall-Rinnen (Eifel) - 3 km south of Kall, 10 km east of Schleiden 70 km south of Aachen. The clear spring-water-well is situated in a little forest of a farmer's ground. Underground pipe.

SWITZERLAND

Montreux - "Source de Montreux" at the entrance of the tourist information pavilion directly on the promenade situated at the border of Lake Geneva in the middle of the town near the bronze monument of Freddy Mercury. Underground pipe leads to fountain.

Montreux - "Fontaine á Lourds" Well water directly beside the road opposite the big old hotel Excelsior 500 m from the old town center under the railway line Geneve-Sion. Water pipe is coming fresh from the mountains.

Montreux - Tap water of Hotel Excelsior – on the border of Lake Geneva. Underground pipeline across from "Fountain á Lourds".

Montreux - Hotel Eden au Lac tap water in the hotel 200 m from the old town on the border of Lake Geneva. Underground pipeline. WARNING: All hotel waters must be freshly tested at time of travel. Ask for sample of cold faucet water.

SPAIN

Calpe (Alicante) - Costa Blanca tap water of the urbanisation "La cometa". Without chlorox coming from the western mountains (Val de Ebo). Calpe is 80 km north of Alicante. "La cometa" is 2 km north of the old town on a hill 800 m from the Mediterranean Sea.

Calpe (Bernia) - Little Mountain spring-water-well 15 km west of Calpe on foot of the 800 m high Bernia Massiv. Take the road Calpe-Benissa-Los Pinos-Caseria Bernia (Little Mountain Road). The spring-well is coming from a rock.

Fontaine del Gel (Val de Laguar) near Fleix - Mountain spring-water-well 30 km north west from Calpe, town in the valley of Laguar (Val de laguar). Flowing out of a rock. Take the road from Calpe-Benissa-Jalon-Murla-Val de Laguar-Freix. 500 m east of Freix

El prado Nuevo (Madrid/El Escoŕial) - Spring water in a wild garden south east of the town El Escoŕial. 5 km from the big castle of Spanish Kings 46 km west of Madrid. The garden belongs to a sanctuary (Marias apparition). Water comes from underground.

La Becea - Mountain spring water 60 km west of Madrid in the mountains. Comes from a rock. (Also sold as "Bezoya" water in bottles).

Lietor (Albacete) - 60 km south of Albacete near Hellin in the mountains, little village with water in the middle of the town opposite the town hall. One of the famous wells of "rio mundo". Underground pipe with a fountain made of tiles.

PORTUGAL

Fatima - Well water fountain exactly in the middle of the Maria's Sanctuary. In the middle of the town 50 m from the Chapel of Apparition. Fatima is 90 km north of Lisboa and 65 km south of Coimbra. Underground pipe.

E. BELGIUM

Banneux - Spring water in the sanctuary (near the forest). 60 km west of Aachen (Autobahn A3), 22 km east of Liege, 17 km west of Verviers. Underground pipe.

YUGOSLAVIA

Medugorje (Bosnia-Herzegowina) - 25 km north of Mostar, 90 km southeast of Split (Airport), 50 km east of Mediteranean Sea (Makarska). Underground pipe of spring water of 2 fountains in front of the main church of Medugorje. Tap water in local houses has Desert Star bleach disinfection.

FRANCE

Lourdes - Spring water comes from a rock near the apparition place. Many water taps and bathrooms in one row. Lourdes (Pyrenäen) south of France, 170 km east of Toulouse, 16 km south of Tarbes. The spring is in the south of the village.

Mont Roucous - Spring water coming from a granite rock (mountains), 145 km east of Toulouse in Natural Park of "Haute Languedoc". The well is in the forest of Lacaune, 60 km west of Montpellier, 50 km south of Milleau.

Evian - Underground pipe fountain coming from the mountains south of Lake Geneva. Near the border of the lake, a fountain spring in "Evian-Les-Bains", 40 km northeast of Geneva after "Thonon-Les-Bains".

ITALY

Lauretana/GRAGLIA - Mountain spring comes from "Monte Rosa Massif", 125 km west of Milano, from Graglia (Piemont), 5 km west of Biella (Piemont). "Lauretana" water is also sold in bottles.

Food And Product Dyes

Numbers after dash are Color Index (CI); Square brackets are CAS numbers

- 4-amino-3-nitrotoluene (S) —37110
- Chlorotoluidines, liquid (S)
- (DAB) 4-dimethyl aminoazobenzene 4-isothiocyanate dye (S) [7612-98-8], D-872
- (DAB) p-dimethylaminoazobenzene [60-11-7], CI 11020, Sigma #D-6760 causes elevated alkaline phosphatase enzyme in blood tests.
- Fast Blue BB Base (S) —37175
- Fast Blue RR Base (S) —37155, [6268-05-9], EEC No 228-441-6, F-0375
- Fast Garnet GBC Base (S) —11160 causes death of T4 helpers; dye is found on most fish, fresh or canned and poultry.
- Fast Green FCF (S) —42053 blocks BUN and creatinine making enzymes, increases rate of mitosis.
- Fast Red 1 TR Salt Practical Grade (S) —37150
- Fast Red AL salt (S) —37275
- Fast Red RC Salt (S) —37120
- Fast Red TR Base (S) —37085
- Fast Red Violet LB Salt (S) —may be 32348-81-5 causes lymph blockage and effusions, inhibits maleic anhydride detoxification
- Fast Scarlet TR Base (S) —37080
- Fast Violet B Base (S) —37165
- Nitrotoluidines, mono (S)
- Sudan Black B Practical Grade (S) —26150, [4197-25-5], Sigma #S-2380 causes elevated lactic dehydrogenase enzyme in blood tests.
- Sudan I—12055
- Sudan II (SP) (S) —12140
- Sudan III (SP) (S) —26100
- Sudan IV (S) —26105, Spectrum #SU120, [85-83-6], Sigma #S-8756
- Sudan Orange G (S) —11920

Tartrazine (acid yellow 23, FD + C #5) (SP)

Testing Laboratories

(For testing heavy metals, including lanthanides, in carbon filters.)
Alchemy Environmental Laboratories, Inc.
315 New York Road
Plattsburgh, NY 12903
(518) 563-1720
www.aelabs.com

(For testing heavy metals, except lanthanides, in carbon filters.)
Braun Intertec Corp.
11001 Hampshire Ave. S.
Bloomington, MN 55483
(952) 995-2000
www.braunintertec.com

The GEL Group, Inc.
2040 Savage Road
Charleston, SC 29407
P.O. Box 30712
Charleston, SC 29417
(843) 556-8171
Fax (843) 766-1178
www.gel.com

Phoenix Environmental Laboratories, Inc.
587 East Middle Turnpike
PO Box 370
Manchester, CT 06040
(860) 645-1102
Fax (860) 645-0823
www.phoenixlabs.com

(For testing benzene, heavy metals, including lanthanides, in carbon filters.)
SRC Analytical Laboratories
422 Downey Road
Saskatoon, Sask. S7N 4N1 Canada
(306) 933-6932
www.src.sk.ca

Index